Fostering Health

Health Care for Children and Adolescents in Foster Care

3rd Edition

Author
American Academy of Pediatrics Council on Foster Care, Adoption, and Kinship Care

Editors in Chief
Camille A. Broussard, MD, MPH, FAAP
Kristine Fortin, MD, MPH, FAAP
Mary V. Greiner, MD, MS, FAAP

Senior Editor
Moira Szilagyi, MD, PhD, FAAP

Associate Editor
Anu Partap, MD, MPH, FAAP

American Academy of Pediatrics
DEDICATED TO THE HEALTH OF ALL CHILDREN®

American Academy of Pediatrics Publishing Staff
Mark Grimes, *Vice President, Publishing*
Jeff Mahony, *Senior Director, Professional and Consumer Publishing*
Chris Wiberg, *Senior Editor, Professional/Clinical Publishing*
Grace Klooster, *Editor, Professional/Clinical Publishing*
Annika Hawkinson, *Editorial Assistant*
Jason Crase, *Senior Manager, Production and Editorial Services*
Leesa Levin-Doroba, *Production Manager, Practice Management*
Soraya Alem, *Manager, Digital Publishing*
Sara Hoerdeman, *Marketing and Acquisitions Manager, Consumer Products*

Published by the American Academy of Pediatrics
345 Park Blvd
Itasca, IL 60143
630/626-6000
www.aap.org

The American Academy of Pediatrics is an organization of 67,000 primary care pediatricians, pediatric medical subspecialists, and pediatric surgical specialists dedicated to the health, safety, and well-being of all infants, children, adolescents, and young adults.

This publication has been developed by the American Academy of Pediatrics. The contributors are expert authorities in the field of pediatrics. No commercial involvement of any kind has been solicited or accepted in the development of the content of this publication. Disclosures: Dr Joseph S. Zickafoose has disclosed a financial relationship as a researcher and consultant to federal and state agencies with Mathematica. Any other disclosures were reviewed and determined not relevant to the work related to *Fostering Health*, 3rd Edition. Disclosures are reviewed and mitigated through a Conflict of Interest process that consists of reviewing pertinent information which is then used to decide what action is required to maintain content integrity. There may be instances where no action is necessary. This process has been approved by the AAP Board of Directors.

Every effort has been made to ensure that the drug selection and dosages set forth in this publication are in accordance with the current recommendations and practice at the time of publication. It is the responsibility of the health care professional to check the package insert of each drug for any change in indications or dosage and for added warnings and precautions.

Every effort is made to keep *Fostering Health* consistent with the most recent advice and information available from the American Academy of Pediatrics.

Please visit www.aap.org/errata for an up-to-date list of any applicable errata for this publication.

Special discounts are available for bulk purchases of this publication. Email Special Sales at nationalaccounts@aap.org for more information.

Printed in the United States of America

9-498/0925 1 2 3 4 5 6 7 8 9 10
MA1216
ISBN: 978-1-61002-874-5
eBook: 978-1-61002-876-9

Cover and publication design by Linda Diamond

Library of Congress Control Number: 2025939009

American Academy of Pediatrics Reviewers

Board of Directors Reviewer

Susan Buttross, MD, FAAP

Committees, Councils, and Sections

Committee on Child Health Financing

Committee on Infectious Diseases

Committee on Pediatric and Adolescent HIV

Committee on Practice and Ambulatory Medicine

Committee on Substance Use and Prevention

Council on Adolescents and Young Adults

Council on Child Abuse and Neglect

Council on Clinical Information Technology

Council on Genetics

Council on School Health

Section on Breastfeeding

Section on Developmental and Behavioral Pediatrics

Section on Lesbian, Gay, Bisexual, and Transgender Health and Wellness

Section on Neurology

Section on Oral Health

Lived Experience Reviewers

Ivory K. Bennett, MEd

Dashaan L. Jennings, BA

Shantell L. Steve, ScM

Ivy-Marie Washington, MSCJ

American Academy of Pediatrics Council on Foster Care, Adoption, and Kinship Care

Contributors

Editors in Chief

Camille A. Broussard, MD, MPH, FAAP
Assistant Professor of Pediatrics
Division of Adolescent and Young Adult Medicine
Johns Hopkins University School of Medicine
Baltimore, MD

Kristine Fortin, MD, MPH, FAAP
Associate Professor of Clinical Pediatrics
Perelman School of Medicine at the University of Pennsylvania
Division of General Pediatrics
Children's Hospital of Philadelphia
Philadelphia, PA

Mary V. Greiner, MD, MS, FAAP
Medical Director
Comprehensive Health Evaluations for Cincinnati's Kids (CHECK) Foster Care Center
Cincinnati Children's Hospital Medical Center
Professor of Pediatrics
University of Cincinnati
Cincinnati, OH

Senior Editor

Moira Szilagyi, MD, PhD, FAAP
Professor of Pediatrics
David Geffen School of Medicine at University of California, Los Angeles
Division Chief, Developmental Behavioral Pediatrics
Peter Shapiro Term Chair for Enhancing Children's Developmental and Behavioral Health
Los Angeles, CA

Associate Editor

Anu Partap, MD, MPH, FAAP
Pediatrician
Fort Worth, TX

Contributing Authors

Kym Ahrens, MD, MPH
Professor of Pediatrics and Adolescent Medicine
Seattle Children's Hospital and Research Institute
Medical Director
Washington State Department of Children, Youth, and Families Juvenile Rehabilitation
Seattle, WA

Katherine A. Ariano, MSN, RN, CCM, SANE-A, SANE-P
Population Health Nurse
Duke Foster Care Program
Duke Population Health Management Office
Duke Health
Durham, NC

Lisa Ayoub-Rodriguez, MD, FAAP
Senior Faculty
Medical Director, Behavioral Health in Pediatric Hospital Medicine
Division of Pediatric Hospital Medicine
Baylor College of Medicine
Houston, TX

Sarah J. Beal, PhD
Associate Professor of Pediatrics
Divisions of Behavioral Medicine and Clinical Psychology and General and Community Pediatrics
Cincinnati Children's Hospital Medical Center
University of Cincinnati College of Medicine
Cincinnati, OH

Colleen E. Bennett, MD, MSHP, FAAP
Assistant Professor of Clinical Pediatrics
Perelman School of Medicine at the University of Pennsylvania
Division of General Pediatrics
Children's Hospital of Philadelphia
Philadelphia, PA

Molly Curtin Berkoff, MD, MPH, FAAP
Professor of Pediatrics
Division of General Pediatrics and Adolescent Medicine
University of North Carolina at Chapel Hill School of Medicine
Chapel Hill, NC

Camille A. Broussard, MD, MPH, FAAP
Assistant Professor of Pediatrics
Division of Adolescent and Young Adult Medicine
Johns Hopkins University School of Medicine
Baltimore, MD

Kristine A. Campbell, MD, MSc, FAAP
Professor of Pediatrics
Center for Safe and Healthy Families
University of Utah
Salt Lake City, UT

Katy Carlsen, MD, FAAP
Associate Clinical Professor of Pediatrics, Volunteer Clinical Faculty
Assistant Medical Director, Comprehensive Integration of Resilience Into Child Life Experiences (CIRCLE) Clinic
University of California, Davis Health
Sacramento, CA

Adrienne W. Carmack, MD, FAAP
Medical Director
Office of Child and Family Services
Maine Department of Health and Human Services
Augusta, ME

Channelle S. Carr, MD, MHS, FAAP
Postdoctoral Fellow
Division of Adolescent Medicine
Johns Hopkins Children's Center
Baltimore, MD

Barbara H. Chaiyachati, MD, PhD, FAAP
Assistant Professor of Pediatrics
Division of General Pediatrics, Children's Hospital of Philadelphia
Perelman School of Medicine at the University of Pennsylvania
Philadelphia, PA

Emmanuel L. Chandler, MD
Division Director and Joseph L. Rauh Chair of Adolescent Medicine
Cincinnati Children's Hospital Medical Center
Associate Professor of Pediatrics
University of Cincinnati College of Medicine
Cincinnati, OH

Ariel Kiyomi Daoud, MD
Resident Physician
Department of Family and Community Medicine
Department of Psychiatry
University of Cincinnati
Cincinnati, OH

Sabrina Darwiche, MD, MPH
Fellow Physician, Child Abuse Pediatrics
Division of General Pediatrics
Children's Hospital of Philadelphia
Philadelphia, PA

Jason Deen, MD, FAAP, FACC
Director
University of Washington Medicine Center for Indigenous Health
Associate Professor of Pediatrics and Medicine
Division of Cardiology
University of Washington
Seattle, WA

Amy Dworsky, PhD, MSW
Senior Research Fellow
Chapin Hall
Chicago, IL

Jennifer Ehrhardt, MD, MPH
Associate Professor of Pediatrics
Division of Developmental and Behavioral Pediatrics
Cincinnati Children's Hospital Medical Center
Cincinnati, OH

Elana A. Feldman, MD, FAAP
Clinical Assistant Professor of Pediatrics
Division of General Pediatrics
University of Washington
Seattle, WA

Heather C. Forkey, MD, FAAP
Professor of Pediatrics
UMass Chan Medical School
Director, Foster Children Evaluation Service
UMass Memorial Health Children's Medical Center
Worcester, MA

Kristine Fortin, MD, MPH, FAAP
Associate Professor of Clinical Pediatrics
Perelman School of Medicine at the University of Pennsylvania
Division of General Pediatrics
Children's Hospital of Philadelphia
Philadelphia, PA

Karla Fredricks, MD, MPH, FAAP
Assistant Professor of Pediatrics
Director, Program for Immigrant and Refugee Child Health
Division of Global Health
Baylor College of Medicine
Texas Children's Hospital
Houston, TX

Abigail Genco, MD, FAAP
Assistant Professor of Pediatrics
University of Cincinnati College of Medicine
Division of Developmental and Behavioral Pediatrics
Cincinnati Children's Hospital Medical Center
Cincinnati, OH

Kari A. Gillenwater, MD, MPH, FAAP
Clinical Professor of Pediatrics
Division of Pediatrics
University of Washington
Seattle, WA

A. Bird H. Gilmartin, MD, FAAP
Associate Professor of Clinical Pediatrics
Director, Kids in Care Settings (KICS) Clinic
Children's Hospital Colorado
University of Colorado School of Medicine
Aurora, CO

Mary V. Greiner, MD, MS, FAAP
Medical Director
Comprehensive Health Evaluations for Cincinnati's Kids (CHECK) Foster Care Center
Cincinnati Children's Hospital Medical Center
Professor of Pediatrics
University of Cincinnati
Cincinnati, OH

Mary Emily C. Haas, MD, FAAP
Public Health Pediatrician
Cincinnati Health Department
Cincinnati, OH

Eric S. Hall, PhD, MBA, FAMIA
Chief Research Informatics Officer
Nemours Children's Health
Jacksonville, FL

Yuan He, MD, MPH, FAAP
Assistant Professor of Clinical Pediatrics
Perelman School of Medicine at the University of Pennsylvania
Children's Hospital of Philadelphia
Philadelphia, PA

John (Jack) Hessburg, MD, PhD, FAAP
Pediatric Hospitalist
Alaska Native Medical Center/ Southcentral Foundation
Anchorage, AK

Sara J. Hills, PhD, IMH-E
Integrated Behavioral Health, Infant, Pediatric, and Obstetrics-Gynecology Mental Health
Denver Health and Hospital Authority
Instructor Faculty, Pediatrics
University of Colorado School of Medicine
Denver, CO

Jeff Hudson, MA
Manager, Child Welfare Initiatives
American Academy of Pediatrics
Itasca, IL

Melissa Jimenez, MD
Associate Professor of Pediatrics
David Geffen School of Medicine at University of California, Los Angeles (UCLA)
Division of Pediatrics
Harbor-UCLA Medical Center
Torrance, CA

V. Faye Jones, MD, PhD, MSPH, FAAP
Professor and Vice Chair of Inclusive Excellence
Department of Pediatrics
Associate Vice President for Health Affairs
University of Louisville
Louisville, KY

James G. Kaferly III, MD, FAAP
Associate Professor of Pediatrics
Director, Connections for Kids Clinic
Department of Pediatrics
Denver Health and Hospital Authority
University of Colorado School of Medicine
Denver, CO

Colleen C. Katz, PhD, LCSW
Associate Professor
Silberman School of Social Work
Hunter College, City University of New York
New York, NY

Rachael J. Keefe, MD, MPH, FAAP
Associate Professor of Pediatrics
Texas Children's Hospital
Baylor College of Medicine
Houston, TX

Brooks Keeshin, MD, FAAP
Professor of Pediatrics
University of Utah
Salt Lake City, UT

Susana Williams Keeshin, MD
Associate Professor of Pediatrics
Division of Infectious Disease
University of Utah
Salt Lake City, UT

Joseph Kiesler, MD
Professor of Family Medicine
Division of Urban, Underserved, and Global Health
Department of Family and Community Medicine
University of Cincinnati College of Medicine
Cincinnati, OH

Bryn King, MSW, PhD
Associate Professor
Factor-Inwentash Faculty of Social Work
University of Toronto
Toronto, ON

Patricia M. Lantis, MD, FAAP
Associate Professor of Pediatrics
Pediatric Hospitalist
Division of General Pediatrics and Adolescent Medicine
Emory University School of Medicine
Atlanta, GA

Zach Laris, MPH
Founder and President
Child Welfare Wonk
Founder and Executive Director
Bolder Horizon
Springfield, VA

Hilda Loria, MD, MPH, FAAP
Associate Professor of Pediatrics
Division of Developmental-Behavioral Pediatrics
University of Texas Southwestern Medical Center
Center Director, Rees-Jones Center for Foster Care Excellence
Children's Health
Dallas, TX

Nathan M. Lutz, PhD
Postdoctoral Research Fellow
Division of General and Community Pediatrics
Division of Behavioral Medicine and Clinical Psychology
Cincinnati Children's Hospital Medical Center
Cincinnati, OH

Keith J. Martin, DO, MS
Assistant Professor of Pediatrics
Johns Hopkins University School of Medicine
Baltimore, MD

Raul J. Martinez-McFaline, MD, PhD
Resident, Pediatrics
UMass Chan Medical School
Worcester, MA

AnnMarie Matusak, DDS, MS
Assistant Professor
University of Cincinnati College of Medicine
Associate Director, Division of Pediatric Dentistry and Orthodontics
Cincinnati Children's Hospital Medical Center
Cincinnati, OH

Molly McHenry, FNP, PMHNP
Comprehensive Health Evaluations for Cincinnati's Kids (CHECK) Foster Care Center
Cincinnati Children's Hospital Medical Center
Cincinnati, OH

LaToya Montgomery, MSW, LCSW-C
Early Childhood Development Expert
Division of General Pediatrics
Johns Hopkins University School of Medicine
Baltimore, MD

Wynne Morgan, MD
Assistant Professor of Psychiatry and Pediatrics
Department of Psychiatry
UMass Chan Medical School
Worcester, MA

Michelle R. Munson, PhD, LMSW
Professor, Silver School of Social Work
New York University
New York, NY

Rachel Murphy, JD
Senior Attorney
Youth Law Center
San Francisco, CA

Lisa Nalven, MD, MA, FAAP
Director, Developmental Pediatrics
Kireker Center for Child Development
Valley Hospital
Paramus, NJ
Clinical Assistant Professor, Pediatrics
Icahn School of Medicine
Mount Sinai Health System
New York, NY

Miguel Nuñez, PhD
Forensic Psychologist
Department of Psychiatry
Dartmouth-Hitchcock Clinic
Lebanon, NH
Forensic Psychologist
Department of Psychology
New Hampshire Hospital
Concord, NH
Assistant Professor of Psychiatry
Geisel School of Medicine
Dartmouth College
Hanover, NH

Jennifer M. Porter, MD, FAAP
Associate Professor of Pediatrics
Division of General Pediatrics
University of Louisville School of Medicine
Louisville, KY

Megan Radenhausen, PhD
Assistant Professor
Department of Pediatrics
University of Cincinnati
Division of Behavioral Medicine and Clinical Psychology
Cincinnati Children's Hospital Medical Center
Cincinnati, OH

Jason Rafferty, MD, MPH, EdM, FAAP
Clinical Assistant Professor
Department of Psychiatry and Human Behavior, Department of Pediatrics
Warren Alpert Medical School of Brown University
Providence, RI

Anish Raj, MD, FAAP
Pediatrician
WakeMed Children's Hospital
SAFEchild Advocacy Center
Raleigh, NC

Margaret Reynolds
Medical Student
UMass Chan Medical School
Worcester, MA

Keri Hope Richmond
CEO, Keri Hope Co
Washington, DC

Jennifer Rodriguez, JD
Executive Director
Youth Law Center
San Francisco, CA

Joseph R. Rojas, MD, MSHPM, FAAP
Assistant Clinical Professor
Department of Pediatrics
David Geffen School of Medicine at University of California, Los Angeles
Olive View–UCLA Medical Center
Los Angeles, CA

Tagrid M. Ruiz-Maldonado, MD, MS, FAAP
Assistant Professor of Pediatrics
Center for Safe and Healthy Families
Division of Child Protection and Family Health
Child Abuse Pediatrics
University of Utah
Salt Lake City, UT

Amanda Scully, MD, MEd, FAAP
Child Abuse Pediatrician
Northwest Permanente
Associate Professor
Oregon Health and Science University
Portland, OR

Rebecca R. Seltzer, MD, MHS, FAAP
Associate Professor of Pediatrics
Division of General Pediatrics
Johns Hopkins University School of Medicine
Baltimore, MD

Kirsten Simonton, MD
Attending Physician, Division of Child Abuse Pediatrics
Ann and Robert H. Lurie Children's Hospital of Chicago
Assistant Professor of Pediatrics
Northwestern University Feinberg School of Medicine
Chicago, IL

Kristen Slaymaker, DO, FAAP
Assistant Professor of Pediatrics
University of Colorado School of Medicine
Department of Developmental Pediatrics
Children's Hospital Colorado
Aurora, CO

Yael Smiley, MD, FAAP
Associate Professor of Pediatrics
George Washington School of Medicine and Health Sciences
Medical Director, Healthy Generations Program
Department of General and Community Pediatrics
Children's National Hospital
Washington, DC

Valerie Borum Smith, MD, MPH, FAAP
Assistant Professor of Pediatrics
University of Texas at Tyler School of Medicine
Tyler, TX

Sarah H. Springer, MD, FAAP
Primary Care Pediatrician
Kids Plus Pediatrics
Pittsburgh, PA

Moira Szilagyi, MD, PhD, FAAP
Professor of Pediatrics
David Geffen School of Medicine at University of California, Los Angeles
Division Chief, Developmental Behavioral Pediatrics
Peter Shapiro Term Chair for Enhancing Children's Developmental and Behavioral Health
Los Angeles, CA

Christelle Tan, MD, FAAP
Associate Professor of Clinical Psychiatry
University of Cincinnati
Cincinnati Children's Hospital Medical Center
Cincinnati, OH

Lindsay Terrell, MD, FAAP
Assistant Professor
Department of Pediatrics
Child Abuse and Neglect
Director
Duke Foster Care Program
Duke University
Durham, NC

S. Thikkurissy, DDS, MS, MA
Professor, Division of Pediatric Dentistry
Cincinnati Children's Hospital Medical Center
Cincinnati, OH

Robin van der Merwe
Foster/Adoptive Parent
Director
North Texas Foster Care Consortium
Dallas, TX

Raquel Vargas-Whale, MD, MSc, FAAP
Medical Director, Child Abuse Resource and Evaluation (CARE) Team
Driscoll Children's Hospital
Corpus Christi, TX

Douglas Waite, MD, FAAP
Division Chief, Developmental Pediatrics
Metropolitan Hospital
Assistant Professor of Pediatrics
Mount Sinai Hospital
New York, NY

Elizabeth Wallis, MD, MSHP
Associate Professor, Departments of Pediatrics and Psychiatry and Behavioral Sciences
Director, Division of Adolescent Medicine
Medical Director, Foster Care Support Clinic (FCSC)
Medical University of South Carolina (MUSC)
Charleston, SC

Lisa Zetley, MD, FAAP
Medical Director, Care4Kids Foster Care Medical Home Program
Children's Wisconsin
Associate Professor of Pediatrics
Division of General and Community Pediatrics
Medical College of Wisconsin
Milwaukee, WI

Joseph S. Zickafoose, MD, MS, FAAP
Principal Researcher, Mathematica
Assistant Professor of Clinical Pediatrics
Vanderbilt University Medical Center
Nashville, TN

This book is dedicated to Mary Crane, PhD, who committed her career at the American Academy of Pediatrics to improving our knowledge about and skills in caring for children who have experienced trauma. Her compassion, kindness, gentleness, wisdom, expertise, and deep insights into the power of relationships to promote healing inspired all of us who had the honor of working with her. As the adoptive parent of her beautiful daughter, Lindy, she walked the generous, generative path of nurturing caregiving she envisioned for all children and families.

This book is also dedicated with our deepest gratitude to the children, youth, and families who have been its inspiration and to the foster care alumni and caregivers and the many professionals across systems who have graced us with their expertise and wisdom.

Equity, Diversity, and Inclusion Statement

The American Academy of Pediatrics is committed to principles of equity, diversity, and inclusion in its publishing program. Editorial boards, author selections, and author transitions (publication succession plans) are designed to include diverse voices that reflect society as a whole. Editor and author teams are encouraged to actively seek out diverse authors and reviewers at all stages of the editorial process. Publishing staff are committed to promoting equity, diversity, and inclusion in all aspects of publication writing, review, and production.

Contents

Part 3. Adolescent-Specific Issues

Part 4. Additional Considerations for Specific Populations

Part 6. Cross-Systems Collaboration

Part 7. Legislation, Policy, and Advocacy

Preface

Moira Szilagyi, MD, PhD, FAAP

A Short Story of Finding One's Path

I began caring for children in foster care a few hours a week as a second-year pediatric resident, an experience that introduced me to a population of children with tremendous health, mental health, and psychosocial needs and to the child welfare system. But it was one particular interaction that changed my career trajectory. I was seeing an adolescent who had grown up in foster care in a stable family and was by any measure "resilient" (highly personable, on the honor roll, a star athlete, good peer relationships, headed to college, future plan to be an engineer). At the end of his visit, I asked him if there was anything else I could do for him that day. After a long, uncomfortable pause, he quietly said, "You can tell me what I did when I was 6 months old to be placed in foster care."

I had the immediate sensation of being in over my head. Somehow I managed to say, "There is nothing you could have done…you were a baby. But I will find the answer to your question about why you were placed in foster care." His question led me on an exploration of his copious child welfare records, his many caseworkers, and the literature on family disruption. I discovered he had been told by several prior caseworkers that his mother was institutionalized because of the neurological effects of chronic alcoholism by the time he was born. When his new caseworker and I met with him a few weeks later, I emphasized to him that his mother was terribly ill and could not have cared for him—that her illness was not his fault; nor was the fact he needed a loving family to care for him.

Caring for this youth taught me many lessons: that for a child to be separated from their family is an abiding and deep loss; that sometimes people do not hear what we say until they are ready to hear it; that children need reassurance they are not to blame when parents cannot care for them because of illness or addiction; that we must listen to hear not only the question but the pain behind it; and, for this youth, the importance of speaking with compassion about the parent he never knew. I am grateful every day to this young man—his courageous question made me a better physician and, I hope, has benefited in some small way the thousands of other children I have had the privilege of caring for over 40 years.[1]

About This New Edition

As I reflect on the past 40 years of being a "foster care doc," I can say that the challenges of providing high-quality, comprehensive health care to children in foster care remain immense but that there have also been tremendous efforts to improve both care and outcomes. These attempts have grown in concert with our understanding of the high burden of trauma and loss these children endure and how we, the professionals who serve them, can intervene to promote healing through trauma-informed relational care. Such care is informed by the sciences of attachment, resilience, stress, epigenetics, neuroscience and brain development, immunology, parenting, and evidence-based trauma-informed mental health interventions. Because we have expertise in science, I believe that pediatricians and mental health professionals have a major responsibility for providing this care and for effectively translating the science that supports it to inform the care practices of caregivers and our professional partners in sectors such as child welfare, the courts, education, early intervention, and care coordination and payment. Trauma-informed care involves both understanding the effects of trauma on children and their families and promoting their physical and emotional well-being by building the safe, stable, and nurturing relationships (SSNRs) that promote healing. Trauma-informed care also supports child welfare in its goals of promoting the safety, permanency, and well-being of children and families.

In this third edition of *Fostering Health: Health Care for Children and Adolescents in Foster Care*, the authors and editors incorporate the principles of trauma-informed relational health care into all aspects of caring for children involved with child welfare, whether still living at home with their families; removed to foster, kinship, or congregate care; or in transition to independent living as young adults. We have stived to incorporate an equity lens into all chapters, given that the child welfare system has not always affected children, families, and communities equitably. In this book, we strive to always use person-first and strengths-based language (eg, *child in foster care* instead of *foster child*) and ask all readers to do the same. Youth and foster care alumni often remind us that there should be "nothing about us without us," and we have strived to include the voices of those with lived experience throughout and incorporated their insightful feedback. This book is designed for use by pediatric, child welfare, mental health, educational, developmental, legal, early childhood, care coordination, and other professionals and by policymakers, insurers, and those who design payment systems for children involved with child welfare. *Children in foster care* includes infants, children, adolescents, and young adults up to 21 years of age served by child welfare regardless of placement type. *Foster parent* includes both foster and kinship caregivers, and *caregiver* includes all foster, kinship, and biological parents.

Evolution of Care

Out-of-home care and health care for children and adolescents involved with child welfare has evolved in fits and starts. In the 1800s, children who were labeled "destitute" or "abandoned" were either left to fend for themselves on the streets or housed in mental health institutions and almshouses designed for adults unless family or neighbors took them in. Early on, the best of care was often provided by religious and charitable groups. The history of child welfare is detailed in Chapter 16, History of Child Welfare in the United States and Issues of Disproportionality, Inequity, and Injustice.

The early pediatric literature in this field emerged from research on child maltreatment—in particular, child physical abuse. Dr John Caffey, a radiologist, first described the multiple unexplained fractures he diagnosed in young children as the result of inflicted trauma.[2] Awareness about child abuse and neglect increased when pediatrician Dr Henry Kempe published an article on "the battered child" in 1962.[3] As a result of this work and growing interest in protecting children, the population of youth removed for maltreatment mushroomed beginning in the late 1960s. By the 1980s, the number of children who spent some time in out-of-home care annually hovered around 850,000. Child welfare had become a complex, under-resourced, overwhelmed system. During the last 2 decades of the 20th century, society was grappling with 2 epidemics, crack cocaine and HIV infection, that were layered onto the intertwined underlying drivers of family disruption: poverty, family violence, and parental mental illness and substance use disorder.

What was less appreciated as the child welfare system evolved was the deeply embedded historical and structural racism woven into the fabric of our institutions and agencies—including child welfare and health care. As far back as the 1970s, the National Association of Black Social Workers pointed out the role of bias, stereotyping, and discrimination in the overrepresentation of Black children in foster care and opposed the placement of Black children in white homes.[4] Recognizing that there were racial and ethnic disparities in reporting, investigation, family disruption, lengths of stay, and achievement of permanency, in the 1990s child welfare began focused work on reducing disproportionality in the child welfare system. Data on health inequities that accrued over the last decades and the recent dual crises of the COVID-19 pandemic and the racial reckoning that followed the murder of George Floyd focused a harsh light on the trauma of racism and its pervasive presence in our structures and institutions, including child welfare and health care. See Chapter 26, American Indian and Alaska Native Youth, for a further exploration of this topic.

Given the overrepresentation of Black and Indigenous populations, all professionals involved with child welfare should recognize that racism is a powerful erosive trauma, whatever form it takes (eg, interpersonal, intergenerational, systemic, stereotyping). Experiencing racism or discrimination, like any other trauma, activates the body's neurohormonal stress responses. It is a unique trauma because individuals most often have repetitive, varied experiences. Systemic or structural racism embedded in policies, laws, regulations, and culture is pervasive. The structures and systems that serve children and families have been on a journey of identifying and modifying policies, procedures, knowledge, and attitudes to promote equity, diversity, and inclusion. Progress has been made, but there is still tremendous work to do within and across all our child- and family-serving systems: child welfare, health care, education, juvenile justice, courts, and others. Although we are all still learning, *Fostering Health* is intended to help inform this work, focused on relational approaches, so we move forward together. Child welfare is a system in which Black and Indigenous families remain overrepresented and, while there has been improvement as child welfare, like health care, explores and attempts to correct the structural and systemic racism, discrimination, and implicit bias that underlie these inequities, much work remains. Although still overrepresented in foster care, Black children make up a smaller percentage of the population now (22% in 2021 versus 38% in 2000).[5]

Another overrepresented group of children are those who are lesbian, gay, bisexual, transgender, and queer or questioning (LGBTQ+), many of whom have experienced family rejection, bullying, and physical and/or sexual assaults. While progress has been made in reducing discrimination and bias, current federal policies limiting access to gender-affirming care reinforce negative stereotypes and behaviors toward this population.

Prevention of Family Disruption

Efforts to reduce family disruption have focused on implementing preventive services. These efforts grew out of the recognition that poverty was often conflated with neglect, especially when investigators and families were of different cultures, and the growing understanding of how deeply traumatizing family disruption is for children and their parents. Two examples of evidence-based interventions are the Nurse-Family Partnership, which has been found to enhance parent understanding of child development, prevent child maltreatment, and improve child development outcomes, and the introduction of evidence-based dyadic parenting interventions grounded in child development science.[6,7]

Child welfare has long advocated for increased preventive resources to stabilize families, improved education of its own workforce and foster families, and services to support youth aging out of care. In recent years, cross-systems advocacy efforts have resulted in significant legislation designed to reduce family disruption. Research indicating that the separation of parents and children is almost always traumatizing led to enactment of the Family First Prevention Services Act of 2018 (Public Law No. 115-123). This potentially transformative legislation shifts funding toward family preservation through the provision of evidence-based preventive services to stabilize families when safe to do so.

Children involved with child welfare live in a system of care riddled with uncertainty, grief, and loss. Earlier legislation requires child welfare to prioritize kinship care, keep sibling groups together, and keep children in their schools when removal from the home is deemed necessary for safety reasons. Other legislation has focused on requiring diligent efforts by child welfare to shorten lengths of stay in foster care and promote permanency through reunification and through legal guardianship or adoption when reunification is unlikely. Enhanced visitation schedules, Medicaid coverage for young adults formerly in foster care until age 26 years, and state oversight of health care and the use of psychotropic medications were all the result of joint advocacy by child welfare, advocacy groups, pediatricians, and others over the last few decades.[8]

Challenges

Child welfare is charged with caring for families who are struggling with multiple stressors and challenges and who are often oppressed by the very systems designed to serve them. Caseloads often exceed recommendations, and child welfare staff may lack the education and supports necessary for their work. Birth families are often dealing with housing, food, and financial insecurity and living in unsafe and even violent neighborhoods. Parents, many of whom have their own history of trauma, may also be struggling with interpersonal violence, substance use, and mental health issues. Involvement with child welfare may also activate parental stress responses that can include externalizing or avoidance behaviors, which can be misinterpreted as uncooperative, nonadherent, or even unsafe. While child welfare has been engaged in familiarizing its personnel with the effects of trauma on individuals, education about trauma-informed responses is variable, just as it is in medicine. Foster and kinship families may lack adequate training, resources, and supports to care for children with histories of significant trauma, grief, and loss.

Placement in foster and kinship care is a journey that is unique to each child and their family and new caregiver. As the journey unfolds, children may sadly have experiences that can reinforce a negative vision of the world, other people, and themselves. Separation from siblings, poor-quality or inconsistent visitation with family, and placement changes are almost always traumatic for children. Children may experience reminders of prior trauma that activate their survival responses, such as being bullied in school because they are separated from their families. Transitions, even minor ones, may evoke deep anxiety and even fear. Even seemingly "small" events such as court hearings, the start or end of the school year, or major holidays can upend progress for a child who is doing well. While being available for adoption by a forever family is viewed as a positive outcome for a child, the final termination of parental rights may result in a deep sense of loss in the child.

Many challenges exist in providing high-quality comprehensive health care that is continuous over time to this population. This is a highly traumatized and mobile population, moving in and out of care or among different placements; health care can become fragmented and important information lost over time. Caring for children in foster care requires close collaboration with child welfare, because the caseworker is the case manager for the family of origin and oversees the child's care. It requires detective work to piece together a child's health and developmental history, collaboration with a network of health and mental health professionals, and diligent care coordination to track children throughout their time in care and ensure their needs are identified and met. Developing advocacy and communication skills can be useful in working on behalf of individual children and in promoting systems change.

Children With Special Health Care Needs

The American Academy of Pediatrics (AAP) has long recognized children in foster care as children with special health care needs because of the high prevalence of health, developmental, mental health, behavioral, educational, and dental problems. Overall, 30% to 80% of children come into foster care with at least 1 medical problem; up to 80% of children enter with a significant mental health need; approximately 60% of children younger than 5 years have developmental health issues; and more than 40% of school-aged children have educational difficulties.[9]

In addition, there are micropopulations within the child welfare population with their own unique needs: infants prenatally exposed to substances, children with medically complex conditions, pregnant and parenting teens, unaccompanied refugee minors, those with complex mental health conditions, and those who have been or are involved with the juvenile justice system. The AAP now recommends that trauma-informed relational care be the universal approach to pediatric care; children in foster care or otherwise involved with child welfare particularly need to receive health care in a centralized trauma-informed medical home that has a working collaborative partnership with child welfare and mental health professionals.

Approaching Children and Families With a Trauma-Informed Relational Health Care Lens

Pediatricians serving children in foster care should be knowledgeable and skilled in trauma-informed care and collaborate closely with their child welfare partners. Child welfare can be envisioned as a unique microculture riddled with uncertainty for children and families; it also imposes complex and sometimes competing demands on its workforce, which often lacks the resources needed for the work. Children have multiple families (birth, foster, and kin), and each is likely involved with multiple systems (eg, child welfare, education, early intervention, mental health, courts, probation). Children often enter care with a high burden of trauma and loss but little health information, which is further compounded by consent and confidentiality barriers. Placement in out-of-home care may deprive a child of the safe, nurturing, protective caregiving that is continuous over time and fundamental to building the child's sense of security and a coherent sense of self. Reminders of loss or prior trauma can lead to behaviors that challenge caregivers and can disrupt placements. A medical home that recognizes the effects of trauma and loss on children can support caregivers by offering trauma-informed caregiving guidance to help children heal, making indicated referrals to services such as mental health and evidence-based treatment, and serving as an educational resource for child welfare and courts to increase understanding the child's needs through a trauma-informed lens. Pediatricians can support families in helping children adjust to placement in care and visitation with their biological family.

It is crucial that we in pediatrics, who understand child development and what is needed to nurture it forward, translate what we know into the care of children involved with child welfare. We must look through the lenses of trauma, resilience, and culture and interpret a child's development, behavior, and symptoms through those lenses for caregivers and others who interact with the child. Separating a child from their family—parents, siblings, and others–can be deeply traumatizing. A child who has been separated from all that is familiar—family, home, school, neighborhood, and culture—is likely to be deeply grieving those losses, be worried about those they love, and even blame themselves for the separation. The first weeks of care may be a period of calm as the child navigates their new world or one of chaos as they scream out their pain. Either should be viewed for what it is—traumatic stress in a grieving child who needs abiding reassurance and tender care.

Many of the conditions that children present with are in fact symptoms of the effects of unbuffered trauma on the developing brain. Recognizing and helping caregivers and youth understand the relationship between trauma and symptoms can reduce stigma and increase adherence to trauma-informed interventions. For example, we can educate caregivers about externalizing behaviors after a visit that may result from activation of the child's neurohormonal stress responses when separation from the birth parent at visit's end reminds the child of the original removal. This information can help a caregiver remain calm, soothing, and reassuring toward the child, thus helping the child to regulate. We can educate all caregivers about child development, trauma effects, and using skills such as routines, reassurance, and co-regulation to help children.

Newer research has confirmed that positive childhood experiences (PCEs) are more powerful than childhood adversities. PCEs, especially those grounded in SSNRs, are not just important; they are necessary for typical brain development. Neuroscience and resilience science have arrived at the same conclusions via different pathways: a child develops resilience and emerges from childhood as an empathic adult ready for life through exposure to an array of PCEs, including at least one safe, stable, nurturing caregiver and a variety of typical experiences and activities. Resilience, like language, is a developmental skill that is built over time in the care of SSNRs and exposure to PCEs. The best PCEs involve exposure to more SSNRs—teachers, child care providers, coaches, extended family, neighbors, and other caring adults. For children in foster care, stability in a safe nurturing home, positive visitation with birth families, exposure to a variety of typical childhood experiences, and the support of professionals who are well-trained and able to provide trauma-informed care have the power to help children heal and even thrive.

Importance and Challenges of Visitation With Family

More than half of children in foster care reunify with their family, and visitation that is consistent and of good quality remains the best predictor of reunification. Visitation with family may be deeply desired by the child but fraught as the child reexperiences separation at the end of each visit. At the other end of the spectrum, depending on what has happened to the child, visitation may remind the child of past trauma and be deeply disturbing. Either can manifest as externalizing and disruptive behaviors. It is thus incumbent that all professionals center the child and view their world through the lenses of trauma, grief, and loss.

The family of origin is more likely to adhere to visitation when their needs for mental health care and substance use treatment are met and when they have a collaborative relationship with child welfare. Specific supports around visitation are also important and include transportation, a safe and child-centered visitation environment, and staff who have knowledge of positive parenting strategies and child development and can provide trauma- and developmentally informed coaching. In some communities, on-site dyadic evidence-based interventions such as Child–Parent Psychotherapy or Parent–Child Interaction Therapy are woven into visitation and have improved reunification rates.[10–12] Pediatricians can advocate for such supports and offer to include birth parents in health visits when deemed safe by child welfare.

How to Use This Book

Readers can, of course, read this entire publication or can use it as a reference when specific questions arise or as a reference source for advocacy. In this edition of *Fostering Health*, Part 1 contains guidance for preventive health care practice and visit frequency, screening, health care coordination, integrated care, and specific types of visits (eg, sexual and reproductive health care, developmental and educational issues, mental health). Part 2 covers the culture of child welfare, including its history, the pervasive presence of trauma, and the importance of stability, nurturing care, and permanency in promoting resilience. Part 3 is devoted to the care of adolescents who are at a unique developmental stage of brain development as they approach independence and need support in achieving it while ideally maintaining a sense of belonging in family and culture. Trauma often fragments one's sense of self so that identifying and supporting a young person's talents and strengths is important in their development of competency and self-efficacy, which can lead to formation of a healthier, more positive personal identity. Topics on adolescents include supporting transition-age youth, substance use, and dual involvement with juvenile justice and child welfare, among others. Further attention is paid to specific populations in foster care in Part 4, including LGBTQ+ youth, American Indian and Alaska Native youth, and those prenatally exposed to substances or with neurodevelopmental or medically complex conditions. Part 5 considers some of the system and practice challenges of providing health care to children in foster care, including the complexities of consent, confidentiality, financing, and psychotropic medication oversight. In Part 6, solutions are described for improving care, cross-systems collaboration, and privacy and information sharing. In Part 7, the importance of pediatrician involvement in policy and advocacy is discussed.

Conclusion

While legislation and regulations governing child welfare have headed in the right direction over my nearly 40 years of being a foster care doc, there remains much work to do. Too many children still find their way into out-of-home placement, the "intensive care unit" of the child welfare system, indicating upstream preventive work is insufficient despite immense increases in our understanding of what helps children and families thrive. Some of that preventive work is advocating with our states and local agencies to implement strategies and interventions funded through Family First, such as home-based mental health care, parenting support, and substance use treatment. In some communities, these services may not even exist, so developing them or taking advantage of remote services will be a major investment and advocacy issue for pediatricians. Child welfare leadership and professionals and all caregivers and congregate care staff also need high-quality education and training in trauma-informed care and practical ways to effectively implement and apply it in their settings.

The sciences of neurobiology, early brain development, epigenetics, resilience, attachment, and developmental psychology have profoundly increased our understanding of the effects of childhood adversity—how trauma in childhood and adolescence literally alters physiology and can derail typical development and erode both physical and mental health over time. Now, scientists are adding to our knowledge of how safe, nurturing caregivers who are stable over time in a child's life nurture typical brain development and the growth of resilience. It turns out that the brain is built to adapt to the world it lives in; children who grow up with safe, stable, nurturing caregiving are more likely to emerge resilient, ready for life, and able to manage adversity. Their brains are powered up and have the neural circuits they need to adapt and grow. Children in foster care are not those children but could be. Working together and using the science to guide us, we can truly help reduce the suffering and build the buffering.

Definitions of Terms Used Throughout This Book

Adoption: Legal process in which a person other than the biological parent becomes the child's legal parent, establishing a permanent legal parental relationship. Adoption requires termination of parental rights. However, adoption may be *open,* under which continued contact with the family of origin is allowed on an agreed-on basis, or *closed,* which terminates all family of origin contact with the child.

Aging out/Emancipation: Youth who have reached the maximum age in their state to be in foster care and have not achieved permanency through reunification, legal guardianship/custodianship, or adoption. All states except Oregon and Utah enable youth to continue receiving foster care services until age 21 years, although youth can opt to emancipate beginning at age 18 years. Oregon and Utah do provide some ongoing supportive services for young adults who emancipate from foster care until age 21 years.

Child in foster care: A child who is under the protective custody of a local child welfare agency and placed in a living situation out of their home of origin. This is person-first language and preferred over *foster child* or *foster youth.* The term is used to include all children, youth, and young adults aged birth to 21 years who are placed by child welfare into out-of-home placement under court jurisdiction.

Child welfare: A continuum of services and systems designed to ensure that children have safety, permanency, and well-being and that families have the necessary support to care for their children. Each state or locality has a local child welfare agency that is responsible for receiving and investigating reports of child maltreatment and administering services that are within the child welfare jurisdiction.

Court Appointed Special Advocate (CASA)/Guardian ad litem (GAL): Trained individuals appointed by the court to advocate within the court system for the best interests of a child who has experienced maltreatment. Typically, CASAs/GALs remain with their assigned child through the case from appointment to permanency. Title and training prerequisites of CASAs and GALs vary by location.

Family of origin: The family that a child grows up with, encompassing primary caregivers such as biological or adoptive parents and other relatives. This is the first social group a person belongs to during childhood.

Foster care: A formal system that provides a temporary living situation for a child when a parent or caregiver cannot safely take care of them.

Foster caregiver: An adult who has received specialized training and is certified to provide temporary care for children who are in the custody of a child welfare agency. Title varies by location but can include *resource parent* and *foster parent.*

Guardianship/Custodianship: Legal process that is established through a court order that grants permanent legal rights and responsibility for the care and well-being of a child to a court-appointed caregiver. This process creates a legal relationship between a child and caregiver without having to terminate parental rights.

Kinship caregiver: An adult, often related or known to the family of origin, who temporarily cares for children who are in the custody of a child welfare agency. This is considered a less restrictive placement than a nonrelative foster home. Some states require that kinship caregivers complete the same or similar training and certification as nonrelative foster caregivers.

Maltreatment: An encompassing term capturing child abuse and neglect, which is any act or failure to act on the part of a parent or caregiver that results in death, serious physical or emotional harm, sexual abuse, or exploitation or an act or failure to act that presents an imminent risk of serious harm.

Permanency: A permanent, stable living situation for a child that includes reunification with the family of origin, guardianship or custodianship, and adoption. Permanency planning is a child welfare process that includes setting a permanency goal for each child and modifying it as circumstances indicate.

Placement/Out-of-home placement: The living situation in which a child is placed on entering foster care. This can include kinship care/relative foster home, nonrelative foster home, pre-adoptive home, congregate care such as a group home or residential facility, or supervised independent living.

Placement stability: The degree to which a child in foster care remains in the same placement for a sustained period with the goal of minimizing frequent moves or disruptions.

Removal: The process of separating a child from their family of origin after child welfare investigation has determined that the child's safety is at imminent risk. *Removal* is preferred to the terms *detention* and *child was detained,* which are regarded as pejorative.

Reunification: Legal process of returning a child to their family of origin when it is deemed safe and in the best interest of the child. It is the most common permanency goal for children in foster care to preserve family connections.

Termination of parental rights: A legal process that ends a family of origin's legal relationship with their child. This allows a child to be placed for adoption.

Trauma/Traumatic event: An experience or witnessed experience that is frightening or dangerous and poses a threat to a person's life or well-being.

Trauma-informed care: Care that assesses, recognizes, and responds to the impacts of traumatic stress on children, families, communities, and professionals while ensuring their safety, both physical and psychological. It is a universal relational health approach that promotes and empowers safe, stable, and nurturing relationships.

Traumatic stress: Events or experiences that elicit reactions that persistently or frequently activate the child's stress response systems and have potentially lasting physiological effects.

References and American Academy of Pediatrics Policy

To view complete, numbered reference lists for all chapters in this book, please visit **aap.org/fosteringhealth**.

For an open-access portal to all current American Academy of Pediatrics policies authored by the Council on Foster Care, Adoption, and Kinship Care, please visit **https://publications.aap.org/pediatrics/collection/561/Council-on-Foster-Care-Adoption-and-Kinship-Care**.

Part 1. Health Care Practice Parameters

CHAPTER

1

Core Components: A General Overview

Kristine Fortin, MD, MPH, FAAP

Introduction

Core components of pediatric health care include history, measurements, developmental/social/behavioral health screening, physical examination, procedures, and anticipatory guidance according to a visit schedule.[1] This chapter highlights aspects of core components that are unique to children in foster care. In addition to more frequent health supervision visits, specific types of assessments are needed to support health care needs throughout transitions in living environments. This chapter also highlights elements of history, physical examination, screenings, and anticipatory guidance that require special consideration when caring for children in foster care at different points during their time in care. One such important element is addressing trauma experiences, including but not limited to transitions in living environments. This chapter provides an overview of medical assessments, while Chapter 2, Health Care Visits: Type and Periodicity; Chapter 11, Screenings; Chapter 12, Mental Health; and Chapter 17, Childhood Trauma and Resilience, can be referenced for in-depth discussion.

Origins of Health Care Standards for Children in Foster Care

On the basis of years of data demonstrating prevalent medical concerns, the American Academy of Pediatrics (AAP) has classified children in foster care as a population with special health care needs. As such, there are special health care recommendations for children in foster care. In consultation with the AAP, the Child Welfare League of America (CWLA) published standards for health care services for children in out-of-home care in 1998, as well as a revised edition in 2007.[2] To develop these standards, CWLA used methods including review of current practices, professional literature search, expert discussions, and review by relevant organizations.[2] The AAP published additional specifications for the health care of children in foster care in a technical report[3] and the previous (second) edition of *Fostering Health*.[4] Standards were developed by the Task Force on Health Care for Children in Foster Care, a multidisciplinary task force convened in 1997 by the AAP Committee on Early Childhood, Adoption, and Dependent Care to define health care practice standards for youth in foster care.[4] These standards are outlined here and detailed in Chapter 2, Health Care Visits: Type and Periodicity.

Visit Types and Schedules

Children need to be seen early and often as they enter foster care, adapt to new living environments, and experience additional transitions such as placement changes and/or reunification. Different visit types and more frequent visits are needed beyond the routine health supervision visits.[3] As detailed in Chapter 2, Health Care Visits: Type and Periodicity, these visits include

- Initial health screening visit within 24 to 72 hours of placement
- Comprehensive health assessment within 30 days of placement
- Follow-up comprehensive health assessment within 90 days of placement
- Periodic primary preventive health care per schedule modified for foster care

Models of Health Care Delivery

The AAP has described different models of health care delivery that can meet the special health care needs of children in foster care; **Table 1-1** presents a summary of these models by Greiner and Beal.[5] Additional factors to consider when selecting a health care delivery model include local resources, needs, and policies.

History

Special considerations when obtaining a history during visits for children in foster care include potential barriers to obtaining history, available sources of information, and elements unique to children in foster care.

As with pediatric visits for children who are not in foster care, components of the history include birth history, past medical history, medications, allergies, family history, parent and child concerns, development, diet, review of

Table 1–1. AAP Models of Health Care Delivery for Children in Foster Care, With Potential Advantages and Disadvantages Noted

Health Delivery Model	Description	Advantages	Disadvantages
Evaluation/consultation	Centralized facility to provide health assessment for child welfare, with referral to primary care	• Standardized evaluation • Access to foster health expertise • Impact on high number of children	• Can have inadequate follow-up • May not establish primary care • Poor chronic disease management
Medical home	Primary care office for children in foster care to include initial evaluations and ongoing sick and well care	• Consistent care over time and placements • More complete health records • Chronic disease management	• Limited number of children can be served • Geographic proximity to placement • Disrupt relationships between caregivers and their PCPs
Preferred provider	Networks for primary care and specialty providers who provide care for children in foster care, tracked with case management	• Foster health trained providers • Larger geographic area served • Collaboration between providers for complex health conditions	• Limited choices for foster caregivers • Variance between providers • Requires high level of coordination
Nurse coordinator	Public health nurse–led care management, sometimes colocated with child welfare	• Convenience of home visitation • Extra supervision of home and caregivers • Less expensive model	• Limited evaluation in home setting • Lack of access to laboratory, radiology, etc • May not establish primary care
Mental health/development-based model	Medical care focused on mental health and/or development, specialized for children in foster care	• Addresses important mental health and/or developmental concerns, common in foster children • Access to mental health/development expertise • Provides specialty care over time	• More expensive and time-consuming model • Limited number of children can be served • Not all children may need same level of care
Special needs/multidisciplinary	Focused care for children in foster care who also have special health needs	• Access to specialized expertise in foster care children with special health care needs • Coordination of care for children with social and medical risks • Consistent care over time and placements	• More expensive and time-consuming model • Limited number of children can be served • Not all children in foster care may need same level of care

Abbreviations: AAP, American Academy of Pediatrics; PCP, primary care provider.

Reproduced from Greiner MV, Beal SJ. Developing a health care system for children in foster care. *Health Promot Pract.* 2018;19(4):621–628.

systems, and social history. Children in foster care may present with a caregiver who is not aware of some of these components, such as past medical and family histories. Youth may also be unaware of elements of their family history, and this could lead to feelings such as anxiety or isolation. Family history forms that list medical diagnoses and ask patients to check "yes or no" should be avoided, if possible, or include an "unknown" answer option. Instead of asking questions that assume family history is known, health care professionals can acknowledge that this information may be unknown and ask more open-ended questions about available history.[6] Once obtained, documentation of family history in the medical record will help inform relevant medical decision-making by health care professionals within the medical home and others to whom the child is referred.

When gathering history, the consultation of various sources of information can help fill information gaps. Examples of such sources include family of origin, child welfare professionals, foster parents, youth, medical records, school professionals, pharmacists, prior clinicians, and immunization registries. Relationships between family of origin, foster/kinship parents, and child welfare professionals differ. In situations where relationships are strained, individuals may feel uncomfortable sharing information openly when all are present at a health supervision visit. Offering the opportunity to provide history individually could facilitate the gathering of different perspectives.

It is also important to provide youth with the opportunity to provide history individually when developmentally appropriate. While some children who have experienced or are experiencing abuse may have findings on their physical examination as detailed in the Examination Findings section, many children will not have any specific signs at the time of their medical evaluation. History provided by children is an important part of evaluating for safety concerns and abuse. In most instances, foster care entry is preceded by a child protective services investigation that can include an investigative interview. While repetitive interviews about an experience of abuse should be avoided, questions about child safety are applicable during health supervision visits for children in foster care because they may have experienced additional instances of abuse that were not disclosed during the investigation preceding placement or that occurred afterward. It is helpful to start by establishing rapport with children, for example, by talking about interests and hobbies.[7] Nonleading, open-ended questions should be used when gathering information. Examples include "Is anything bothering you?"; "Tell me about your home"; "Tell me about your caregiver"; and "Is there something you are worried about?" Avoid questions that are beyond the child's development level and questions that are leading or suggestive, such as "You were abused by your parent, right?" If a child makes a disclosure of abuse, open-ended follow-up statements, such as "Tell me more" or simply "Uh-huh," can be used to gather information needed for medical decision-making. Thorough documentation of questions asked by the health care professional and the child's responses, including quotes when possible, is important. Additional resources on interviewing children can be found in publications by the AAP[7] and the American Professional Society on the Abuse of Children.[8]

Additional topics to address with youth individually when developmentally appropriate include sexual and reproductive health, mental health, and substance use. Chapter 9, Sexual and Reproductive Health Care, addresses confidentiality of medical information for youth in foster care. Lesbian, gay, bisexual, transgender, questioning, or queer (LGBTQ+) youth are overrepresented in the foster care system,[9] and it is important to use inclusive and affirming language when obtaining history as outlined in Chapter 9; Chapter 27, Children and Youth who Identify as LGBTQ+; and Chapter 28, Additional Considerations for Transgender and Gender-Diverse Children and Youth. Important sexual health history content and sample questions can be found in Chapter 9.

The prevalence of suicidal ideation and attempts is higher among youth in foster care compared with peers who are not in foster care.[10] Therefore, routine screening for suicidality is indicated when developmentally appropriate. Chapter 12, Mental Health, details an approach to suicidality screening that includes standardized screeners, tools to aid in following up on positive screens, and the gathering of collateral information. Chapter 12 details other important components of history related to mental health, including assessment for symptoms related to trauma experiences, depression, and anxiety. Foster care placement is associated with increased odds of engaging in substance use and earlier age at time of initiation.[11] Chapter 21, Substance Use, details an approach to screening for and responding to substance use.

It is also important to ask children and caregivers about manifestations of prior trauma experiences. Trauma experiences can negatively affect sleep (difficulty falling or staying asleep, nightmares), eating (hoarding, loss of appetite, lack of satiety), and toileting (encopresis, enuresis, constipation). Trauma experiences can also manifest in children's behaviors. For example, children may experience hypervigilance, dysregulation, or avoidance behaviors. Attachment can be affected by trauma experiences prior to placement as well as by placement instability. Clinicians can use open-ended questions to facilitate discussion about concerns related to symptoms associated with prior trauma experiences. It is also important to ask about factors that promote resilience, such as observed coping skills, strengths, family supports, access to normalizing activities, and community services in place.[12] Chapter 17, Childhood Trauma and Resilience, provides a detailed discussion of this important component of health care for children in foster care.

Trauma experiences can affect development, and it is important to obtain a comprehensive developmental history, as detailed in Chapter 13, Developmental and Educational Issues, and Chapter 30, Neurodevelopmental Disorders: Identification and Intervention.

Social factors impact child health and are another component of the history. Components of the social history unique to children in foster care can include

- Reason for foster care placement
- Age at initial placement
- History of placement instability
- Length of time in current placement
- Characteristics of current placement, including type (eg, nonrelative, kinship, group home, independent living)
- Visitation with family of origin, including whether visits have been established, whether the child has been separated from siblings, who is present at visits, type (ie, supervised versus unsupervised), location, and child's adaptation
- Name and contact information for child welfare professionals, guardian ad litem/Court Appointed Special Advocate, family of origin, and caregivers, including how the child refers to their caregivers (ensuring this information is kept up to date in medical documentation can help other health care professionals involved in the child's care to identify if a placement change has occurred and to reach necessary parties)
- Available information about permanency plan and upcoming court dates

Social history can also address the need for concrete supports. Caring for children involves multiple expenses. Children in foster care often have multiple appointments to meet their health care needs, which require transportation. Foster caregivers include kinship caregivers who may become primary caregivers without opportunity for advanced planning. In addition to assuming new expenses, becoming a primary caregiver can affect one's ability to sustain work hours. Seventeen percent of American grandparent caregivers older than 60 years experience food insecurity.[13] Youth transitioning out of foster care are also at risk for food insecurity.[14] It is important to consider and assess for the social needs of older youth in care, which are detailed in Chapter 20, Transition-Age Youth. These youth may be in independent-living placements and need to figure out how to attend health care appointments on their own. In addition to assessing for concrete needs of youth and families, clinicians can evaluate if there are available sources of assistance that have not yet been accessed. See Chapter 11, Screenings, and Chapter 35, Supports for Foster and Kinship Caregivers and Families of Origin, for additional discussion.

Measurements

The Bright Futures/AAP Periodicity Schedule shows recommended measurements (length/height, weight, head circumference, weight for length, body mass index [BMI], blood pressure) by patient age.[1] While studies of health status of children in foster care conducted in the 1990s noted the prevalence of failure to thrive,[15,16] a 2008 study found that overweight or obesity was the most common health condition.[17] Useful resources include the Centers for Disease Control and Prevention BMI category definitions[18] and the AAP Institute for Healthy Childhood Weight page, which has materials for professionals and patients.[19]

Bright Futures/AAP note that periodicity schedule recommendations were designed for children without manifestations of health problems and that components not completed at the suggested age should be caught up.[1] The measurements mentioned in the previous paragraph are applicable to children in foster care who have increased prevalence of both chronic health problems and fragmented care.[3] For example, head circumference measurement is recommended at newborn through 24-month visits. Head circumference measurement may be needed in children older than 2 years who have not had the prior recommended measurements or for whom there are manifestations of health problems such as fetal alcohol spectrum disorders (FASD), a diagnosis that is associated with microcephaly[20] and commonly missed among children in foster care.[21]

Physical Examination

Trauma-Informed Approach

It is important to consider how prior trauma experiences such as neglect, physical abuse, sexual abuse, discrimination, and medical trauma could affect children's perceptions of and responses to a physical examination. A trauma-informed approach to physical examination is important and, as discussed in an *American Medical Association Journal of Ethics* article,[22] congruent with ethical principles. These principles include

- Respect for autonomy: in accordance with the patient's developmental level, provide explanations about procedures to inform assent/consent and allow children to exercise control.
- Beneficence and nonmaleficence: aim to provide care that does not cause distress and employ strategies to reduce distress during necessary procedures.
- Justice: recognize and address disparities in experiences with medical care.

Some specific measures to consider as part of a trauma-informed approach to physical examination[23,24] are outlined in **Table 1-2**. Other chapters in this book provide in-depth discussion of medical home practice readiness to provide trauma-informed care (Chapter 3, Medical Home Readiness), including through training of all staff members about childhood trauma and resilience (Chapter 17, Childhood Trauma and Resilience).

Chaperones

The AAP has published policy statements regarding the use of chaperones during the physical examination.[25,26] A policy statement on protecting children from abuse in the health care setting discusses how nonfamily medical professional chaperones can provide additional safeguards over family member presence alone during sensitive examinations.[26] Recommendations from these policy statements include development of clinic policies[22] in accordance with state medical board regulations and documentation about chaperone use in the medical record.

Examination Findings

A seminal paper on the health status of children entering foster care found that 92% of children had at least one abnormal finding on physical examination.[15] Abnormal findings could be manifestations of known chronic medical conditions; chronic medical conditions that have not yet been diagnosed or fully treated; acute medical conditions, such as infections; or injuries.

Table 1–2. Examples of Measures to Consider as Part of a Trauma-Informed Approach to Physical Examination

Stage of the visit	Measures to consider
Preparing for the examination	Be cognizant that prior traumas may impact how children experience a physical examination. Create and highlight opportunities for choice. • For example, when developmentally appropriate, ask patients whom they would like to be present during the examination in addition to clinicians. Create a safe physical environment for the examination. • Considerations include privacy, avoidance of loud noises, and people present in the examination room (as noted previously in this chapter). Explain the physical examination. • For example, explain examination procedures and their purpose and estimated duration. Give patients control. Allow space for patients to ask questions and express concerns. Ask patients what could make them more comfortable and provide some options. • Potential distraction strategies include music and the presence of a supportive person. Offer the use of hospital gowns. • Hospital gowns facilitate important components of the examination, such as a skin examination. • If patients are comfortable wearing a hospital gown after explanation of its purpose, allow the patient privacy to change and minimize their time in the gown. • If a patient is uncomfortable wearing a gown, collaborate to develop alternative strategies to complete accepted portions of the examination. Exhibit cultural sensitivity

(continues)

Table 1–2 *(continued)*

Stage of the visit	Measures to consider
During the examination	Explain steps of the examination and their purpose. Ask permission before proceeding with elements of the examination. Avoid unnecessary touching. • For example, verbally explain examination positions instead of moving patients. Stay in the patient's line of sight. Observe for nonverbal signs of discomfort. Ask the patient how they are doing during the examination. Use developmentally appropriate distraction techniques per patient preference and acceptability. • Examples of distraction techniques include a patient-identified support person and music. Stop when requested by the patient.
After the examination	Discuss results of the examination. • If the patient was in a gown, provide time and privacy for them to change before discussing the results. Allow patients to ask questions. For portions of the examination not completed, ask about circumstances that could make future examinations more comfortable. • For example, future examinations may be more comfortable when a patient-identified support person can be present or when the patient is more familiar with the clinic setting and clinicians.

Examples of clinical manifestations of medical conditions that could be observed in a head-to-toe examination include

- General appearance: Features of some genetic conditions and prenatal exposures to infections or substances may be identified. A meta-analysis found the prevalence of fetal alcohol spectrum disorder (FASD) among children in out-of-home care was 17%.[27] The AAP has resources for assessment of FASD, including a diagram of distinctive features that may be present.[28]
- Head, neck, ears, nose, throat: Dental problems were present in more than one-third of patients entering foster care.[15]
- Heart, lungs, abdomen: Among children evaluated at a California clinic serving children younger than 12 years, the percentage of children with disorders of respiratory, digestive, and cardiovascular systems was 38%, 18%, and 9%, respectively.[16]

- Neurological: Approximately one-third of children in the California study had a nervous system disorder.[16]
- Skin: Of all body systems, skin had the highest percentage of abnormal findings on physical examinations completed at the time of foster care entry (61%).[15] Examples of findings that could be identified are infections, eczema, acne, manifestations of chronic disease such as acanthosis nigricans, injuries associated with self-harm, and injuries associated with abuse. The clinical decision rule TEN-4-FACESp was validated in children younger than 4 years and highlights characteristics that distinguish abusive and accidental bruising: body region (injuries to the Torso, Ear, Neck Frenulum, Angle of jaw, fleshy part of face Cheeks, Eyelids and Subconjunctivae), patient age (bruising anywhere on an infant 4.99 months or younger), and patterned bruising.[29]
- Musculoskeletal: Injuries could also be identified on musculoskeletal examination; the AAP provides guidance on evaluating children with fractures for physical abuse.[30]
- External anogenital examination: Resources pertinent to anogenital examination and interpretation of findings can be found in **Table 1–3** and AAP policy statements.[7,26,31,32] Factors to consider when determining timing of examination include clinical concerns and patient comfort. Possible findings could include congenital abnormalities missed in the context of fragmented care, issues of pubertal development, signs of some sexually transmitted infections, and injury (although it is important to note that most children who have experienced sexual abuse have normal physical examination findings[33]).

Health encounters present an opportunity to screen for signs of abuse.[3] Circumstances associated with foster care placement include physical abuse and sexual abuse for 12% and 4% of children, respectively.[34] Abuse can also occur during a child's time in foster care.[35,36] Most children who have experienced sexual abuse have normal physical examination findings,[33] and a review article categorized examination findings as those that are normal variants, commonly caused by medical conditions, and traumatic.[31] Children who experience abuse can have visible injuries; photographic documentation is helpful in addition to detailed written documentation in the medical record. In addition to visible injuries, children, especially infants and young children, can have clinically occult injuries detected on studies such as skeletal surveys, head imaging, and laboratory tests to screen for abdominal trauma. An AAP clinical report provides guidance on evaluation of children with suspected physical abuse, including indications for radiology and laboratory tests to evaluate for occult injuries and differential diagnoses.[37] **Table 1–3** displays resources pertinent to medical evaluation of concerns for physical and sexual abuse. Consultation with a child abuse pediatrician also may be helpful when questions arise.

Table 1–3. References for Pediatricians Evaluating Children for Suspected Abuse

Reference	Comment
Physical abuse—general	
Christian CW, Committee on Child Abuse and Neglect. The evaluation of suspected physical abuse. *Pediatrics.* 2015;135(5): e20150356. https://publications.aap.org/pediatrics/article/135/5/e20150356/33747/The-Evaluation-of-Suspected-Child-Physical-Abuse	This AAP clinical report provides guidance on evaluating children for suspected physical abuse, including medical history, physical examination, and diagnostic tests. See Table 3 (page 12) for an overview of tests that may be used.
Physical abuse—skin injuries	
Pierce MC, Kaczor K, Lorenz DJ et al. Validation of a clinical decision rule to predict abuse in young children based on bruising characteristics. *JAMA Netw Open.* 2021;14(4):e215823. https://jamanetwork.com/journals/jamanetworkopen/fullarticle/2778559	Investigators conducted a study of a clinical decision rule to help differentiate bruises caused by accident and abuse in children < 4 years of age (TEN-4-FACESp – torso, ear, neck, infant < 4.99 months, frenulum, angle of the jaw, cheeks, eyelids, subconjunctivae, patterned). Figure 2 on page 6 lists the frequency of bruising for each body region and the percentage of bruises attributed to abuse versus nonabuse.
Lurie Children's Child Injury Plausibility Assessment Support Tool (LCAST) app. Stanley Manne Children's Research Institute. (Updated October 7, 2024)	This free mobile app was designed to support recognition of abuse in young children with bruises. Users can view injury plausibility assessments after entering skin examination findings, clinical decision rules, and likelihood ratios for abuse with bruising to specific body regions.
Physical abuse—fractures	
Haney S, Scherl S, DiMeglio L, Perez-Rossello J, Servaes S, Merchant N; American Academy of Pediatrics Council on Child Abuse and Neglect, Section on Radiology, Section on Endocrinology; Society for Pediatric Radiology. Evaluating young children with fractures for child abuse: clinical report. *Pediatrics.* 2025;155(2):e2024070074	This AAP clinical report reviews factors to consider in evaluating causes of fractures, including fracture characteristics, history, and differential diagnoses. Components of clinical, laboratory, and radiology evaluations are reviewed.
Sexual abuse	
Jenny C, Crawford-Jakubiak JE, Committee on Child Abuse and Neglect. The evaluation of children in the primary care setting when sexual abuse is suspected. *Pediatrics.* 2013;132(2):e558–567	This AAP clinical report outlines steps in responding to concerns for sexual abuse. Evaluation components, including history, interviewing children, physical examination, and sexually transmitted infection testing, are reviewed. Management of acute alleged sexual assault is also discussed.

(continues)

Table 1–3 *(continued)*

Reference	Comment
Adams JA, Farst KJ, Kellogg ND. Interpretation of medical findings in suspected abuse: an update for 2018. *J Pediatr Adolesc Gynecol.* 2018;31(3):225–231 and Kellogg ND, Farst KJ, Adams JA. Interpretation of medical findings in suspected child sexual abuse: an update for 2023. *Child Abuse Neglect.* 2023;145:106283	Most children who have experienced abuse do not have injury or infection. These articles discuss how to interpret medical findings. Adams et al. review medical examination and documentation. Kellogg et al. provide updated information on sexually transmitted testing and an updated table categorizing examination findings as those that are normal variants, commonly caused by medical conditions, and caused by trauma. Interpretation of infections with respect to concern for sexual abuse is also outlined.
Berkoff MC, Zolotor AJ, Makoroff KL, Thackeray JD, Shapiro RA, Runyan DK. Has this prepubertal girl been sexually abused? *JAMA.* 2008;300(23):2779–2792	This article outlines the purpose and procedures for physical examination in prepubertal girls presenting with concern for nonacute sexual abuse. See page 2781 for an illustration of genito-urinary examination positions and techniques. See page 2782 for a figure detailing normal anatomy.

Screenings

Sensory Screening

Abnormal vision and hearing screening results were noted for 25% and 16% of children entering foster care, respectively.[15] The frequency of speech and language delays among children served by a clinic for children in foster care (20%)[16] further highlights the importance of sensory screens, because hearing assessment is indicated with such concerns.[38] Hearing and vision screening procedures are outlined in the Bright Futures/AAP periodicity schedule and AAP clinical reports.[1,38,39] Visual acuity screening strategies for children with developmental delays affecting use of optotype screening are outlined, including the use of developmentally appropriate symbol optotypes and instrument-based screening. Further information about vision screening technology can be found in the AAP policy statement on instrument-based pediatric vision screening.[40]

Developmental, Social, Behavioral, and Mental Health Screening

In-depth discussions of screening and response to developmental, social, behavioral, and mental health needs can be found in Chapter 11, Screenings; Chapter 12, Mental Health; Chapter 13, Developmental and Educational Issues; Chapter 21, Substance Use; Chapter 30, Neurodevelopmental Disorders: Identification and Intervention; and Chapter 35, Supports for Foster and Kinship Caregivers and Families of Origin.

The prevalence of developmental delays among children in foster care is as high as 67% to 68% in some studies,[40,41] highlighting the importance of developmental screening and surveillance. As outlined in an AAP technical report,[3] developmental surveillance and screening are recommended components of initial health screening, comprehensive and follow-up health assessment, and periodic health supervision visits. AAP resources for developmental screening include Bright Futures,[1] the Developmental Surveillance and Screening Initiatives web page,[42] and clinical reports on promoting optimal development, autism spectrum disorder, and motor delays.[43–45] Considerations specific to children in foster care include that initial health visits can occur prior to new caregivers fully observing developmental skills or to children becoming familiar with a new environment. Longitudinal follow-up is important. Fragmented care can impede developmental screenings from occurring per the Bright Futures/AAP periodicity schedule, and missed screenings can be caught up. For example, the M-CHAT-R/F is applicable to children aged 16 to 30 months,[44] so it could be administered to children in this age group who were not screened at 18 and 24 months per the periodicity schedule.[1]

Mental and behavioral health screening and assessment are also a component of all health care visits for children in foster care. Pertinent AAP resources include the clinical report on screening for behavioral and emotional problems[46] and the policy statement on mental health competencies for pediatric practice.[47] The clinical report reviews the low sensitivity of clinical assessment alone without standardized screening tools for identification of behavioral problems in primary care.[46] The report reviews steps for implementing behavioral and emotional screening tools as well as characteristics of multiple screening measures. Domains that can be screened for include depression, anxiety, attention-deficit/hyperactivity disorder (ADHD), depression, substance use, suicidality, and trauma-related symptoms. Some screening measures evaluate single domains of behavioral and mental health, while others evaluate multiple domains. In addition to domain(s) addressed by the screening tool, factors to consider in the context of clinic demographics and resources when selecting measures for pediatric practice include

- Psychometrics (populations included in validation studies, sensitivity, specificity)
- Length of time needed to complete and score
- Languages available
- Administered by staff or self-administered by patient/caregiver
- Modes of administration (verbal, written, electronic)

- Applicable age range
- Associated costs

The National Traumatic Stress Network measure review database is an additional resource pertinent to selecting standardized behavioral and mental health measures.[48]

Social Needs

The importance of screening for social needs is detailed in the last paragraph of the History section in this chapter. Organizations including the AAP and Health Leads have references on approaches to standardized screening and available tools.[49,50]

Procedures

In addition to laboratory studies ordered based on history and physical examination findings, there are special considerations for screening laboratory studies when evaluating children in foster care. Chapter 11, Screenings, focuses on screening tests for children in foster care.

A trauma-informed approach to discussing and performing blood work is needed, and many measures in **Table 1–2** are also applicable to these procedures. Additional resources for children who have anxiety or fear of needles can be found at Healthychildren.org[51] and the Meg Foundation, whose mission is to help manage pain and medical anxiety.[52]

Immunizations

An immunization schedule recommended by the Advisory Committee on Immunization Practices and approved by the US Centers for Disease Control and Prevention, AAP, American Academy of Family Physicians, American College of Obstetricians and Gynecologists, American College of Nurse-Midwives, American Academy of Physician Associates, and National Association of Pediatric Nurse Practitioners is published annually.[53,54]

Special considerations for youth in foster care include challenges locating immunization records for some children. Potential sources of information include

- Local immunization registries
- Medical records from past and current health care professionals, birth hospital, and medical centers where the child was treated

- History from youth and caregivers about when and where immunizations were received and any name changes or alternate spellings that could help with immunization registry searches
- Schools
- Day care centers, preschools, and Early Intervention programs
- Past and current foster care and child welfare agencies

Obtaining antibody titers may also be beneficial when records are not available. The Advisory Committee on Immunization Practices catch-up immunization schedule can be referenced when children are behind on immunizations or when immunization status cannot be determined despite thorough efforts.[55]

Policies and procedures regarding consent for immunizations vary by jurisdiction. In some areas vaccine administration may be covered under general medical consent.[3] See Chapter 34, Medical Consents, for additional discussion about consent.

Family Education and Anticipatory Guidance

Bright Futures outlines anticipatory guidance by periodic visit age.[56] Topics in Bright Futures such as car seat safety, safe sleep, sunscreen, oral health, and nutrition are important for all families, including those involved with foster care. There is also a need for additional guidance on topics related to foster care (**Table 1–4**).

Table 1–4. Examples of Additional Anticipatory Guidance for Families Involved With Foster Care

Topic	Resources
Trauma • Information about how trauma experiences can affect children's brain and behaviors as well as guidance on how to respond.	• Chapter 17, Childhood Trauma and Resilience • Safe and Sound: Resources for helping children who have experienced trauma and adversity developed by the AAP and Dave Thomas Foundation for parents and other adults involved in the lives of children who are in foster care or adopted (https://www.aap.org/en/patient-care/foster-care/safe-and-sound-helping-children-who-have-experience-trauma-and-adversity/).

(continues)

Table 1–4 *(continued)*

Topic	Resources
Communicating about foster care placement • Parents may seek guidance on how to talk to children about being in foster care, and guidance will vary based on the child's age and developmental level. Pediatricians and mental health professionals can guide parents in having open and early discussions using positive language.[57]	• AAP Clinical Report "Pediatrician Guidance in Supporting Families of Children Who Are Adopted, Fostered or in Kinship Care"[57] contains recommendations, such as having natural conversations about foster care even when children are too young to understand these words, creating a "life book" of positive and challenging experiences, and developing rituals to honor the child's family of origin on special occasions. • Sesame Workshop, the nonprofit organization associated with Sesame Street, has resources on foster care including videos with Karli, a Muppet who is in foster care, and coloring pages (https://sesameworkshop.org/topics/foster-care/). • The Creating a Family nonprofit organization has a list of children's books about foster care (https://creatingafamily.org/foster-care/foster-care-suggested-books/books-for-kids-in-foster-care/).
Racism and family differences • Families with members of different race/ethnicity can face additional challenges including confusion about racial/ethnic origins and parents with different personal experiences with racism than those of their children.[58]	• The AAP policy statement on the impact of racism on child and adolescent health outlines an approach to providing anticipatory guidance for all children and families experiencing racism.[58] • AAP Bright Futures has a resource repository for caregivers to help families talk with children about race and racism. (https://downloads.aap.org/AAP/PDF/AAP_BF_HealthEquityTipSheet_FamilyRepository.pdf) • The Adopted Life video series includes discussions about transracial adoption by people with lived experience expertise (https://www.youtube.com/watch?v=gNH71bnLjxA). • Adoptive and Foster Family Coalition New York Transracial and Transcultural Families page links to resources for families (https://affcny.org/family-supports/transracial-transcultural/). • AdoptUSKids transracial parenting resources page includes a list of books on transracial parenting (https://blog.adoptuskids.org/transracial-parenting-resources/).
Transitions • Children in foster care experience many transitions, including new home environments and primary caregivers. Visiting their family of origin and then returning to the foster home are also transitions that can occur regularly. Foster parents may notice changes in behavior related to transitions.	• Healthy Children has a "Tips for Helping Children and Teens Before and After Visitation" page. Tips include collaborating with the child to identify a transitional item that is comforting and establishing a return from visit routine. (https://www.healthychildren.org/English/family-life/family-dynamics/adoption-and-foster-care/Pages/Tips-for-Helping-Children-and-Teens-Before-and-After-Visitation.aspx).

Key Takeaways

- » Children in foster care need to be seen early and often at visit types specific to their stage in care and on an enhanced periodic visit schedule.
- » Children in foster care have special health care needs and may have missed laboratory, mental health, and developmental health screenings due to fragmented care.
- » Children in foster care experience trauma that could affect their interactions in the health care setting.
- » Special considerations are needed for each core component of pediatric visits to deliver trauma-informed care that meets the needs of children in foster care.

CHAPTER 2

Health Care Visits: Type and Periodicity

Kari A. Gillenwater, MD, MPH, FAAP
Elana A. Feldman, MD, FAAP

Overview and Guiding Principles

Because of the many factors affecting the health of children in foster care, this population has special health care needs and is seen on an accelerated schedule.[1] The increased care schedule provides more opportunities to identify health care needs, offer treatments and referrals to support services, and support maintenance of the care plan if a placement transition occurs.

Following the American Academy of Pediatrics (AAP) guidelines, children in foster care should be seen early, often, and comprehensively.[1] The initial screening examination should occur within the first few days of placement, and a comprehensive health assessment should be performed within 30 days of placement. Future follow-up and health supervision visits should be completed on an advanced schedule, including a follow-up visit for the comprehensive health assessment around 90 days after placement and periodic health supervision visits for children in care, approximately twice as often as the AAP recommends for children who are not in foster care. Additional assessments should be provided for any change in placement (any change in caregiver including reunification or a move to a kinship placement). The purpose of these recommendations is to ensure that physical and psychological health needs are addressed and that resources and support are provided both to the child and to the current caregivers. Each visit is an opportunity to promote well-being for the child and continuity of care during the child's journey in the foster care system. This may be accomplished through ensuring follow-up with the same physicians or through a warm handoff with appropriate sharing of data (see **Box 2-1**).

Box 2–1

Guiding Principles of Care Delivery

- See early, see often (advanced schedule), see comprehensively.
- Provide trauma-informed care.
- Maintain continuity of care during a child's journey, either through the same clinic or via a warm handoff to the future pediatrician or clinician.
- Know and follow your state's requirements for periodic examinations and the AAP advanced care schedule for children in foster care.
- Know your state's child welfare and tribal laws and policies.
- Help children connect to their communities and promote resilience.

Most states have established requirements for health care when a child is in foster care. Maintaining an awareness of these requirements for periodic examinations and a familiarity with child welfare laws and tribal laws and policies will help direct care. The Child Welfare Information Gateway maintains a helpful database at https://www.childwelfare.gov/resources/states-territories-tribes.

Entry to Care/Initial Period

Children should be seen as soon as possible after any entry into foster care, even if they have previously been in care. Per the AAP policy statement on Health Care Issues for Children and Adolescents in Foster Care and Kinship Care, children should have 3 separate pediatrician visits upon entry into care (see **Box 2–2**).[1]

Box 2–2

Schedule of Visits Upon Entry Into Foster Care

- Acute visit within 24 to 72 hours
- Comprehensive health assessment visit within 30 days
- Follow-up health assessment within 60 to 90 days

Initial Visit (Within 24 to 72 hours of Entry Into Care)

Many states mandate that children should be seen within 24 to 72 hours after entry into foster care. Children with complex or chronic medical conditions should be seen within 24 hours. In many circumstances, a child will not be in a long-term placement at the time of this visit and may be in an emergency placement or a shelter. The primary purposes of this visit are to address any acute medical issues, identify chronic conditions that require treatment (such as asthma), refill medications, and ensure that the child is medically stable and does not require urgent hospitalization or other care. The secondary purposes are to address any possibly contagious conditions (such as lice or scabies), document any physical examination findings that might indicate abuse or neglect, and update immunizations, if appropriate (see **Table 2–1**).

Table 2–1. Initial Health Supervision Visit

Health Visit Type	Time After Entry to Foster/ Kinship Care	Purpose	Components	Actions
Initial health supervision visit	Within 72 h[a]	1. Identify health conditions requiring prompt attention: acute/ chronic illness, child abuse/neglect, mental health disturbance, pregnancy	1. Review of health information	1. Appropriate treatment and referral
			2. Review of trauma history	
			3. Review of systems	
			4. Symptom-targeted examination	
		2. Identify health conditions important in making placement decisions	5. Child abuse screen: growth parameters, vitals, skin, joints/ extremities, external genitalia	2. Communication with caseworker
			6. Developmental surveillance or screen	
			7. Mental health screen: suicidality, homicidality, violent behaviors, trauma exposures	
		3. Identify significant behavior issues important in making placement decisions	8. Adolescent health screen: pregnancy screen for sexually mature girls and sexually transmitted infection testing for all adolescents	3. Anticipatory guidance related to transition into foster care, parenting the traumatized child, specific health issues

[a] Some children should have their initial health screen within 24 hours: children younger than 3 years; any child with a complex chronic health condition or significant developmental delays, or on medication, or with an acute illness or infestation; any child with known mental health or behavioral problems; or any child for whom a more immediate examination for suspected child abuse and neglect is indicated.

Reproduced from Szilagyi MA, Rosen DS, Rubin D, et al. Health care issues for children and adolescents in foster care and kinship care. *Pediatrics*. 2015;136(4):e1142-e1166. doi:10.1542/peds.2015-2656.

History should be elicited from all available historians who may help create a better understanding of the child's history and needs, as well as any available medical and state record systems. Common historians may include the foster caregiver, the family of origin, the Court Appointed Special Advocate or guardian ad litem, therapists, teachers, and previous pediatricians and other clinicians.

It can be helpful to know about the circumstances that led to the child's placement in foster care; however, this should be limited to what is medically needed to care for the child. Ideally, this history should be obtained from the caregiver or caseworker separate from the child, either during the visit or by telephone. It is very important not to ask the child specific or leading questions about abuse or neglect because this can both interfere with an ongoing investigation and retraumatize the child. If the child is in care due to physical or sexual abuse, the history should include whether they were seen acutely for their injuries and whether an appropriate child abuse workup was done. If a workup was not performed, the clinician should consider consulting a child abuse pediatrician or the AAP guidelines on the evaluation of physical and sexual abuse in children.[2]

Past medical history should include any previous pediatricians and other physicians and clinics so records can be requested before the next visit. Social history should include caseworker's name and contact information, school name, and grade in school, if known. Current living arrangements should be assessed, including members of the current household, as well as the visitation schedule with their family of origin. Social history should also include whether the current caseworker will be assigned to the child long-term.

The physical examination should be as complete as possible while remaining trauma informed. Growth parameters and nutrition status should be assessed. If severe malnutrition is diagnosed, then the possibility of refeeding syndrome should be considered. Any skin findings should be documented, photographed, and entered into the medical record. Caries and tooth decay are common in this population, so all children should be examined for evidence of any dental abscess or infection and referred to a dentist for treatment, accordingly. See Chapter 1, Core Components: A General Overview, for more detailed information on the physical examination.

Evaluate medications and doses prescribed for appropriateness. Explore questions about medications from the sources available, including the child welfare case worker and using any accessible information-sharing electronic systems that may provide such information. Refills should be ordered for all long-term medications. Consider prescribing common over-the-counter medications such as acetaminophen and ibuprofen if this would improve caregiver access and is covered by Medicaid in the state where the child is being seen.

Comprehensive Wellness Examination

A comprehensive wellness examination should be completed within 30 days of each entry into foster care, regardless of whether the child has had a recent prior wellness examination. The purpose of this visit is to assess how the caregiver and child are adjusting to the new living situation, assess the child's developmental and educational milestones and mental health, and provide a referral to resources (see **Table 2–2**). Validated screening tools (discussed in more detail in other chapters) should be used to evaluate mental and behavioral health and assess for substance use.

Ideally, medical records will be requested before this visit to ensure that medical and immunization histories are available.

In addition to routine wellness history questions, screening for trauma-related behavioral concerns, such as problematic eating or sleeping behaviors, providing education related to these concerns, and referring for support are important components of the comprehensive health assessment (see Chapter 12, Mental Health, and Chapter 17, Childhood Trauma and Resilience, for more specific information on how to assess and refer) (see **Box 2–3**). The social history should include the number of placements the child has had since their prior visit and any caseworker changes.

A confidential adolescent assessment using a standardized tool should be conducted with any child who is in the appropriate developmental stage in order to provide appropriate preventive care and anticipatory guidance. (See Chapter 11, Screenings; Chapter 12, Mental Health; and Chapter 21, Substance Use.) Clinicians should be aware of adolescent confidentiality laws in their state and inform the adolescent about the specifics of confidentiality in their office before the discussion.

Many adolescents in foster care have had negative previous experiences with authority figures, which can lead to wariness regarding the sharing of any confidential or personal information. An open and honest discussion of the limits of confidentiality in the medical office can help develop the relationship. The AAP recommends screening for substance use disorders for all adolescents.[3] In addition, some centers routinely screen adolescents for commercial sexual exploitation of children (CSEC) risk factors using standardized screening tools (see Chapter 23, Commercial Sexual Exploitation of Children, for more specific information on how to screen and specific tools to use).

Table 2–2. Comprehensive Health Assessment

Health Visit Type	Time After Entry to Foster/Kinship Care	Purpose	Components	Actions
Comprehensive health assessment	Within 30 days	1. Review available health information	1. Review of available health information including trauma history	1. Appropriate treatment and referral (mental health, developmental, educational, dental)
			2. Review of systems	
			3. Complete physical examination	
		2. Identify acute and chronic health conditions	4. Child abuse and neglect screen	
			5. Contraceptive and sexual safety counseling for adolescents	2. Communication with caseworker
		3. Identify developmental and mental health conditions	6. Developmental screen and referral for evaluation	
			7. Mental health screen and referral for evaluation	3. Anticipatory guidance particularly around parenting traumatized child
		4. Trauma assessment	8. Adolescent health survey	
			9. Review of school performance	
		5. Develop an individualized treatment plan	10. Immunization review	4. Schedule follow-up visit
			11. Dental screen and referral	
			12. Hearing and vision screening	
			13. HIV risk assessment	
			14. Laboratory studies[a]	
			15. Anticipatory guidance[a]	

[a] See recommendations in AAP technical report cited in text.

Reproduced from Szilagyi MA, Rosen DS, Rubin D, et al. Health care issues for children and adolescents in foster care and kinship care. *Pediatrics*. 2015;136(4):e1142-e1166. doi:10.1542/peds.2015-2656.

Box 2–3

Additional Components of Behavioral History for a Child Who Has Experienced Trauma

- Eating behaviors: picky eating, bingeing, hording, food refusal
- Sleep disruptions: nightmares, insomnia, night terrors
- Anxiety and hypervigilance
- Attention and impulse control
- Mood symptoms
- Oppositional behaviors
- Peer interactions
- Behavior related to visits with family of origin

Some clinicians also recommend offering private discussion with younger children who are amenable to talking with the clinician independently to provide them with an opportunity to share any questions or concerns.

Physical examinations should be as comprehensive as possible and performed in a trauma-informed manner. Laboratory studies should be ordered as indicated by AAP guidelines or by history and physical examination (see Chapter 11, Screenings, for specific guidance).

Vaccines should be updated in accordance with Centers for Disease Control and Prevention guidelines. No change to the routine vaccination schedule is needed for children in foster care; however, some practitioners prioritize vaccination for human papillomavirus for children at age 9 years because this has been shown to increase the series completion.[4,5] Given the complexity of vaccine requirements and consent for children in foster care, it is important to remain up to date on state-specific vaccine-related policies and laws. This topic is further discussed in Chapter 34, Medical Consents.

Follow-up Health Assessment Within 60 to 90 Days

Some caregivers and children experience a "honeymoon phase" when entering a new placement; while adjustment can initially seem smooth, difficulties may appear after the first weeks. A comprehensive follow-up assessment after several weeks in care is important to inquire about this adjustment period and refer to resources (see **Box 2–4**).

Box 2–4

Goals of Follow-up Health Assessment

- ▲ Assess adjustment of both child and caregiver.
- ▲ Follow up on any referrals made and ensure that those appointments have been completed.
- ▲ Assess academic progress and determine whether additional educational supports are needed.
- ▲ Update vaccinations.
- ▲ Provide anticipatory guidance.

This visit is also to monitor for any ongoing stressors and develop the relationship with the pediatrician as a source of consistency for the child. Further mental health and behavioral resources may need to be provided to both the child and caregiver at this visit.

If the child starts attending a new school at the time of entry into care, this visit should also assess their adjustment to the new school and their educational progress. For school-age children, it is important to ensure that children have a 504b plan or individualized education program (IEP), when appropriate, to provide academic support. Pediatricians and other physicians may send a letter of request to the school including a qualifying diagnosis (regarding a 504b plan) or request for an assessment (regarding an IEP) for children, when indicated. See Chapter 13, Developmental and Educational Issues, for more details.

Maintenance Phase of Care

Since placement in foster care is, by definition, temporary, it is important to remember that the maintenance phase is likely to be brief and still dynamic. Due to traumas leading to and resulting from removal into foster care and further disruptions while in care, these children have higher rates of chronic illnesses, both physical (for example, asthma) and psychological (posttraumatic stress disorder, for example), which can develop or be diagnosed while in foster care.[1]

In addition to following all the routine AAP guidelines, pediatricians should address some additional items during each health supervision visit with a child in care. The current caseworker should be updated and entered into the electronic medical record (EMR) at each visit, given that they act as the legal representative for the child. Communication with the caseworker should also occur after each visit, as would happen with a parent. These conversations and updates should occur directly with the caseworker, not via the caregivers. When the feature is available in the EMR, the chart should be flagged to alert other physicians across the medical system of the child's foster care status (see **Box 2–5**).

Box 2–5

Administrative Items to Address at Each Health Supervision Visit

- Update contact Information for current caseworker and placement.
- Update the legal medical decision-maker.
- Place a flag in the electronic medical record to indicate the child is in care.
- Update the caseworker directly on all medical findings and plans.

In many situations, physicians will have difficulty accessing past information and family history during the routine health supervision visit. When able, physicians should assess the child's past medical history and obtain releases (through the case worker) to access prior health records. Height and weight for all children, head circumference for children younger than 3 years, and blood pressure for those older than 3 years should be updated. Sensory measurements, as appropriate for age (vision for >3 years and hearing for >4 years of age), should be conducted if not completed at the prior visit.
Remember that children in care often have greater physical, developmental, and emotional health care needs than children not in care; therefore, screening should be performed for these issues regularly using age-appropriate tools and a trauma-focused history.[6] Also, pediatricians should continue to have age-appropriate conversations, as noted in the acute phase, at each visit. Pediatricians also should have a low threshold to refer for mental health care and ensure that each child has ongoing, consistent, and appropriate mental health care.

Pediatricians and other clinicians must be aware of and utilize local resources to support children in care, including caregiver and peer support programs for school-age children and adolescents, transition support services for those transitioning from adolescence to adult care, care coordination services to ensure connections occur, and educational support.

Laboratory assessments should generally follow the schedule recommended by the AAP,[1,7] with consideration for local and individual risk factors.

Involving the Family of Origin

Since reunification with the family of origin is almost always the goal on entry to care and occurs in approximately half of cases, ensuring that the family of origin is involved in medical appointments for routine care and counseling is important. When reunification is the goal, regular visits should be maintained with the family of origin, including siblings, during this phase. Moreover, connections to family and culture continue to be important for children even after termination of parental rights has occurred.

It is important that physicians inquire about visits with family during routine follow-up and provide support for the child and foster caregivers in managing these transitions. Provide the caregiver with tools to help with emotional regulation and routines before and after visits with the family of origin if this is a difficult time for the child.

The child's biological parents should be included in medical care whenever and as early as possible when the goal is reunification and contact is not restricted, which can be informed by the child welfare case worker.[8]

Including the family of origin can give the clinician more information about child and family history and can help provide the family of origin with the skills to manage medical or developmental care concerns prior to reunification. This may mean taking additional measures to make joint appointments possible, such as providing additional outreach, including parents through telemedicine, or performing outreach after visits. When a child has medical complexity, this is a critical step to help with this transition and to empower the parent to ask questions and take on the caregiving role. Birth parents may have their own trauma history, emotions related to the removal of their child (such as frustration, guilt, or anger), and varying abilities, involvement, and cooperation that may affect the visit. It is important to provide adequate time and a supportive environment that encourages cooperation between the family of origin and the foster caregivers during the visit (see **Box 2–6**).

Box 2–6

Ways the Pediatrician Can Support Reunification

- Include the family of origin in medical appointments as soon as is appropriate, either in person or via telemedicine, especially for children with medical complexity, using the support of the caseworker.
- Identify any training the family needs before reunification (eg, training on tube feedings or medical devices), and help coordinate this.
- Support the family of origin in understanding a child's behavioral and mental health needs before reunification; ensure that services are in place and can continue after reunification.

Placement Changes and Disruptions

Placement changes affect most children in care. On average, children are in foster care 1 to 2 years before exiting care, and one-third of children will experience more than 2 placement changes per year.[9] Sometimes placement changes result from behavioral challenges, but many times they are due to systems-related issues. Multiple placements are associated with delayed permanency, academic difficulties, and challenges in developing meaningful relationships and attachments.[10,11]

Children should be seen for a comprehensive wellness examination with any placement change to counsel and support the child and new caregivers during the adjustment phase. It is important to maintain contact with the child's caseworker to help maintain continuity if and when a placement change occurs. Ideally, the medical visit should be conducted by their current pediatrician to provide continuity for the child during a time of disruption and dysregulation. Pediatricians and other physicians should advocate for continuity through placement changes whenever possible, though limitations may exist due to geography and other factors. A stable pediatrician is sometimes the only point of continuity for a child who has experienced placement changes.

Placement changes are disruptive to a child's education, support services, medical care, and mental health care and often lead to challenges with adjustment and dysregulation. The pediatrician's role is to ensure that services remain in place for the child, ensure that there are no gaps in medical care, educate and support the new caregiver about the child's needs, and rescreen for adjustment reactions and dysregulation (see **Box 2–7**).

Box 2–7

The Role of the Pediatrician During a Placement Change

- Advocate that the child remain with the same pediatrician through placement changes.
- Ensure that the child's medical care, services, and supports continue uninterrupted.
- Rescreen for adjustment reactions and dysregulation.
- If the child needs to change pediatricians due to a placement change, complete a warm handoff with the new physician.

Unexpected disruptions are especially dysregulating for children in care, and they will need additional support during this time. Pediatricians should promote the use of the "3 Rs" (reassurance, routines, and regulation), as noted in Chapter 17, Childhood Trauma and Resilience.

Elopement from Care

It is not uncommon for adolescents to elope from care. There are often policies that require a health supervision visit when an adolescent returns to care. The clinic should always be a safe and supportive place for the adolescent. During these visits, clinicians should assess children for CSEC and other high-risk behaviors while missing from care, such as substance use. Clinicians should also do appropriate screening tests, as well as determine the need for and, when indicated, provide emergency contraception. Mental health, school, and employment supports, as well as age-appropriate anticipatory guidance on safety and future planning, should also be offered during these visits.

Transitioning to Permanency and Aging Out of Foster Care

Transitioning to permanency is a high priority at all points when a child is in foster care, and placement status should be reviewed regularly. Nationally, the outcomes for children in foster care in the most recent report from the Adoption and Foster Care Analysis and Reporting System, known as AFCARS, showed that 47% of children were reunified with 1 or both parents, 25% were adopted, 18% had permanent legal custodianship, and 9% aged out of foster care without finding permanency.[12] See Chapter 42, Advocacy and Public Policy, for more information on pertinent policies.

It is important to maintain awareness of the stage of a child's case to help support the child and caregivers through this process, particularly if the case moves from reunification to concurrent planning, where adoption or an alternative option to permanency is being considered, as well as when termination of parental rights occurs for either parent. The pediatrician should consider the impact this may have on the child and determine how to support the child through this transition. Mental health assessments and additional therapeutic supports also may be indicated (see **Box 2–8**).

Also, given that children in care have higher rates of developmental delays and that birth parents may have missed different developmental stages, it is an important opportunity to support them in understanding current developmental stages and needs and how to support their child. This can be a very important relationship-building opportunity with long-standing benefits to the caregiver and the child, as trust is built through providing a safe space to receive care. A resource regarding reunification and supports to provide to families can be accessed through the Child Information Gateway at https://www.childwelfare.gov/resources/reunification-foster-care-guide-parents/.

Box 2-8

Role of the Clinician in Transition to Permanency

- Be aware of the stage of the child's case to provide appropriate support.
- Keep in mind that reunification with birth parents is the plan for almost all children on entry to care.
  - Involve the birth parents in medical appointments and care when possible, to prepare for reunification.
  - Support birth parents around developmental stages they may have missed.
- Prepare for adoption if that is the next step in the case.
  - Be aware of when termination of parental rights occurs and the impact that this might have on the child.
  - Advocate for the child to receive adoption support for needs that may arise in the future.
- Prepare for aging out of care, as this is a high-risk time for youth.
  - Advocate for extended foster care if available.
  - Find supportive resources for adult life skills.
  - Provide a warm handoff to a new primary care provider.

Termination of Parental Rights and Adoption

When reunification appears less likely, then concurrent planning for alternative permanency options is considered. Priority will be given to placements with kinship caregivers who may be an adoptive or permanent guardianship option. States must notify relatives on both sides of the family when a child is removed within 30 days of placement. States are also mandated to try to keep siblings together. If the child is not placed with siblings, then maintaining visits with siblings and ongoing visits with birth parents will remain a priority.

Pediatricians should be aware that when the parental rights of a child have been terminated by the courts and a child is legally free for adoption, the child may experience big emotions, confusion, or complex and possibly conflicted feelings during this time. Pediatricians may help prepare for and provide support both for the caregivers and children during this time of transition, reinforcing the message that adoption does not mean replacing the people they have known and loved before; rather, it is growing their family. It is important for pediatricians to create an accurate reconstruction of the child's history in an age-appropriate fashion (for example, a life book), remain truthful about information that is shared, and keep an open discussion. Adoptive families and children should be encouraged to create traditions to acknowledge the adoption day while recognizing that it may bring mixed emotions around love and loss. Children may need additional support around the trauma of grief related to loss.[13]

Extended Foster Care and Aging Out of Care

Extended foster care and aging out of foster care are situations that occur when permanency is not established for a child before they transition to adulthood on their 18th birthday. This is when they lose the financial, social, and educational support that they previously had through the state. This transition is extraordinarily challenging and high risk for youth (for example, increased risks of homelessness, incarceration, and unintended pregnancies), as many are not equipped with the skills to make the transition to independent living. This challenging stage is often associated with deterioration of chronic health conditions. Additional transition support is essential for youth as they enter young adulthood. Pediatricians should stay updated on resources and programs available to support youth during this transition and begin these conversations well in advance. Helpful resource lists can be found online, including https://www.acf.hhs.gov/cb/faq/foster-care7; https://www.childwelfare.gov/resources/extension-foster-care-beyond-age-18/; and https://www.childwelfare.gov/topics/permanency/independent-living-and-transitioning-foster-care/.

Post-Permanency (Adoption, Reunification)

After foster care, children need continued behavioral health support and educational advocacy. Caregivers often need additional support and may not be aware that the child's experiences and exposures in foster care may continue to influence them throughout their life. Times when additional support may be needed include early adolescence, times of increased academic demand, and during the transition to adulthood.

Almost half of children in care are ultimately reunified with their biological parents. Ideally, the foster caregivers and parents can discuss how best to support the child's transition smoothly, including their health needs; however, this is not always possible. The family of origin may or may not be aware of any developments in their child's health needs while the child was in foster care. A comprehensive health assessment should be provided at the time of reunification to review any developmental or health needs. Ideally, this visit should be completed by a physician who has had continuity with the child; however, if this is not possible, then the child's medical records should be requested and a warm handoff from the previous pediatrician or other physician should be requested, if feasible. As the child adjusts to the reunification, additional supports might be necessary, including family therapy and behavioral supports.

If a child is being adopted, a comprehensive health assessment should be provided near the time of the adoption to review the medical history and prior diagnoses, perform a complete physical examination, order indicated screening laboratory tests, and provide appropriate referrals. This initial visit should be comprehensive but may happen over a series of visits, if indicated, to keep them manageable and supportive for the family and child. Also, when possible, a preadoption health supervision visit may be helpful to allow the pediatrician to review medical records and provide information and counsel families on adoption-related issues, support services, and resources.[14]

Adoption support services and guardianship assistance are available in many states and can help financially and logistically support both children and caregivers. Consider evidence-based parenting interventions for families and mental health services for children during times of need.

Key Takeaways

- » Children in foster care should be seen early, often, and comprehensively, especially around periods of transition in and out of care and between placements.
- » Even in stable placements, children should be seen frequently to assess for new needs and to develop a continuity relationship with their pediatrician.
- » The role of the pediatrician for children in foster care includes the provision of direct medical care as well as education to caregivers and caseworkers about the child's medical needs to ensure medical information is appropriately transferred when a child transitions or moves placements.

CHAPTER 3

Medical Home Readiness

Sarah H. Springer, MD, FAAP

A patient- and family-centered medical home (PFCMH), an approach to providing high-quality and comprehensive health care, is defined by the American Academy of Pediatrics (AAP) as being accessible, child- and family-centered, continuous, comprehensive, coordinated, compassionate, and culturally effective.[1] The AAP has identified the PFCMH as the optimal means for providing high quality and equitable care to all children and youth, especially those with complex health care needs.[2–4] Children who are involved with the child welfare system have experienced significant trauma and adversity and are by definition children with special health care needs.[5]

A comprehensive, trauma-informed, medical home approach to care is ideal for helping children and youth experiencing foster care and child welfare system involvement to heal. Optimally, a PFCMH can help prevent abuse and neglect and subsequent child welfare involvement by helping families to access the resources, supports, and services they need to thrive.[6–8] But even when a child has already experienced involvement in the child welfare system, the comprehensive, coordinated, compassionate, and culturally sensitive care offered in a PFCMH can help address those complex needs and help children heal and thrive. The principles outlined in this chapter can be applied by pediatricians and clinicians working in either a general primary care medical home or a specialty medical home specifically for children and youth in foster care. See Chapter 1, Core Components: A General Overview, for a discussion of different models of health care delivery for children in foster care. The remainder of this chapter will outline some of the unique aspects of caring for children and youth in foster care and offer strategies that medical practices can use to help children and youth to thrive.

Practice Environment

Culturally competent care means being knowledgeable about the cultures, traditions, languages, health care beliefs, and life experiences of the patients and communities one serves. A vital part of that care for children and youth in foster care is to provide trauma-informed care. Because family separation is an adverse childhood experience, every child who enters the child welfare system has experienced trauma and adversity. Every staff member, including front-desk staff, nurses, medical assistants, social workers, and care coordinators—even the billing department—can have positive effects on patients and families by using a trauma-informed approach to all interactions.[9,10]

Words matter.[11,12] When talking with children, youth, and families with histories of foster care, kinship care, and adoption, using respectful terms for birth families and families of origin, foster and kinship caregivers, and adoptive parents lets individuals know that they and their role in the child's life are respected.[5,13] All individuals who interact with this population must recognize and respect that families come in a wide variety of constellations and make the office welcoming to them. Office decor and websites should feature families from diverse backgrounds, children with single parents, grandparents, same-sex parents, and parents who are of a different race than the child. Office forms should ask for information about "parent/caregiver" rather than "mother" and "father." Depending on the child's circumstances, it may be appropriate for office visits to be attended by the current caregivers as well as the family of origin. Including the family of origin can help parents remain knowledgeable about the child's care and be better prepared to resume their parental role effectively.

While the needs of children and youth in foster care are often myriad, it is critically important to recognize, celebrate, and build on their strengths as well. Helping children develop talents and pursue interests can help restore some normalcy to life and build resilience. Recognizing a parent's love for their child, even when they are struggling to parent safely and effectively, can begin to promote healing.

Recognizing Foster, Kinship, and Adoptive Families

Recognizing and identifying children and youth who are experiencing foster care, kinship care, and other child welfare involvement is an important first step in being able to address their unique needs. One approach is to use the flagging system in the electronic health record to create an alert for this special need that would allow for extra time to be planned, when needed, and facilitate tracking of outcomes and quality measures.

Identify the adults who accompany the child or youth to each visit and their role (such as biological parent, kinship caregiver, foster parent, or caseworker). Different types of foster care placements and caregivers are detailed in Chapter 18, Out-of-Home Placements. Have a system to keep track of the names, contact information, and roles of the caregivers and other professionals who are part of the child's team. Each of these individuals has an important role to play in the child's safety and well-being and can be an important collaborator with a PFCMH to help the child be healthy and well.

It is also important to know the child's current status in the child welfare system and the current child welfare goals; for example, is the goal reunification with the child's family of origin or permanent legal guardianship with a relative, or have the parental rights been terminated and the goal is adoption? Considerations for medical care by stage of child welfare system service are detailed in Chapter 2, Health Care Visits: Type and Periodicity. Keeping all of the aforementioned information current is extremely challenging for the pediatrician, whether running a general PFCMH and seeing a few children in foster care or working in a specialized PFCMH for children and youth with child welfare involvement. This could be facilitated by information sharing between the child welfare and medical systems, which is discussed in Chapter 41, Privacy and Information Sharing.

Collaboration With Child Welfare Professionals

Collaboration and communication with local child welfare professionals is critical to providing the best possible care to this population. Child welfare systems vary by state or county.[14] Understanding local structures, laws, and processes will allow clinicians to most effectively collaborate and advocate for the children and youth in their care.

Cultivating relationships with child welfare and related professionals in the community can help build trust, which in turn enhances the abilities of all involved to support the health, safety, and well-being of children, youth, and families. Pediatricians should get to know child welfare leadership, supervisors, and caseworkers, as well as family court judges, legal professionals, and court-appointed special advocate volunteer groups. These contacts and relationships are helpful when there is a need to connect urgently in the midst of a busy clinical day. Chapter 40, Systems Involved in the Life of a Child in Foster Care: An Overview, is a helpful reference on these systems. Pediatricians should know their local child abuse specialized medical teams and child advocacy center and recognize that children and youth involved with the child welfare system will often need to see medical, developmental, and mental health specialists. This population will often also need support and advocacy within the educational system. Developing rapid referral processes can help to address the needs of children and families in a timely fashion.

Medical Records and Information Sharing

Obtaining and maintaining complete, accurate, and up-to-date medical records when children move into, through, and out of the child welfare system can be very challenging.[5] It is important to try to gather as much information as possible as early as possible. Sources of information may be lost to follow-up over time, and details of a child's health history and personal life story can be helpful to that child for the remainder of their life.

It is important to gather more than just vaccine and growth records, though those are also important. Prenatal exposure to alcohol and other toxic substances; physical, sexual, and emotional abuse; neglect; household and community violence; and parental substance use disorders are common contributing factors to child welfare system involvement. Medical history should ideally include prenatal and birth histories, including any known details about prenatal substance exposure and maternal stresses and trauma during the pregnancy.[5] Chapter 30, Neurodevelopmental Disorders: Identification and Intervention, outlines important details to gather from the birth history. Details of the child's developmental and educational histories can help guide evaluations and ongoing supports. Details of the traumas experienced by a child can help caregivers provide a safe and healing space for the child, and a detailed mental health history can guide ongoing mental health care. A detailed family medical history from the child's biological family can also be critically important to the child's long-term preventive care, well into adulthood.

Gathering all of this information can be challenging and time-consuming. Clinical care coordinators, a key role in any PFCMH, are critical to this effort; see Chapter 7, Care Coordination and Case Management, for a detailed discussion. As noted previously, relationships facilitate this information gathering. It is helpful to know not only local child welfare professionals but also case managers with both Medicaid and private health insurance companies, other regional clinicians, and local vaccine registries. Health information exchanges are discussed in Chapter 41, Privacy and Information Sharing. The child's family of origin may be the most important source of information that is helpful for all aspects of their life, including health care. Welcoming families of origin, who may feel ostracized by or angry at the child welfare system, can help gather key information and provide a safe space for their involvement and mutual concern for the child.

Collaborative record sharing between child welfare and health care systems can facilitate the delivery of better care by both systems. While privacy, technical, and logistical concerns abound, there are now examples of health information exchange and data-sharing systems that hold great promise.[15,16] Participating in such information-sharing systems can be enormously helpful for the PFCMH caring for children and youth in foster care. See Chapter 41, Privacy and Information Sharing, for additional information.

Complexities With Consent and Access to Records

Obtaining consent for care can be challenging for children and youth in foster care, starting with understanding who has the legal authority to consent. There may be 1 or 2 individuals who legally have authority to consent for any and all care, or different individuals may be authorized to consent for different things. For example, different parties could be authorized to consent for medical procedures and education decisions. Consent procedures can also vary based on the nature of the medical care required (routine, nonurgent, or emergent).

Who has consenting authority may change as the child's legal status in the child welfare system changes. Norms for all consent rules are highly variable by state and county. For example, immunizations may be considered routine health care in one state but may require separate consenting authority in another.

Consenting authority for teens also varies by state, with states allowing teens to have input or complete authority at differing ages, particularly regarding decisions about sexual and mental health care. Maintaining confidentiality for teens can be challenging, with the teen's rights to autonomy and confidentiality sometimes clashing with the need for foster parents, caseworkers, legal advocates, judges, and others to understand and accommodate all of a teen's needs as other decisions are made. See Chapter 34, Medical Consents, for adolescent-specific issues.

Access to patient portals is a particularly vexing dilemma. While having equitable access to health records is important, maintaining confidentiality is also critical. The challenges of keeping information up to date and accurate regarding who has access to the medical records can lead to privacy breaches that are both undesirable and illegal.[17] The AAP page on the Health Insurance

Portability and Accountability Act (HIPPA) provides general guidance for pediatric practices on managing protected health information.[17] Here too, health information and data exchange systems between child welfare and health care systems hold great promise.[16]

Understanding local laws is critical,[18] as is ongoing communication with child welfare professionals in accordance with those laws. It is important to review and update consenting authority at every visit and to keep the child's chart updated with names and contact information for each adult who has consenting authority. Lack of clarity on who has consenting authority can cause delays in care, which could range from being minor inconveniences to life-threatening situations.

Health Care Financing and the Medical Home

Chapter 37, Health Care Financing, provides a detailed discussion of this topic. Most children and youth in foster care are eligible for Medicaid in the state in which they reside.[19] Under amendments to the Affordable Care Act made in 2014 and 2018,[19] young adults who have previously been in foster care are eligible for Medicaid coverage until they are 26 years old, even if they were in foster care in another state.[19] Many Medicaid managed care organizations have specialized teams to coordinate care for children with medical complexities, and many children and youth in foster care are eligible for those supports as well. Knowing and collaborating with those teams can be an enormous help in meeting the needs of children with complex needs.

In the PFCMH setting, children and youth in foster care will require more than just an annual health supervision visit to address their often complex physical, mental, and developmental health needs and educational needs. Chapter 2, Health Care Visits: Type and Periodicity, details visits recommended for children in foster care. The first visit is really about identifying any urgent or emergency needs, developing and prioritizing a list of needs to be addressed, identifying screenings that will be helpful, and identifying protective factors that can help mitigate the effects of trauma. Follow-up visits can be scheduled frequently and with enough time at each visit to (1) allow for appropriate developmental and mental health screenings, (2) address each item on the problem list, (3) address school needs, and (4) support caregivers as they work to help the child begin to heal. These visits are appropriately coded as "sick visits," using standard evaluation and management coding for time and complexity.[20]

Conclusion

Caring for children and youth in foster care can be challenging, given the complex needs and sometimes limited information available, especially at early visits. However, foster care can and always should be a time for healing. The opportunity to help children and youth, their caregivers, and their families of origin to heal and to thrive is among the most rewarding experiences in pediatric medicine.

Key Takeaways

» A PFCMH is ideally structured to help meet the needs of children and youth with child welfare system involvement.

» Every staff member, including front-desk staff, nurses, medical assistants, physicians, social workers, and care coordinators, can have positive effects on patients and families by using a trauma-informed approach to all interactions.

» Planning ahead and developing relationships with local child welfare professionals can greatly facilitate the provision of high-quality care to children and youth with child welfare involvement.

» Having a tracking system to identify children with child welfare involvement will allow extra time to be scheduled, when needed, to address complex needs.

» Recognizing and encouraging strengths in children and families can help promote healing.

CHAPTER

4

Emergency Department and Inpatient Care: Practice Readiness

Patricia M. Lantis, MD, FAAP

Introduction

Clinicians working in emergency departments (EDs) and hospital inpatient settings have unique opportunities to care for children in foster care. Children in foster care have high rates of health care utilization and may present for scheduled or unscheduled care.[1,2] ED and inpatient settings vary widely in resources from rural to more urban centers. However, knowledgeable clinicians can optimize the well-being of children in foster care in any of these environments. Allowing extra time for this care is critical to keeping children thriving in safe, stable, nurturing families. This chapter describes general principles of practice to guide the delivery of health care to children and adolescents encountered in ED and inpatient settings.

Consent

Children in foster care often present to the ED with an adult who is not their legal guardian. Staff should clarify custody status as soon as life-threatening emergencies are stabilized. This ensures that appropriate informed consent is obtained and that the diagnostic evaluation and treatment program is discussed with the family of origin as well as with current caregivers.[3] Adolescents presenting for sexual or reproductive care may be able to consent individually without a guardian or parent. Consult local state regulations for guidance[4] (see Chapter 34, Medical Consents).

History

Often, the caregiver who brings the child to the hospital may not have full details of the chief complaint or the medical history. Children may present with relatives, new foster caregivers, or child welfare workers who have little knowledge of the child. Pediatricians who refer children for emergency services should attempt to call ahead and provide any relevant history to the treating team. The history should be obtained from the individual who has the best knowledge of the patient's medical history. Efforts to contact the family of origin may be appropriate if supported by the child welfare organization. Clinicians should review all available records in a timely manner, including electronic medical record (EMR) systems. If information sharing is available, inquire through these platforms (for example, Epic's Care Everywhere or Cerner's Community View) as well as any institution-specific data-sharing platforms.[5] Historical information needed for immediate treatment should be the focus of the initial inquiry (eg, allergies in a child who needs an urgent antibiotic). Birth records, prior medications, previous ED or inpatient encounters, allergies, and immunizations should be updated and verified. In-person medical interpreters (or phone/video-enabled interpretation services if necessary) should be used to ensure accurate communication with those with a first language other than English. Children and caregivers should be approached with cultural awareness during all encounters. A confidential adolescent history is critical for ongoing diagnostic and treatment planning (see Part 3, Adolescent-Specific Issues). Suicidal ideation or plans should be asked about with all children 11 years or older and with those under 11 years who have warning signs (see Chapter 12, Mental Health). For acute cases of sexual abuse, follow protocols and defer forensic interviewing to legal authorities or their designees.

Physical Examination

The physical examination should be performed in response to the chief complaint. If a child presents to the ED for a placement screening examination or concern for maltreatment, a full examination can be conducted to ascertain injuries (including self-inflicted), bruising, and other signs of neglect or abuse. Acute oral health needs may also be identified; these are often overlooked in children in protective custody.[2,6] An external genitourinary inspection should be conducted in young children and in older children when indicated. A chaperone should be used during any sensitive examinations (the caregiver does not qualify as a chaperone). Asymptomatic testing for sexually transmitted infections has a low yield other than nucleic acid amplification testing for gonorrhea and chlamydia, for which a speculum examination is unnecessary.[7] The medical examination should be conducted sensitively to minimize further trauma to the child and to maintain the child's privacy and dignity (see Table 1–2 in Chapter 1, Core Components: A General Overview, for measures to consider). The child's physical comfort should be considered during the examination as well, such as the provision of a warm blanket or fresh undergarments. Clinicians should consider limiting learner participation in some scenarios while also instructing learners on the unique health care needs of children in protective custody.

Diagnostic Data

Diagnostic data should be sought based on chief complaint. If the child has presented for a placement screening examination or evaluation for maltreatment, follow American Academy of Pediatrics recommendations for laboratory or radiographic testing.[8] If the child is a neonate, state systems should be used, if possible, to review the screening results. If the child has a chronic illness with or without an exacerbation, appropriate testing should be sent (such as antiepileptic drug levels in a seizing child) to assess and optimize chronic disease management.

Strongly consider additional diagnostic workup of the following:

- Malnutrition
- Fractures
- Unexplained bleeding or bruising
- Seizures
- Burns
- Altered mental status (eg, delirium, catatonia, acute psychosis)
- Abrupt behavioral change (eg, food refusal, sudden change in toileting habits)

Medical Record

The EMR should be consistently updated during the encounter to ensure accuracy. This includes resolving old problems, reviewing the growth chart, updating allergies and immunizations, and adding new medical problems, if indicated. Relevant photographs are appropriate and helpful if they can be taken and uploaded to the chart confidentially. Some EMRs have confidential tabs visible to hospital staff where helpful information (for example, the foster caregiver's name and phone number) can be shared with the multidisciplinary team. Legal custody status, medical decision-making rights, and visiting rights should be clarified regularly. Ensuring updated insurance provider and outpatient pharmacy information is also helpful.

Admission Criteria

Careful consideration of medical admission for children in foster care is necessary. Indications may include but are not limited to

- Concern for medical neglect or abuse in current placement
- Serious medical condition
- Significant exacerbation of a chronic condition
- Mental health concerns (eating disorders, suicidal ideation/homicidal ideation, altered mentation)
- Current caregiver unwilling or deemed unable to care for the patient
- Need for education of caregiver about serious medical condition
- Concern by medical professionals about the safety and well-being of the child

In some states (eg, Georgia[9]), physicians can determine to take temporary protective custody of a child deemed to be in imminent danger. Hospital risk management experts and individual state laws should be consulted in such situations.

Care Coordination

Once a child in foster care is admitted, care coordination is helpful to ensure a safe and timely discharge. Daily formal rounds with a multidisciplinary team can facilitate this goal. Children may be admitted to the hospital due to lack of resources or other issues that are readily addressed by knowledgeable case managers. Equipment and medication needs and subspecialty access are often problematic for families. Child welfare workers may be part of this multidisciplinary team as well. If a new placement is necessary, updating child welfare workers on anticipated discharge date and need for skilled caregivers (eg, to place a child with a tracheostomy) will prevent prolonged hospitalizations for this reason alone.[10] Additional care coordination is necessary for children with chronic conditions such as sickle cell anemia or diabetes who are being placed in a group home or in residential care.

Medical Needs During Hospitalization

The guiding principles of trauma-informed care should be used in all encounters with children in foster care in the hospital.[11,12] Loss of control is often extremely frustrating to the patient as well as the caregivers. Giving "voice and choice" when possible and using positive reinforcement should be the goal. Implement current best practices for withholding food and drink prior to a procedure to minimize prolonged unnecessary fasting. Ensure appropriate anxiolysis and careful pain management during hospitalization to limit further traumatic experiences. Help children and caregivers understand each team member's role in the child's care. Consideration should be taken to limit the number of team members who round in the room. Child life services are helpful for procedural preparation and diversional activities. Canine therapy has been demonstrated to provide emotional support and alleviate pain during hospitalization.[13]

Consider giving catch-up immunizations and removing other barriers to enrolling in school that families may have encountered. Consider subspecialty consultation during admission for exacerbations of chronic conditions (such as asthma) or to expedite needed procedures after discharge (such as tonsillectomy for obstructive sleep apnea). Review all previous medications and adjust dosages if necessary. Consult appropriate clinicians for assistance if the indication for any medication is uncertain.

Assess urgent educational needs and make referrals for outpatient psychoeducational evaluation if indicated. Provide caregivers with any needed information about educational rights for children with learning differences. If a confidential adolescent history was not performed on admission, ensure it is done during the hospital stay and that appropriate referrals for mental health care needs are made. Ethical considerations may also arise with other decisions that need to be made, including consents for blood transfusions, surgical procedures, end-of-life care, and certain treatments (such as bone marrow transplantation).[3] Medical needs should be shared in a timely way with the child welfare system. All information relevant to posthospital care ideally should be provided to the family of origin (when deemed appropriate by the child welfare system) as well as the fostering caregivers. Providing holistic care during a medical crisis ultimately alleviates further stress on the child and caregivers by minimizing interruptions to education and decreasing the stress of multiple follow-up appointments.

Social Needs During Admission

When possible, involving social workers and or case managers can support a child in foster care during their admission. Social workers can help update legal custody and placement status, facilitate communication with child welfare, and make arrangements for safe visitation with the family of origin when appropriate, as well as with foster and kinship caregivers. Additionally, social workers may refer children and families to appropriate community support groups (such as teens with chronic illnesses, postpartum depression support, bereavement support) with approval from the child welfare system. Social workers are also critical members of the discharge planning team.

Health Education

The patient should receive age-appropriate education about their own medical diagnosis and care. This is especially critical for youth who are close to aging out of the foster care system.[14] Youth in protective custody have higher rates of risk-taking behaviors and should be counseled based on the needs identified in their confidential history.[15] Parents and caregivers also should be educated on the child's medical condition and care during hospital stays. Common topics for which families need education include

- Formula preparation
- Medication administration and scheduling (eg, tapering pain or respiratory medications)
- Feeding tube use and care
- Apnea monitor
- Cardiopulmonary resuscitation training
- Use of epinephrine for anaphylaxis
- Use of rescue medication for seizures or narcotic overdose
- Sickle cell emergencies
- Asthma management
- Diabetes management
- Behavioral health emergencies

Discharge Planning

Discharge planning should include feedback from the child or teen when appropriate, as well as the caseworker and the guardian to allow adaptation as necessary. Children in foster care often have delays during discharge that are not under the control of the hospital care team.[10] However, to avoid further delays, the hospital team can work toward ensuring the following:

- Discharge medications are on the patient's insurance formulary
- Specialty formulas are located, and relevant caregiver education completed
- Medications and equipment are ready to pick up or are delivered to the home or hospital
- Medical home has been identified and discharge plan communicated effectively
- Community resources, if needed, are identified
- Subspecialty referrals are made or appointments scheduled
- Written forms are signed for medication administration at school (eg, asthma inhalers, epinephrine autoinjector)
- Speech, physical, or occupational therapy referrals are provided
- Early-intervention services referral is provided
- Developmental evaluations (eg, autism screening or services) are completed
- Caregivers are comfortable with equipment use and medication administration; consider "rooming in" before discharge

Strong communication, early and often during hospitalization, with the child welfare team regarding anticipated needs and discharge date can assist with timely discharge.

Follow-up

All children in foster care should be considered "high-risk" discharges, with careful attention given to postdischarge communication to the medical home to prevent adverse events during the transition.[16] Ideally, the attending physician or another member of the health care team should try to communicate discharge follow-up needs with the medical home clinician verbally. Common discharge diagnoses requiring close and frequent follow-up include mental health crises, malnutrition, and poorly controlled chronic illnesses. Ideally, the patient will be cared for in a medical home with expanded resources for children in foster care (a foster care clinic).[17]

Discharge plans and goals should be meticulously documented in the EMR and communicated in writing as well as verbally to the caregivers and child welfare team in plain language. The caregivers should also have a clear understanding of the necessary actions for the child's recovery and safety, such as weekly feeding adjustments or adherence to subspecialty follow-up care. Specific instructions for return to care (for example, "please return to the hospital should fever over 101°F recur while taking oral antibiotics") as well as for the timeliness of care (such as "your pediatrician should see your child tomorrow to recheck her asthma") ensures closed-loop communication between the guardian and the medical and child welfare teams.

Team Support

Caring for special-needs populations, such as children in foster care, with a high incidence of complex chronic conditions is often emotionally charged work. Staff including nurses, social workers, case managers, and child life specialists should be adequately trained in trauma-informed care practices and have a basic understanding of the child welfare system and the intersection of the child welfare and pediatric health care systems.[18] Empowering staff to feel prepared to treat these children and caregivers will hopefully prevent staff turnover and staffing shortages. Additionally, health care trainees should be educated in these principles. Support of all members of the health care team will help each member recognize and respond to trauma effectively as professionals.[19]

Key Takeaways

- ED and inpatient clinicians will encounter children in foster care frequently and can become skilled in their care.
- Extra time is necessary for optimizing the health, safety, and well-being of children in foster care.
- Assess and address medical, educational, and mental health needs for children in foster care in a holistic manner.
- Effective communication among the health care team and with child welfare professionals prevents delays in discharge.
- Assess and address necessary resources and barriers to care for families prior to discharge.
- Staff and trainees should have regular education and support in their mission to care for children in protective custody.

CHAPTER 5

Specialty Care: Practice Readiness

Abigail Genco, MD, FAAP
Jennifer Ehrhardt, MD, MPH

Children in the foster care system have unique circumstances that can predispose them to needing specialty care. Research has shown that these children, when compared with children not in foster care, are more likely to have chronic conditions, including growth failure, asthma, obesity, vision impairment, hearing loss, neurological problems, and sexually transmitted infections. Additionally, those children in foster care who require a higher complexity of care are more likely to experience frequent placement changes.[1–4]

Given the potential difficulties with obtaining consistent care, children in foster care may not have received needed specialty care. The specialist's role in providing care should be to act as a partner to the patient's primary care physician to manage acute and chronic conditions. The specialist may need to communicate more frequently with the primary care physician, given the difficulties with obtaining information about and services for these children. Beyond the child's health conditions, the specialist may need to consider factors that interplay with physical health, such as prenatal (maternal) substance exposure and access to health care both prenatally and during early childhood.[1] [1]

Finally, the specialist should provide care with cultural competency and humility. Children in foster care often have diverse racial, cultural, economic, and linguistic backgrounds, which may differ from those of their foster family.[5] The specialist should keep these in mind when collecting medical histories and providing treatment and patient and caregiver education. This may require asking more clarifying questions of both the child and the foster family to better understand their experiences.

Comprehensive Medical History

Children in foster care often have fragmented care, going periods of time without care or receiving care at multiple locations.[3] The history-taking may be more targeted with this population, given the likely gaps in care. However, the history should be expanded to screen for barriers to care commonly seen in the foster care system, such as poverty, housing insecurity, placement changes, and previous trauma.[1] Given the complexity of the social situation and the degree of medical support needed, the specialist may need to consider closer follow-up of this population. This may need to be coordinated with other appointments; if this is not possible, frequent outreach with nurses or social workers may be appropriate.

Specialists should also consider how to obtain supplemental information to fill in gaps or discrepancies in the medical history. Every effort should be made to ensure that the history is objective; however, it may be difficult for foster parents to give a comprehensive, factual medical history of the child. When possible, the history should be obtained either directly from the child's family of origin or, when appropriate for age and developmental stage, from the child. Interfacing with the child's previous foster families may also be helpful. Additional sources of this information include[1,4]

- Child protective services
- Guardian ad litem (GAL)
- Court Appointed Special Advocate (CASA)
- State or community immunization registry
- Previous places of medical care
  - Hospitals
  - Emergency departments
  - Urgent care facilities
- Schools
- Early intervention services

Further, when accessible, platforms that allow patient record sharing across institutions and electronic health record systems, such as Epic's Care Everywhere, should be used for ascertaining the past and recent specialty care the child has received.

Lastly, consideration should be given to barriers to accessing care. Distance to specialty centers may be addressed by comanagement of chronic conditions by specialists and primary care physicians. Primary care clinics that treat a large volume of children in foster care and foster care consultative clinics may develop collaborations with highly sought-after specialists to circumvent the long wait times often experienced with these physicians. Examples of such collaborations include colocation of specialist and primary care clinics, priority access visits within a specialty clinic for children in foster care, and e-consultations.

Consent

Obtaining consent for specialty care can be difficult when caring for children in foster care. Physicians often must navigate complex social situations when considering who is the most appropriate person to give consent to deliver care. The consenting party can vary by state, and several parties may be involved in this process, including birth parents, the commissioner/director of child welfare, or a GAL.[1] Given the higher complexity of care offered in specialty clinics, it is advisable that specialty clinicians familiarize themselves with the procedures or treatments that require additional consent. Often, routine health care, including well-child visits and immunizations, are covered under general medical consents. Procedures that are more likely to require consent from a guardian include[1]

- Surgical procedures
- Prescription of certain medications
  - Psychotropic medications
  - Chemotherapy
- Mental health evaluations

It is also important to consider confidentiality when discussing sensitive topics, such as reproductive and sexual health, mental health, and substance use. These topics are discussed in more detail within Part III, Adolescent-Specific Issues, and Chapter 34, Medical Consents.

Education and Information Sharing

Caregiver education is key for managing a child's chronic health conditions. The specialist should consider which caregivers are most involved in the day-to-day care of the child and ensure they receive the necessary education. It is also helpful to have a written treatment plan that can be distributed to all caregivers. Involved parties who may benefit from information sharing include[1]

- Family of origin
- Foster family/kinship caregiver
- Child welfare agencies
- CASA/GAL
- Schools

Given the number of people involved in the child's care, additional visits may be needed to communicate the plan going forward. It is also important to involve the child in their own education and treatment, as they will be important self-advocates as they enter young adulthood. Effective care coordination is important; see Chapter 7, Care Coordination and Case Management.

Telehealth can be a powerful tool for communicating information about the child's health condition and treatment plan to all parties who need this information. It allows parties in different physical locations, such as the child welfare agency, GAL, and foster family, to join the same visit virtually, thereby promoting a shared understanding of the treatment plan while facilitating more integrated care coordination for the child. Integration of technology in coordinating care across multiple systems is vital, especially in cases where children move frequently between different placements and physicians. However, while telehealth can be helpful for mitigating access issues, pediatricians and other physicians should be cognizant of barriers to care that children in foster care can experience that telehealth cannot address, including difficulty obtaining necessary laboratory tests and imaging. In those instances, in-person visits may be more appropriate.

It is important to help caregivers prioritize which services and treatments would be most beneficial and determine which setting would offer the most consistent utilization of those services. For example, children with disabilities may qualify for an individualized education program (IEP) through their local school district. Through an IEP, a child may receive additional support in school through various nonphysician clinicians. Additionally, children with medical conditions may qualify for a 504 plan, which allows additional accommodation within the classroom, such as preferential seating, medication administration support, or break periods during the school day. While the educational system is separate from the health care system, additional efforts to collaborate with schools may be necessary for children in foster care. This could be done by obtaining consent to share records and visit notes between pediatricians and other physicians and schools, providing written communications to the school with specific recommendations for educational plans, or attending meetings with school officials to discuss the needs of a child.

The process of obtaining these plans is outlined in more detail in Chapter 13, Developmental and Educational Issues.

Insurance Coverage

As specialists may recommend additional services, medications, or therapies, they must consider the insurance status of each patient. State Medicaid insures most children in foster care.[1] Insurance reimbursement may not adequately reflect the time and effort clinicians spend treating a patient. Additional information concerning insurance coverage can be found in Chapter 37, Health Care Financing.

Conclusion

Given the higher rates of chronic health conditions and medical complexity for children in foster care compared with those not in foster care, the specialist may play a key role in their medical care. Involving multiple parties in obtaining the child's medical history, consenting for treatment, and ensuring that all parties know the child's treatment plan are important components to consider when providing specialty care to this population.

Key Takeaways

» Children in foster care are at higher risk for chronic conditions that may require specialty care but have unique barriers to care, such as previous trauma and discontinuity of care.

» Taking a medical history in a specialty setting for children in foster care should be comprehensive and may require multiple sources of information to account for gaps in care.

» Information-gathering, education, and treatment should be discussed with the child's various caregivers and, when developmentally appropriate, the child themself to ensure continuity of care.

Chapter 6

Staff Training and Resources

V. Faye Jones, MD, PhD, MSPH, FAAP
Jennifer M. Porter, MD, FAAP

Introduction

Navigating the complexities of the foster care system can be challenging for pediatricians, families, and youth. Children and adolescents who are or have been in foster care have often experienced trauma secondary to exposure to multiple adverse childhood experiences (ACEs).[1] ACEs can take many forms, including child maltreatment and disruptions in a child's environment, placing them at increased risk for medical, developmental, and psychiatric issues. Often these problems remain either unaddressed or untreated. Pediatricians can support other health professionals and families of children in foster care by providing appropriate resources while optimizing children's medical care and helping each child reach their full potential.[2] Wraparound support services are critical components in delivering high-quality, outcome-focused, and culturally sensitive care. Pediatricians, other clinicians, and foster families must be familiar with available trauma-informed resources that best support the overall care of children in foster care. This chapter provides insight, evidence-based resources, and best practices for pediatricians to navigate the challenges faced by foster families related to health care. The evidence-based resources mentioned cover topics on the provision of care, policy and education, support for families, and local and national agencies.

Trauma-Informed Care

Traumatic experiences are common among children with experience in the foster care system. Research on the epigenetics of trauma has contributed to our understanding of the negative outcomes these children may face.[3] However, an area of recent exploration is the epigenetic transfer of resilience.[4,5] *Resilience* is defined as "a dynamic process or complex function of numerous individual (such as genetic) and social-environmental (such as social support) factors that allows an individual to maintain good psychological health despite significant adversity."[4–6] Resilience develops in the interaction of each individual's genetic code with their environment. Medical systems and clinicians can play a role in the process of building resilience by being knowledgeable about the impact of trauma and by using a trauma-informed care (TIC) approach within their environment.[7]

Hopper and associates[8] defined TIC as "a strengths-based framework that is grounded in an understanding of and responsiveness to the impact of trauma, that emphasizes physical, psychological, and emotional safety for both providers and survivors, and that creates opportunities for survivors to rebuild a sense of control and empowerment." Though this concept originated in behavioral health organizations, TIC is recognized as an essential component in pediatric health practices.[9]

Several reports are available to describe the importance of TIC and how to incorporate these principles into practice. A multilevel systems approach is necessary to change the way organizations and practices support families.[9] In 2021, the American Academy of Pediatrics (AAP) published a policy statement and a clinical report entitled "Trauma-informed Care in Child Systems" and "Trauma-Informed Care," respectively.[10,11] The policy statement describes the resources needed for financial support and infrastructure development with the implementation of TIC principles into all pediatric points of care.[10] The clinical report translates the science of trauma and resilience by informing care from prevention to treatment.[11] TIC reframes the question, "What's *wrong* with you?" into "What *happened* to you?" Going beyond this, assessing the youth's strengths with questions such as "'What unique qualities or skills have you developed through your experiences," "What special skills or talents have you gained from your experiences," "What personal strengths have you discovered," or "What makes you feel proud" may be appropriate.

Creating a Trauma-Informed Environment in the Clinical Setting

It is crucial to train all members of the medical office about the importance of a trauma-informed environment.[12–14] Training enables all members, from front-office staff to pediatricians and other clinicians to discharge planners, to understand the nature of trauma and its triggers within the health care setting. This understanding equips them with the necessary tools to create a safe and nurturing setting that fosters healing and recovery for patients who have experienced trauma.[12] Creating a safe atmosphere can be exemplified by the implementation of inclusive language on signage. Consistently maintaining respectful, open, and empathetic communication with families serves as a demonstration of a secure social and emotional environment.[12]

Personnel training should prioritize the development of affiliate skills including empathic engagement, identifying trauma symptoms, responding to triggers, and providing appropriate care.[14] Moreover, personnel should be trained to recognize the impact of trauma on patients' physical, emotional, and psychological well-being. This training will enhance the quality of care provided to patients and promote their overall health and well-being.[14] The National Child Traumatic Stress Network offers both online and in-person training. Featured topics include general trauma education, assessment measures, intervention techniques, and a series focused on systems change.[14] The AAP offers free online training resources for members, including for pediatric clinicians and staff, at https://aap.org/trauma.

Pediatricians can provide patients and their families with the necessary resources and support when trauma is identified or suspected. One effective approach is to identify referral sources in the community and partner with various organizations to create a coordinated response to situations that may arise during the screening process. BOUNCE (https://bouncecoalition.org) serves as a prime illustration of a community organization dedicated to fostering resilience. Its mission revolves around enhancing the resilience of individuals and families, encompassing children and adults, by disseminating knowledge on the repercussions of ACEs and equipping them with the necessary skills to effectively rebound from adversity. Support for families should involve a team of experts, such as mental health professionals, medical practitioners, social workers, and community partners, to provide patients and their families with the necessary resources to recover from their experiences. The goal of this approach is to provide a holistic and integrated response to trauma, addressing patients' physical, emotional, and social needs. Specific screening tools are discussed in Chapter 11, Screenings, and Chapter 12, Mental Health.

Actively involving the patient and their family in their own care plan and decision-making process is critical.[12–14] This approach not only fosters a collaborative environment but also creates an atmosphere of trust and respect, which are crucial components of effective TIC and patient well-being. Patients and their families can provide valuable insights into their experiences, which can help pediatricians and other clinicians improve the quality of care they provide. In addition, involving families in the health care process can reduce anxiety and improve patient outcomes. One way to involve families and patients is by incorporating a Patient and Family Advisory Council (PFAC)[15,16] within the clinical practice. The PFAC is composed of clinicians, office staff, patients, and family members. Patients and their families are viewed as valuable partners and essential resources to the practice. A PFAC can provide valuable input in various areas, including communication, care coordination, and patient education. Moreover, by involving patients and family members in the clinical processes, a practice can enhance its responsiveness to the needs of patients and their families. This can lead to better outcomes and help to build trust between patients, their families, and clinicians. The National Partnership for Women and Families[15] and the American Hospital Association[16] provide a blueprint for initiating and sustaining an effective PFAC.

Health care leaders need to be aware of the negative effects that learning about trauma histories can have on the emotional well-being of the workforce, especially for those with their own trauma experiences. *Secondary traumatic stress* refers to "the emotional duress that results when an individual hears about the firsthand trauma experiences of another."[17] It is important to provide effective strategies focusing on self-care within the practice. This promotes a healthy work environment, builds resilience for health care workers, and ensures that they are equipped with the necessary tools to manage negative effects that may arise from their work.[17]

Healing Centered Engagement

Another approach to understanding the effects of trauma is healing centered engagement (HCE).[18] This holistic approach, introduced by Shawn Ginwright, is "strength-based, advances a collective view of healing, and re-centers culture as a central feature in well-being.... [HCE] requires a different question that moves beyond 'what happened to you' to 'what's right with you' and views those exposed to trauma as agents in the creation of their own well-being rather than victims of traumatic events."[19] HCE consists of 4 components[18]:

- Bring awareness and actions through policy and opportunities, addressing conditions that created the trauma to enhance well-being and healing.
- Be grounded in culture and identity.
- Use asset-driven strategies that focus on collective strengths and possibilities.
- Support adult clinicians with their own healing.

HCE adopts a comprehensive outlook on health and wellness, going beyond merely treating symptoms and addressing trauma by considering all the factors contributing to a child's overall health and recovery. This holistic approach is consistent with the practices of pediatricians.

Healing centered engagement emphasizes a strength-asset model that provides clinicians with opportunities to play a vital role in promoting child well-being, especially when working with children who have experienced trauma. Components of HCE align with the Youth Thrive framework.[18,19] By identifying and building on the strengths of children and their families, pediatricians can foster resilience.

Pediatricians play an important role in promoting positive youth identity, which is crucial to a child's overall development. One way they can do this is by gathering comprehensive information on the child's past and present social connections. This includes their family, community, and natural networks such as friends and peers. By gaining a deeper understanding of these connections, pediatricians can identify potential sources of support and strengthen positive relationships that can contribute to the child's sense of identity and well-being. Supporting relational connections is crucial because experiencing trauma can lead to social thinning.

Additionally, pediatricians can help address any social or emotional challenges that the child may encounter and provide guidance on how to nurture positive relationships and build a strong social support system. To achieve this goal, clinicians should inquire about various domains, including living conditions, access to quality education, food insecurity, economic stability, literacy or language barriers, racism or discrimination, and environmental injustices that may affect children's health.

Clinicians should also inquire about strengths and promotive factors. Questions might include "Who helps you feel supported at home or where you stay?"; "What helps you do your best learning, even when things feel tough?"; "What are things that inspire a sense of pride in your culture, background, or identity?"; "What do you wish people understood you or your family are good at handling, even when times are hard?"; and "What makes a friend feel like a safe person to you?"

To reduce stressors on caregivers and families, pediatricians should support referrals based on social drivers of health, necessitating the implementation of a closed-loop referral system. It is imperative to verify the dispatch and processing of the referral, and subsequently document its completion, in a manner analogous to closing the loop for a referral to a specialist physician. Obtaining consent to share information between the clinician and the referral source will provide valuable information that may not have been shared previously.

Pediatricians must be aware that individuals from different cultures may have different perceptions of health, healing, medical care, and traumatic experiences. For example, different cultures may have unique beliefs about illness, its causes, and how it can be treated. By acknowledging and respecting these beliefs, pediatricians can provide culturally appropriate care that is sensitive to the needs of the patient and their family.

Online certification in HCE techniques is available through Flourish Agenda.[20] Components of the training include videos, scenarios, interactive and reflective learning activities, and supplemental learning resources.[20]

AAP Evidenced-Based Policy Statements, Clinical Reports, and Technical Guidelines

The AAP provides evidence-based policy statements, clinical reports, and technical guidelines to enhance the health and well-being of children and youth.

In 2015, the AAP Council on Foster Care, Adoption, and Kinship Care provided both a policy statement and a technical report entitled "Health Care Issues for Children and Adolescents in Foster Care and Kinship Care."[21,22] These provided background information about and described trends in foster care. Health needs, as well as barriers, are also described. The authors illustrate and discuss the following key components of basic health services for children and adolescents involved with child welfare:

- Establish a proper pediatric medical home.
- Coordinate care to improve health outcomes by communicating with caregivers, child welfare professionals, health and mental health specialists, and other involved parties.
- Assess overall health status upon entry into foster care.
- Implement guidelines for health services with an enhanced visitation schedule.

Using data from the US Census Bureau from 2022 through 2024, the Annie E. Casey Foundation Kids Data Center found that 3% of children in the United States experience some form of kinship care.[23] Federal and state legislation have been instrumental in protecting and supporting families providing kinship care. Pediatricians can improve their care of children and adolescents placed in kinship care by understanding the needs of each family. While every foster and kinship care situation is unique, research on kin caregivers shows significant differences from nonkinship foster caregivers. For example, kinship caregivers tend to be older, have less formal education, be poorer, report more chronic conditions, and care for larger sibling groups compared with nonkinship caregivers.[24] The AAP offers additional recommendations for pediatric practice as it relates to treating children in kinship care families.[24]

Pediatric practices can assist in the care of children experiencing kinship arrangements by

- Being familiar with laws regarding guardianship and consent and routinely documenting and updating guardianship arrangements in the medical records
- Standardizing developmental and behavioral health screening
- Providing information about community resources for kinship families[24]

The clinical report "Pediatrician Guidance in Supporting Families of Children Who Are Adopted, Fostered, or in Kinship Care" offers guidance on a wide range of foster and kinship areas.[2] The report outlines the significance of the Family First Prevention Services Act of 2018 and other federal mandates for children in adoptive and foster environments. Other critical information for pediatricians includes common medical concerns; issues specific to kinship care; communication related to placement and permanency; loss, grief, and trauma during and following foster care placement; differences across the spectrum of adoptive, foster, and kinship families; challenges with maintaining consistent education and educational attainment; barriers and opportunities as children transition into adulthood; and child and adolescent resilience.[2]

Additionally, the AAP provides tools and resources that pediatricians and other clinicians can use to assist in the care of children who have experienced foster care.[25] Examples of resources include health information and health summary forms, consent to obtain or release confidential information, referral and feedback forms, and visit discharge and referral summary for the family.[25]

Educational Opportunities

Health disparities and health equity remain central foci in the field of health care, particularly for children affected by foster care. A comprehensive review encompassing studies published between January 1, 2017, and July 21, 2022, revealed that racially and ethnically minoritized children received poorer health care services relative to their white counterparts.[26] This disparity is postulated to stem from contributors such as implicit bias from health care practitioners and structural inequities.[26,27] These factors are particularly relevant when addressing the health care needs of children affected by foster care. Notably, data have shown that children of color, especially those who identify as Black or American Indian/Native American, are overrepresented in the child welfare system.[28] Furthermore, according to a study conducted by Baams and associates,[29] approximately 30% of youth age 10 to 18 years residing in foster care and 25% of those in unstable housing self-identify as lesbian, gay, bisexual, transgender, and questioning or queer (LGBTQ+). LGBTQ+ youth subjected to foster care placement or unstable housing exhibit a higher prevalence of mental health issues compared with their heterosexual counterparts who reside in foster care or stable housing.[29]

Little progress has been made in mitigating these health disparities, despite their being documented for many years. As stated previously, research indicates that barriers to achieving health equity may be linked to racism and discrimination. As a result, recent efforts have been directed toward educating pediatricians and other clinicians on topics such as unconscious bias, microaggressions, structural racism, and LGBTQ+ health and how these factors can significantly impact health outcomes. Pediatricians should pursue continuing education on all of these topics to provide holistic and responsive patient care.

Unconscious Bias

Unconscious bias has been identified as a significant contributor to the overrepresentation of minoritized groups within the child welfare system, as well as the disparities in health outcomes for children who have been involved in foster care.[30] *Unconscious bias*, or *implicit bias*, is defined as "the process of unconscious societal attitudes affecting our individual understanding, actions, and decisions, thus leading to assumptions about groups."[31] The Harvard Implicit Association Test (IAT) is a tool that helps to measure unconscious attitudes and beliefs.[32] The test is designed to uncover hidden biases and prejudices toward different social groups and categories. The IAT provides insight into how collective unconscious perceptions influence behaviors and decision-making.[33] Pediatricians can deepen their understanding of this topic by taking the IAT. The recognition of one's own biases can enhance clinician–patient interactions and foster more equitable and effective health care delivery.

Microaggressions

Initially described in 1970 by Chester M. Pierce and later refined by Derald W. Sue, *microaggressions* are defined as "daily commonplace, subtle behaviors and attitudes toward others that arise from conscious or unconscious bias."[34] The accumulation of microaggressions can significantly affect the overall well-being of youth, particularly marginalized populations in foster care. Microaggressions can have adverse effects on both physical and mental health, as well as the general sense of well-being. Clinicians can support children and adolescents, as well as staff and colleagues, by raising awareness about the impact of microaggressions and implementing strategies to mitigate their effects.[35]

Racism

The concept of race as a social construct is an important aspect to consider when examining the pervasive impact of racism. Racism itself can be defined as "a system of power that structures opportunity (education, housing, jobs, and justice, for example) and assigns value (worthy or unworthy, full of potential or full of menace) based on the social interpretation of how one looks (which we call "race"). This system unfairly disadvantages some individuals and communities and unfairly advantages other individuals."[36] Jones[37] described three levels of racism: personally mediated, institutional/structural, and internalized. Personally mediated racism involves prejudice, assumptions, and discriminatory actions based on race. Institutional racism refers to differential access to goods, services, and opportunities by race.[37] Structural racism fosters discrimination through inequitable systems, while institutional racism specifically involves discriminatory policies and practices within institutions.[37] Internalized racism is the acceptance of negative messages about one's worth based on race.[37] Racism, while not exclusive to youth of color, can significantly impact the physiological and psychological health of young individuals, particularly those who have experienced foster care.

As health professionals, pediatricians play a vital role in engaging with youth to understand their historical backgrounds and how these relate to both collective and individual trauma. By doing this, pediatricians can guide youth toward empowerment and encourage their involvement in addressing the effects of racism and eliminating race-based medicine.[38–43] Pediatricians can discover evidence-based strategies to combat the effects of racism highlighted in the 2023 article titled "Health Equity and the Impact of Racism on Adolescent Health" by Coyne-Beasley.[18,38]

LGBTQ+ Health

Pediatricians play a vital role in providing comprehensive and inclusive health care to LGBTQ+ youth as they navigate their sexual and gender identities. Unfortunately, LGBTQ+ youth frequently face discrimination and lack of understanding within the health care system, leading to significant negative impacts on their overall well-being and ability to access essential care. Limited awareness and understanding of LGBTQ+ issues could hinder the ability of a pediatrician or clinician to effectively cater to the specific needs of LGBTQ+ youth. Consequently, this impedes youth access to suitable and supportive health care services, leading to significant health disparities.[44]

The available data indicates that LGBTQ+ youth are disproportionately represented in the foster care system, with the highest prevalence found among LGBTQ+ youth of color and those who identify as transgender and nonbinary. Studies indicate that LGBTQ+ youth who have experienced foster care are almost four times more likely to report instances of being expelled or deserted or running away, particularly among transgender and nonbinary individuals, due to their LGBTQ+ identity.[45] Additionally, studies show that LGBTQ+ youth affected by foster care are 3 times more likely to report a past-year suicide attempt compared to those who have not experienced foster care.[45] These examples underscore the need for health care systems to support patients who are aligned to the margins of society. This support begins with the education of pediatricians and other clinicians. The AAP provides a collection of professional tools and resources for pediatricians, entitled "LQBTQ+ Health and Wellness."[46] The website includes policy statements and technical reports, as well as AAP guidance on inclusive language.[46] Other components include a guide for LGBTQ+ friendly practice, effective communication, cultural competence, patient- and family-centered care, and other resources.[46] Resources for families are also available, including gender identity development and support resources for families of gender-diverse youth.[46] The American Medical Association has partnered with the Fenway Institute to provide continuing medical education activities with topics ranging from skill development, such as combating explicit and implicit bias toward transgender and gender-diverse people, to implementing a culturally responsive environment.[25,31,47]

Patient-Centered Medical Home

Pediatricians can take the necessary steps to be recognized as a patient-centered medical home (PCMH). A PCMH is "an approach to providing comprehensive and high-quality primary care with a focus on building and developing partnerships with families, pediatric clinicians, early childhood professionals, community organizations, educational systems and other key agencies within the system of care."[48] It can include a case management program that provides information on local and national resources available to support children in the foster care system. By working together with other clinicians, families, case managers, and the community, pediatricians can help to create a comprehensive and effective system of care for children in foster care.[48-50] See Chapter 3, Medical Home Readiness, for a detailed discussion.

Support Groups

Many resources exist to support families who care for children in foster care, including national support groups. These groups provide opportunities to share information and resources and to network with individuals with shared experiences.

Foster Care Alumni of America, a national support group, focuses on 2 main areas: 1) connecting alumni and 2) policy and practice transformation within the child welfare system. Its mission is to eliminate the gap between the outcomes of children who have experienced foster care and the outcomes of those who have not. Multiple states have active chapters, which can be found on the group's website (https://fostercarealumni.org).[51]

AdoptUSKids (www.adoptuskids.org) has identified support groups and wraparound service partners for each state and many US territories, including respite care, referral information, group activities, and training. However, different states have varying levels of support based on whether an adoption was completed through the state system or a private agency.[52]

Culture

When children are placed in out-of-home care through foster care or with kinship caregivers, an important area of focus for pediatricians is to prioritize maintaining the child's sense of culture. Stafanson[53] states, "Strong cultural identity contributes to mental health resilience, higher levels of social well-being, and improved coping skills, among other benefits." Children from minoritized communities may be more at risk of feeling disconnected from their culture due to systemic factors already at play. As a result, it is important for pediatricians to actively seek ways to maintain or even promote children's sense of culture. This may include

- Educating caregivers on the importance of maintaining the child's cultural practices and traditions
- Encouraging the child to participate in cultural events and activities
- Providing resources and support to help the child explore and connect with their cultural heritage

By prioritizing the child's cultural identity, pediatricians and families can promote a sense of belonging and connectedness, which can have a positive impact on the child's overall well-being.

Medical–Legal Partnership

A medical–legal partnership (MLP) is "a health care delivery model that formally includes lawyers on a care team to address legal issues that drive poor health and contribute to population health inequities."[54] These partnerships are available in health systems, hospitals, and medical offices in 49 states and the District of Columbia.[55] The goal of MLPs is to screen families for health-related social and legal needs and subsequently develop strategies to address identified issues when appropriate. Areas may include, but are not limited to, guardianship, housing, insurance, and child education. The MLP not only addresses family concerns but also assists clinical and nonclinical staff with navigating system and policy barriers that may hinder the health and well-being of the family. An interactive map is available to locate programs within specific states.[55] Pediatricians can partner with local legal experts to establish an MLP in their practice. A toolkit developed by the National Center for Medical–Legal Partnership, a project of the Milken Institute School of Public Health at the George Washington University, was developed and updated in 2015 to assist practices with implementing an effective program.[56]

Task-Specific Forms in Electronic Health Records

Electronic health records (EHRs) can provide sections in which to place information specific to children and adolescents in foster or out-of-home care. A dedicated section can contain information about guardianship, treatment consent, foster care status and type (foster home, kinship care, or preadoptive home), agency involvement, and emergency contacts. This information can easily be updated during each health supervision visit to ensure the medical team has accurate information. Guardianship information can contain the legal guardian's name, relationship to the child (such as foster/kinship parent, birth parents, legal guardian, case worker), contact information, date of court-ordered guardianship, and status of guardianship (temporary or permanent). Although guardianship is a vital component, consent for medical treatment may be more complex, particularly if parental rights have not been terminated.[57] Authority to consent may vary by state; therefore, becoming familiar with the laws specific to the clinician's jurisdiction is essential.

Other information in the EHR can include details of the child welfare and foster care agency, such as name, assigned caseworker, and contact details, as well as court-ordered restrictions, such as parental consent limitations or any medical decision-making rights. Consult institutional legal counsel for managing compliance challenges effectively. Engaging legal counsel provides an opportunity to enhance knowledge of laws, regulations, and policy requirements.

Summary

Foster care can be difficult to navigate for children, caregivers, and clinicians. To help all involved, important steps and actions include the following:

- Understand the impact of trauma on families and clinical staff.
- Have access to clinical guidelines and policies.
- Provide education and training for the health care workforce.
- Connect children and caregivers to community resources.

With this comprehensive approach, barriers encountered by children and families in the foster care system can be managed and mitigated. This knowledge and active engagement will help move forward the effort to support resilience in the face of trauma.

Key Takeaways

- A patient-centered approach to care in the medical home and other practice settings, such as specialty care and the emergency department, is important for all children, but especially for children who may have experienced trauma, which is more prevalent in children who are placed in foster care.
- Practice settings should be fully equipped to provide a trauma-informed environment for all patients, using strategies described in this chapter.
- Pediatricians and other clinicians should stay updated on AAP evidence-based policy statements, clinical reports, and technical guidelines to ensure the highest standard of care.
- Pediatricians should continuously educate themselves and their office personnel about the impact of unconscious bias, microaggressions, and racism experienced by children placed in foster care to better support these children in a safe and nurturing environment.
- Recognize that children identifying as LGBTQ+ may have specific health care needs that require the implementation of a culturally responsive environment to provide inclusive and supportive care.
- Establishing MLPs can be extremely helpful in navigating complex legal issues related to guardianship and consent for treatment, ensuring the best interests of the children are upheld while addressing their health care needs.

CHAPTER

7

Care Coordination and Case Management

Lisa Zetley, MD, FAAP

Introduction

Given that children in foster care are designated as a population with special health care needs,[1] it is understandable that pediatricians and other clinicians may feel overwhelmed when trying to address their unmet needs during a health supervision visit. Incorporating care coordination or case management into clinical practice can help to meet the complex needs of children and families who are served by the child welfare system. This chapter will define health care coordination and provide a rationale for its use with children in foster care, explain the differences between care coordination and case management in the health care setting, and differentiate these processes from child welfare case management. This chapter will also discuss possible strategies for building care coordination into a practice or community.

Definition

The terms *care coordination* and *case management* are often used interchangeably in health care systems. However, there are significant differences between them, and it is important to define each role.

Case management is a patient-centered process that prioritizes the health needs and goals of the patient (and caregiver) and works with them to find available resources and clinicians.[2] While the process is collaborative in nature, the focus is often on promoting cost-effective (and high-quality) outcomes. Using building a house as a metaphor, case managers often provide the tools necessary to "build the house" or support success, such as giving clinic phone numbers to caregivers and encouraging the caregiver to call or sharing websites.

Care coordination is a process that involves reviewing the overall health of a patient or client and assessing and prioritizing their needs and goals, in collaboration with the patient, caregiver, and health care team.[3] In addition to creating and implementing the plan, there is a focus on accessing resources and monitoring the plan with added support, education, and advocacy when barriers arise. Care coordinators help stakeholders develop a shared understanding of the plan and work collaboratively to prioritize health care needs. Care coordination can occur across multiple systems and may include physical health, mental and behavioral health, dental health, and educational advocacy related to health needs. When care coordination models are implemented to serve families of children with special health care needs, improved outcomes occur.[4] For children in foster care, the goals of promoting continuity of care, placement stability, and enhancing permanency are also very important. Care coordinators not only provide the tools necessary to "build the house," but they also arrange for the delivery of the raw materials, obtain the blueprint for the house, and find the contractors to do the work. They also check back often to be ensure the house is being built safely and in a timely fashion.

The remainder of this chapter will focus on care coordination, as this benefit provides the most comprehensive support for families and youth involved in the foster care system.[1] The term *health care coordinator* will be used because the focus of the coordination is on the child's health, as defined broadly to include physical, developmental, behavioral, and dental health.

Rationale for Care Coordination for Youth in Foster Care

Children in foster care have complex health needs[1]: approximately 50% of this population has one chronic physical health condition, and 10% are considered medically complex.[5] Many have behavioral health needs that can be long-standing and multifactorial and often require multiple modalities to address. In addition to the child's needs, caregivers (particularly kinship caregivers) may have their own needs, such as transportation, child care, or housing. These caregiver needs may affect their ability to support the youth in their home. Access to resources, such as therapies or specialty clinicians, may be more challenging due to limited network options, long wait times, and geographic (long distance) barriers. Children in foster care face unique barriers to health care access, which can include presentation to care with a caregiver who is not aware of the child's past medical history, prior fragmented care, and lack of access to prior health care records.[1]

Health care coordination can serve as a strategy for ensuring that health care needs are met and foster parents are supported. There is often great frustration when a caregiver identifies a need for health care or counseling yet the issue is not addressed in a timely fashion. This may lead to the caregiver feeling overwhelmed and unheard, and a subsequent placement change may be the result. Even if there is not a quick solution to the health issue, health care coordinators can help to ease frustrations by serving as a sounding board. Resource identification and persistence are critical skills for this role. See **Box 7-1** for a vignette illustrating an example of a caregiver facing barriers when an infant is placed into kinship care.

Placement changes affect access to health care.[6] If placement disruption occurs, health care coordination can help to ensure that health care is not also disrupted. Sharing of health care information can be critical to supporting youth during transitions. The cost associated with transitions can be decreased if medication and equipment can travel with the child. Appointment information can also be shared to prevent missed appointments. Achieving permanency may have a greater likelihood of success when a youth has all their health needs met. Chapter 19, Factors Associated With Placement Stability and Permanency Outcomes, details the negative effects of placement instability on child health.

Box 7-1

Case Scenario, Part 1

HM, a 6-month-old who was born at 30 weeks' gestation, was recently discharged into foster care in her grandmother's home. HM's mother has begun treatment for schizophrenia and a substance use disorder. HM has bronchopulmonary dysplasia and requires nebulizer treatments twice daily. She had medical necrotizing enterocolitis and has some difficulty with feeding. She requires a specialty formula and uses a nasogastric tube for supplemental nutrition. She requires outpatient therapies and follow-up in 4 specialty clinics and is on 3 medications.

HM's grandmother received training prior to discharge and has identified a pediatrician for HM. Although follow-up appointments with the specialty clinic have already been scheduled, the grandmother would prefer them to be scheduled at a satellite clinic closer to her home. She has the phone numbers to call to set up speech and physical therapies.

The grandmother also cares for HM's 2-year-old brother and recently moved into a new apartment to make room for HM.

How could a care coordinator help support HM and her grandmother?

Child Welfare Case Management and Health Care Coordination: Roles and Partnerships

The relationship between child welfare case manager and health care coordinator should be symbiotic. While child welfare has a focus on assessing safety, addressing court requirements, and achieving permanency, the health care coordinator is focused on health. Child welfare and health care coordination professionals have shared goals of ensuring the child's health care needs are addressed in a timely fashion and making certain that caregivers and birth parents are knowledgeable about the needs and services for the child. Exact responsibilities related to health care may vary by jurisdiction, program, and payer. It is critical that communication between the child welfare case manager and the health care coordinator is clear and consistent, because a strong working relationship is important in ensuring the priorities and messaging to all stakeholders (eg, birth parent, foster parent, clinicians, therapists) are unified. It is helpful for health care coordinators to have access to child welfare information systems (eg, Statewide Automated Child Welfare Information System) to review case updates and placement changes and understand who can provide consent. Recent advances in shared medical record/child welfare record platforms allow for information sharing between information systems in real time, which enhances care coordination. See Chapter 41, Privacy and Information Sharing, for an in-depth discussion.

Health care coordinators and child welfare case managers should partner to overcome barriers to meeting the health needs of a child. Communication with the child welfare team should be clear and standardized, avoiding medical jargon and abbreviations. Documentation should include who received the communication, methods and dates of communication, and what strategies were recommended for resolution of any barriers. When barriers persist that affect the health and well-being of a child in a significant manner, communication to the child welfare manager and supervisor should delineate the risks of not meeting the child's health care needs. At times, the needs of the child may require additional supports that cannot be provided in the current placement or with the available resources in the community. In either instance, the health care coordinator and the child welfare case manager need a strong partnership to prioritize and support the needs of the child. In some instances when timely resolution does not occur and unmet needs persist despite supports, consideration should be given to filing a new child maltreatment report back to the jurisdiction responsible for the child's case.

Meeting the medical needs of medically complex children and those with high-level behavioral health needs in foster care can present particular challenges. Child welfare agencies often lack a clear and consistent method for identifying medically complex children whom they serve.[7] This could result in children being placed with foster parents who are not prepared for or equipped to address the child's medical needs. Foster parents may feel singularly responsible for accessing and navigating the array of services needed.[8] Health care coordination services can bridge these gaps by identifying which children meet the agency's definition of medically complex and providing an array of possible services and resources to meet the child's needs. Health care coordinators can also support justification of exceptional foster care monthly rates based on the care the child requires in the home.

Issues with consent for medical care are another potential barrier requiring a collaborative approach between child welfare professionals and health care coordinators. For example, clinicians may be unaware of who is authorized to provide consent. Procedures for consent can vary by jurisdiction, status of parental rights, and type of care (routine versus nonroutine, emergency); health care coordinators can develop knowledge about what consent is required for clinical care in different settings. They can facilitate collaboration and information sharing between clinicians, child welfare agency professionals, and birth parents/guardians. Supporting and communicating with birth parents can build allyship and enhance the birth parent's knowledge about their child, which may facilitate obtaining timely consent for needed medical, dental, and behavioral health services. See Chapter 34, Medical Consents, for a detailed discussion of consent.

Roles and Responsibilities of Health Care Coordinators

Box 7-2 continues the vignette, illustrating the role of the health care coordinator in supporting the kinship caregiver. **Table 7–1** outlines roles and responsibilities that care coordination models should consider addressing along with illustrative examples. Of note, these examples are not exhaustive.

Box 7–2

Case Scenario, Part 2

Let's revisit HM's situation after she has been living with her grandmother for 1 month.

The health care coordinator was successful in rescheduling the specialty clinic appointments at the satellite clinic and advocated to ensure the time to appointment was not too long. Medication management was set up with a pharmacy that delivers the medication to the home. Finding the specialty formula was difficult; however, the health care coordinator called all of the distributors in a 3-county region until they found one that was willing to ship the formula to the grandmother.

When HM's weight gain is noted to significantly drop off at a health supervision visit, the health care coordinator calls the grandmother to offer support. HM's grandmother shares that she is exhausted and often sleeps through the alarm for HM's nighttime feeding. The health care coordinator asks permission to share this information with HM's team. The child welfare team is able to find respite twice monthly, and the feeding team adjusts the schedule to allow a longer overnight pause in feedings.

As the weather gets cold, HM's grandmother realizes that the heat is spotty in the new apartment. The health care coordinator encourages the grandmother to speak to the landlord and also connects her with the regional kinship navigator program to help her advocate for her tenant's rights.

Table 7–1. Roles and Responsibilities of Health Care Coordinators

Role/Responsibility	Examples
Gather records at entry into foster care program	• Review past medical records (primary and specialty care, dental, developmental and psychological evaluations), immunization records, medication claims, allergies, educational support documents[a] (individualized education program or 504).
Summarize health information and share with care team	• Review allergies, past medical history, and recent medication claims with foster parent and child welfare team upon placement or as part of initial case review. • Communicate health and mental health diagnoses with child welfare and other stakeholders[b] using a care plan (see example in following section of text). • Ensure foster parent understands medication dosing and has medication in home. • Ensure new stakeholders (eg, new case manager or new foster parent) are informed about child's diagnoses and needs.
Review health visit records and support and facilitate follow-up	• Review notes from medical visit and follow up with foster parent on next steps and new medications. • Ensure follow-up appointments are scheduled and communicate with care team (may include birth parent). • Review urgent treatment plans with foster parent (eg, anaphylaxis, asthma, mental health crisis). • Review emergency visits or admissions for mental health conditions and ensure timely follow-up appointments are scheduled.

(continues)

Table 7–1 *(continued)*

Role/Responsibility	Examples
Address unique health needs for foster youth	• Ensure specialized foster care assessments occur in timely fashion, if eligible (comprehensive examinations upon entry into care or at time of transition). • Ensure enhanced periodicity and timeliness of health supervision and dental care visits in a medical home. • Ensure developmental and mental health screenings occur regularly. • Facilitate reproductive health visits (if indicated) or substance use treatment.
Support access to network or community resources	• Specialized needs: formula, developmental therapy, non-traditional mental health therapies • Specialized equipment and training (orthotics, feeding pump) • Home nursing services • Intensive mental health support services (may include partial hospitalization or residential care) • Orthodontia • Respite care or crisis supports
Identify and resolve barriers (problem-solving)	• Transportation, need to obtain consent, waitlist for services, out-of-network service needs, prior authorization for services and medications
Ensure quality of care measures	• HEDIS (Healthcare Effectiveness Data Information Set) measures such as lead screening, timely immunizations, follow-up after mental health admission • Unique care measures specific to foster care plan contract
Provide support and education to foster parents	• Build relationship with foster parent. • Ensure foster parent is aware of appointments and understands plan of care and follow-up priorities. • Utilize care plan as one tool of communication. • Support placement stability through active listening, empathizing, and resource sharing.
Provide support and education to birth parents or guardian	• Build relationship with birth parents (if within scope). • Ensure birth parents are aware of appointments and understand outcome of appointments and plan of care. • Utilize care plan as one tool of communication
Provide support and education to young adults enrolled in program	• Build relationship with transition-age or emancipated young adults who are enrolled in program. • Ensure young adult is aware of supports and resources (may include housing, transportation, food, employment, education). • Ensure young adult understands their own health diagnoses, needs, and medications.
Provide support and education to clinician team	• Ensure that clinician team is familiar with trauma-informed practices and unique needs of youth who are in foster care.

[a] Depending on health care coordination model and jurisdiction laws, education records may or may not be available for review.

[b] Stakeholder definition: Current clinicians (and upcoming clinicians scheduled), child welfare professionals, foster parent, birth parent or guardian, other professionals (crisis team, therapists).

Care Plan

The care plan (see **Figure 7–1** for an example) may serve as one key tool for communication regarding the child's health needs. The primary goal of the care plan is to ensure that the child's caregivers, guardians, and clinicians have a shared understanding of the child's current health status, important health history, upcoming appointments, and unmet needs. While the care plan template will likely be standardized, accommodations or redactions will need to be made if confidentiality issues exist. For example, if the caregiver's address is confidential, it should be listed on the care plans of clinicians but not those of the guardian. Succinct care plans are best, with limited jargon used. Accurate translation should be available, in the event a stakeholder's primary language is different than the care plan's template language. Programs must decide whether care plans are electronically shared documents, paper documents, or platform-based websites or applications where the care plan can be accessed. Because care plans contain health information, measures must be taken to ensure they are shared in a manner that respects confidentiality and privacy while balancing the preferred method for the stakeholder to access the information.

Care plan completion should occur within 1 to 2 months after entry into foster care and should also occur at the time of discharge from the health care coordination program, exit from foster care, or other significant transition. The frequency of care plan creation should be based on the intensity of the child's needs, with a maximum interval of every 6 months.[9] Each jurisdiction should determine with whom the care plan is shared.

Health passports are another tool that can provide a summary of important health information, such as diagnoses of chronic conditions, immunizations, allergies, and past illnesses. A number of states have implemented a health passport to summarize important health information, which can be available to medical stakeholders, foster parents, guardians, and the child once they reach adulthood.[10,11]

Care Plan

Care Plan Date:	Child Name:	Child Date of Birth:
Date of Removal:	Time Frame Care Plan Covers:	Length of Time in Current Placement:
Name of Current Foster Parent:	**Address:**	**Phone Number:** **Email:** **Preferred Communication Method** *(PCM)*:
Parent 1:	**Address:**	**Phone Number:** **Email:** *PCM:*
Parent 2:	**Address:**	**Phone Number:** **Email:** *PCM:*
Legal Guardian for Medical Decisions:	**Address:**	**Phone Number:** **Email:** *PCM:*
Foster Program Health Care Coordinator:		Phone Number: Email: *PCM:*

Active or Recent Health Problems/Diagnoses/Surgical History

Medical Diagnosis or Problem	Source of Information	Date Identified
Persistent Asthma	*Clinician's Medical Record*	*01/25/23 (New Diagnosis)*

Current Medications

Medication Name	Dosage	Frequency	Last Fill Date	Prescriber
Medications: *None*				
Immunization Status: *Up to date*				

Figure 7–1. Example of care plan. Italicized text represents sample input. *(continues)*

Care Team

Name	Agency	Phone	Role	Email
			Child Welfare Case Manager	
			Child Welfare Supervisor	
			Primary Care Pediatrician	
			Dentist	
			Psychiatrist	
			Therapist	

Medical, Dental, Behavioral Health Goals

Long-term Goal	Short-term Goal	Date	Possible Barrier
MW will have routine health checkups to ensure optimal health and wellness	*MW will attend well exams every 6 months* *-Asthma follow-up visits every 3 months*	*Last checkup appointment: 4/22/23* *Next due for asthma visit: July, 2023* *Next due for check-up: October, 2023*	*Transportation:* ***Please contact us if you need help scheduling a ride***
MW will practice good dental hygiene and attend routine dental exams	*MW will attend dental exams every 6 months*	*Last dental appointment: 9/5/22* ***Due now, please schedule***	*This clinic has long wait list; please schedule now*
MW demonstrates healthy coping skills and habits and will continue to thrive in current placement	*MW will participate in mental health therapy. MW will attend psychiatry appointments every 3 months*	*Attends weekly therapy appointment* *Last psychiatry appointment: 4/26/23* *Next appointment: 8/3/23*	*Transportation:* ***Please contact us if you need help scheduling a ride***

Priorities & Identified Unmet Needs

Stakeholder	Priority	Unmet Need	Resource Provided
Foster parent name	*"MW is healthy and successful in school"*	*Does not currently have an individualized education program (IEP) for special learning needs*	*Encouraged foster parent to talk to child welfare manager about this need*
Adolescent member	*"I want to get braces"*	*Orthodontia*	*Provided foster parent with network resources for orthodontia; offered to schedule appointment*
Parent #1:	*"MW is healthy and happy and answers my text messages"*	*MW does not have a working phone at this time*	*Updated child welfare manager that MW lost phone and does not have way to communicate with parents*
Parent #2:	*Unable to reach parent*		

Attach asthma management plan, eczema management plan, behavior crisis intervention plan, or emergency allergy plan.

Figure 7–1 *(continued)*

Strategies for Building a Care Coordination Model

Health care coordination is an important asset in ensuring health care needs are addressed, yet developing a strategy to access these services can be challenging. While health care coordinators often are available via programs for children with complex health needs, other avenues must be explored to provide every child in out-of-home care with a health care coordinator. Many children are covered by a Medicaid managed care delivery model,[12] and most of these models require the managed care plan to include care coordination. The degree and intensity of care coordination vary and include strategies such as targeted case management, specialized care coordination based on diagnosis or need, integrated care coordination, and intensive care coordination. Another approach is to utilize grant funding, philanthropy, or community health care funding to secure a health care coordinator within a clinic that focuses primarily on serving youth in foster care. Some child welfare agencies have embedded nurses who can provide targeted care coordination for some children. Demonstration of improved outcomes, such as an improvement in the rates of children attending appointments for health supervision visits and dental care in a timely fashion or qualitative surveys completed by caregivers, can garner support and growth of care coordination programs. See Chapter 37, Health Care Financing, for additional discussion.

When filling the role of health care coordinator, an important trait is to be an effective communicator in multiple settings and using a variety of modalities. Strategic thinking, strong organizational skills, and resourcefulness are also very important. While nurses may be a natural fit for providing health care coordination for children with complex medical needs, social workers and professionals familiar with mental health care delivery also can bring important knowledge to this work. Health care coordinators should have competencies to successfully navigate across the many child-serving systems.

The key to a successful program is for caseloads to be kept to a level that allows adequate time to develop relationships and follow up with stakeholders. There is often a significant investment of health care coordination that occurs in the first 2 to 3 months of entry into foster care, attributable to the greater number of appointments and assessments and the need for medical record collection. The optimal ratio of children to health care coordinator may vary based on a number of factors, including health complexity, intensity of unmet needs of the child, degree of placement support required, frequency of placement change, and depth of support provided by the professional.[9]

Key Takeaways

» Health care coordination is an important asset in ensuring health care needs are addressed in a timely fashion.

» Health care coordination can serve to support foster parents in addressing the needs of a child and can support birth parents by keeping them informed and engaged in their child's health.

» Health care coordination can decrease the fragmentation of health care delivery by ensuring that all stakeholders, including child welfare partners, receive a care plan specific to the child.

» Ensuring continuity of care and access to health care resources and specialized clinicians should be a priority for health care coordinators.

Acknowledgment: The example of the care plan (**Figure 7-1**) is based on the care plan used by Wisconsin's Care4Kids Program (https://www.dhs.wisconsin.gov/care4kids/index.htm). Care4Kids provides care coordination as part of a Medicaid benefit package for youth in foster care in southeastern Wisconsin. The author of this chapter serves as the medical director for Care4Kids.

CHAPTER

8

Integrated Models of Care

Katy Carlsen, MD, FAAP
Hilda Loria, MD, MPH, FAAP

Introduction: Case Example

Jaden is a 5-year-old boy who has experienced significant trauma with his family of origin including physical and emotional abuse and neglect. He has had severe behavioral problems in all his foster care placements, and the child welfare social worker can tell he needs trauma-focused cognitive behavioral therapy (TF-CBT) and mental health support; however, she cannot find services adequate to meet his needs. It has become challenging to find foster homes willing to accept Jaden, and the next step under consideration is a group/residential treatment facility due to his severe behavioral issues. The social worker hears of a new integrated care clinic for children in foster care nearby and reaches out to schedule an appointment for Jaden.

The intake includes a full assessment of Jaden's trauma symptoms and risk factors by a mental health specialist, who links him directly in a warm hand-off to TF-CBT services. Care is established in this integrated care medical home, Jaden's placement stabilizes, and he is enrolled in school with an individualized education program. He is also assessed by a developmental pediatric specialist who consults in the clinic; they recommend help with sleep management and ADHD symptoms. The referrals are coordinated by the medical home, and long-term follow-up is ongoing. Jaden's behaviors improve in this stable foster-adopt placement with the collaboration of the integrated care team members and cross-sector partners.

Overview of Integrated Care

Integrated care is defined as "the care that results from a practice team of primary care and behavioral health clinicians, working together with patients and families, using a systematic and cost-effective approach to provide patient-centered care for a defined population."[1] For children in foster, kinship, and adoptive care, integrated care that is timely and trauma-informed is the ideal approach to address the complex health effects of trauma.

Integrated care can be achieved in several ways: through streamlined communication with mental health clinicians, colocation, or onsite fully collaborative joint care and treatment planning. Integrated care within the pediatric medical home setting is a promising model for the care of children in foster and kinship care.[2] In this setting, social and emotional issues during periods of transition (eg, entry into foster care, placement change, reunification, adoption) and multiple complex health care needs can be best addressed by an interdisciplinary team to optimize a child's well-being. Integrated care models also support caregivers in understanding and managing current and future medical, developmental, and mental health problems.[3–6] Evidence has shown that these models of care reduce per capita health care costs; improve access to and communication among medical, mental health, and social services professionals[7]; enhance care coordination and treatment adherence[1,3,7]; and reduce stigma associated with seeking mental health services.[7]

A key principle of integrated care is coordination among the various professionals involved in a patient's health care (see **Figure 8–1**). The current child welfare system is overwhelmed with many complex families, a population of children and youth who are highly mobile, and consent and confidentiality barriers that inhibit communication and collaboration, all of which contribute to fragmentation of health care services and challenges in managing all aspects of care for a child and family.[6]

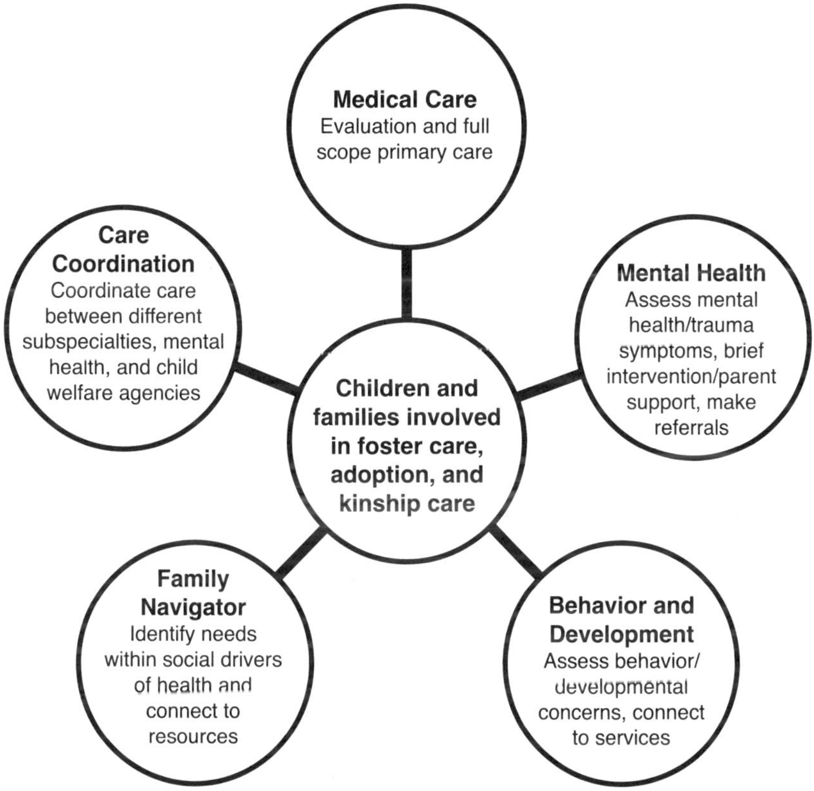

Figure 8–1. Example of integrated care model components in a pediatric medical home (Comprehensive Integration of Resilience Into Child Life Experiences [CIRCLE] Clinic in Sacramento County, CA).

This chapter describes the aspects of integrated care that can improve care coordination and overall health care quality for children and youth in foster care. Health care coordination by the medical home (see Chapter 7, Care Coordination and Case Management) can facilitate linkages among medical, mental health, and developmental services located in a single location or nearby, enabling more efficient communication and collaboration among clinicians, child welfare partners, caregivers, and community organizations. Care coordination is ideally a team- and family-driven process that improves family and clinician satisfaction, facilitates access to services, improves health care outcomes, and reduces costs that occur with fragmented health services by reducing under- and overutilization of care. It is imperative that well-defined care coordination is integrated into the care of children involved with child welfare.[4]

Types of Integrated Care Models

The Center for Integrated Health Solutions (a program of the Substance Abuse and Mental Health Services Administration and Health Resources and Services Administration) developed "A Standard Framework for Levels of Integrated Healthcare" to describe the levels of integration, resources needed, and essential elements with regard to communication, proximity, and practice change.[8] (See **Tables 8–1** and **8–2**.)

Examples of Integrated Care Models for Children in Foster Care

The American Academy of Pediatrics (AAP) has a webpage (https://www.aap.org/en/patient-care/foster-care/models-of-care-for-children-in-foster-care) with examples of various models, programs, and projects that specifically provide care for children in the US foster care system. Examples of Level 6 integration include the Rees-Jones Center for Foster Care Excellence (RJC)[9] in Texas and the Comprehensive Integration of Resilience Into Child Life Experiences (CIRCLE) in California. These clinics serve as primary care medical homes for children involved with the child welfare system and provide services from entry through permanency (eg, reunification, kinship, adoption). Pediatricians, including developmental-behavioral specialists, and mental health clinicians work collaboratively to address the medical, developmental, and mental health needs of patients and their families and partner with child welfare professionals. Patients are screened for trauma-related symptoms and referred as needed to evidence-based, trauma-informed treatment. For example, mental health clinicians at RJC can provide psychiatric evaluation and treatment, trauma-focused play therapy, trauma-focused cognitive behavioral therapy, and parent-child interaction therapy to their patients. At CIRCLE, child-caregiver dyads are offered access to Parent-Child Care (PC Care), an in-home dyadic program over a 6-week period to nurture the caregiver-child relationship and build parenting skills, or connected to clinicians in the community for mental health services. Essential to both are care coordinators (eg, nurse coordinators at RJC, care coordinator and family navigator at CIRCLE), who serve as liaisons among the clinic, child welfare, subspecialists, and community resources. Partnership with child welfare allows for access to trauma histories and care coordination. Finally, at RJC, a shared electronic medical record among medical and behavioral clinicians and child welfare professionals allows for enhanced care coordination and communication.

Table 8–1. Levels of Collaboration/Integration

COORDINATED KEY ELEMENT: COMMUNICATION		COLOCATED KEY ELEMENT: PHYSICAL PROXIMITY		INTEGRATED KEY ELEMENT: PRACTICE CHANGE	
LEVEL 1 Minimal Collaboration	LEVEL 2 Basic Collaboration at a Distance	LEVEL 3 Basic Collaboration Onsite	LEVEL 4 Close Collaboration Onsite With Some System Integration	LEVEL 5 Close Collaboration Approaching an Integrated Practice	LEVEL 6 Full Collaboration in a Transformed/ Merged Integrated Practice
Behavioral health, primary care, and other health care providers work:					
In separate facilities, where they:	In separate facilities, where they:	In same facility (not necessarily same offices) where they:	In same space within the same facility, where they:	In same space within the same facility (some shared space), where they:	In same space within the same facility, sharing all practice space, where they:
• Have separate systems • Communicate about cases only rarely and under compelling circumstances • Communicate, driven by provider need • May never meet in person • Have limited understanding of each other's roles	• Have separate systems • Communicate periodically about shared patients • Communicate, driven by specific patient issues • May meet as part of larger community • Appreciate each other's roles as resources	• Have separate systems • Communicate regularly about shared patients, by phone or email • Collaborate, driven by need for each other's services and more reliable referral • Meet occasionally to discuss cases due to close proximity • Feel part of a larger yet non-formal team	• Share some systems, like scheduling or medical records • Communicate in person as needed • Collaborate, driven by need for consultation and coordinated plans for difficult patients • Have regular face-to-face interactions about some patients • Have a basic understanding of roles and culture	• Actively seek system solutions together or develop work-arounds • Communicate frequently in person • Collaborate, driven by desire to be a member of the care team • Have regular team meetings to discuss overall patient care and specific patient issues • Have an in-depth understanding of roles and culture	• Have resolved most or all system issues, functioning as one integrated system • Communicate consistently at the system, team, and individual levels • Collaborate, driven by shared concept of team care • Have formal and informal meetings to support integrated model of care • Have roles and cultures that blur or blend

Reproduced from Heath B, Wise Romero P, and Reynolds K. *A Standard Framework for Levels of Integrated Healthcare.* Washington, D.C.SAMHSA-HRSA Center for Integrated Health Solutions. March 2013. https://archive.thepcc.org/sites/default/files/resources/SAMHSA-HRSA%202013%20Framework%20for%20Levels%20of%20Integrated%20Healthcare.pdf

Table 8–2. Advantages and Weaknesses at Each Level of Collaboration/Integration

COORDINATED		COLOCATED		INTEGRATED	
LEVEL 1 Minimal Collaboration	LEVEL 2 Basic Collaboration at a Distance	LEVEL 3 Basic Collaboration Onsite	LEVEL 4 Close Collaboration Onsite With Some System Integration	LEVEL 5 Close Collaboration Approaching an Integrated Practice	LEVEL 6 Full Collaboration in a Transformed/ Merged Integrated Practice
Advantages					
• Each practice can make timely and autonomous decisions about care • Readily understood as a practice model by patients and providers	• Maintains each practice's basic operating structure, so change is not a disruptive factor • Provides some coordination and information-sharing that is helpful to both patients and providers	• Colocation allows for more direct interaction and communication among professionals to impact patient care • Referrals more successful due to proximity • Opportunity to develop closer professional relationships	• Removal of some system barriers, like separate records, allows closer collaboration to occur • Both behavioral health and medical providers can become more well- informed about what each can provide • Patients are viewed as shared, which facilitates more complete treatment plans	• High level of collaboration leads to more responsive patient care, increasing engagement and adherence to treatment plans • Provider flexibility increases as system issues and barriers are resolved • Both provider and patient satisfaction may increase	• Opportunity to truly treat whole person • All or almost all system barriers resolved, allowing providers to practice as high-functioning team • All patient needs addressed as they occur • Shared knowledge base of providers increases and allows each professional to respond more broadly and adequately to any issue
Weaknesses					
• Services may overlap, be duplicated, or even work against each other • Important aspects of care may not be addressed or take a long time to be diagnosed	• Sharing of information may not be systematic enough to affect overall patient care • No guarantee that information will change plan or strategy of each provider • Referrals may fail due to barriers, leading to patient and provider frustration	• Proximity may not lead to greater collaboration, limiting value • Effort is required to develop relationships • Limited flexibility, if traditional roles are maintained	• System issues may limit collaboration • Potential for tension and conflicting agendas among providers as practice boundaries loosen	• Practice changes may create lack of fit for some established providers • Time is needed to collaborate at this high level and may affect practice productivity or cadence of care	• Sustainability issues may stress the practice • Few models at this level with enough experience to support value • Outcome expectations not yet established

Reproduced from Heath B, Wise Romero P, and Reynolds K. *A Standard Framework for Levels of Integrated Healthcare.* Washington, D.C.SAMHSA-HRSA Center for Integrated Health Solutions. March 2013. https://archive.thepcc.org/sites/default/files/resources/SAMHSA-HRSA%202013%20Framework%20for%20Levels%20of%20Integrated%20Healthcare.pdf

An example of Level 5 integration is the Comprehensive Health Evaluations for Cincinnati's Kids (CHECK) Foster Care Center at Cincinnati Children's Hospital.[10] A multidisciplinary team colocated in the same clinical space provides diagnostic and therapeutic interventions for the first few months of placement. Patients are then connected to a pediatric clinic in the community for continuity and other community-based resources for families, if needed. The program provides compassionate assistance, education, training, and support for foster and kinship families and is unique in foster parents attending an integrated care appointment credit as part of their training hours.

Considerations in the Development and Implementation of Integrated Care Models

Partnership, collaboration, and care coordination are fundamental tenets of integrated care to improve health care access, services, and health outcomes for children with complex health issues. **Box 8-1** lists some of the partners and stakeholders to consider when designing such a model.

Box 8-1

Essential Partners and Stakeholders to Consider

- **Patients and families:** Including youth/alumni with lived experience, family (birth, foster, kin) as part of an advisory council
- **Child welfare agencies:** State or county agency leaders
- **Community organizations:** Child-placing agencies, Court Appointed Special Advocates, and/or other family support organizations, parenting education and supports, Boys and Girls Clubs, YMCAs
- **Regional centers/developmental support agencies:** Early Intervention and autism supports
- **Education, teachers, counselors:** Local schools, counselors, foster care liaisons, child care, after school programs
- **Medical/mental health clinicians:** Subspecialists and mental health clinicians, especially those experienced in providing care for children/youth in foster care
- **Funders (Medicaid, philanthropic, or academic/government):** Funding of clinical operations and integrated services

Obtaining Buy-In from Stakeholders

One of the most challenging aspects of establishing and maintaining an integrated care model for children and youth in foster care is identifying and gathering external partners to launch the model and sustain its work. Initially, it is essential to learn how child welfare works in one's specific county and what regional and state-level legislation and regulations govern child welfare. In addition, it is important to develop an understanding of the local agencies and partners involved with children and families involved with child welfare. The next step is identifying key leaders and reaching out to these organizations within the county to set up meetings and establish partnerships.

Continued collaboration and communication with all partners and stakeholders in a consistent and predictable manner is crucial, as there is typically high staff turnover in child welfare. At least monthly communication with child welfare partners on topics such as outcomes, remaining gaps and unmet needs, and improving collaboration is ideal. More formal meetings may occur quarterly with the entire cross-sector leadership team.

Other important partners in supporting families include community services such as early childhood intervention programs, parent support groups, financial assistance, respite care, trauma-informed mental health services, substance use disorder services, and social services including local child welfare agencies. As described by Jones et al, some children and youth in foster care show incredible resilience to adverse circumstances. Resilience is supported by having "more than one strong network (biological family, peers, foster care) with multiple strong social networks ameliorating the psychological stress of life struggles."[11] A truly integrated clinic is one approach to providing those networks of support for the youth in foster or kinship care.

National organizations such as the Child Welfare League of America and Generations United may be valuable resources for pediatricians and practices for guidance on understanding the child welfare system and using an intergenerational lens on child welfare, both of which are needed to be effective partners in building resilience for children and families.

Integrated Care Teams and Trauma-Informed Care

Trauma-informed care is necessary for the population of children involved with child welfare because of the high prevalence of childhood trauma, including experiences of child abuse and neglect and chaotic caregiving prior to care, and the uncertainty and ongoing losses of being involved with child welfare. Every professional involved with this population should have intensive training in trauma-informed care. The transient nature of the population also means that intensive care coordination is a vital component of trauma-informed health care. Such care coordination includes collaboration with child welfare to obtain necessary consents for health care and patient historical information, sharing comprehensive treatment plan summaries with child welfare and caregivers, partnering with community agencies to link children to services, coordinating and monitoring services and referrals, and following up on the care plan as it evolves for children and families. See Chapter 7, Care Coordination and Case Management, for a detailed discussion.

Components of Fully Integrated Care Model Visit

In addition to evidence-based guidelines for preventive pediatric care, such as those described in *Bright Futures: Guidelines for Health Supervision of Infants, Children, and Adolescents*,[12] **Box 8–2** describes the unique visit components in a fully integrated care model.[5,8,12] **Figure 8–2** shows the proposed clinic flow in an integrated care model setting. Follow-up is an often overlooked but very important component of trauma-informed care. For more information and resources on trauma-informed pediatric care, see Chapter 17, Childhood Trauma and Resilience.

Information Sharing

The authors of the AAP *Bright Futures Pocket Guide* describe how "[a] public health approach to child welfare can be informed by sharing data and situating child protective services (CPS) within a broader continuum of family support and the efforts of multiple agencies. Utilizing summary data across systems—such as vital records, health care, housing, public benefits, education, and the courts—can help communities better understand areas of strength and need, informing community-based approaches to increase child safety."[12] As an example, California has a centralized website (www.chhs.ca.gov)[13] with a breakdown and guide to laws governing data sharing (State Health Information Guidance [SHIG]). Documents specific to youth in foster care and young adults involved with child welfare may include

- Medical records, including mental health evaluations and treatments
- Child welfare records (eg, trauma history, previous placements)
- Education records
- Legal records
- Health and education passports provided by child welfare partners (available in some states)

Box 8–2

Unique Components of Fully Integrated Care Model Visit[5,8,12]

Preparation for Clinic Visit

- **Gather available information** from sources such as child welfare, primary care physician, school, and immunization registry to obtain health background, trauma histories, previous birth/medical records, and school records.
- **Gather consent documentation from child welfare** to include release of information/authorization to treat (ie, JCE 365 order).
- **Conduct a pre-visit huddle process** including purpose of visit, review of recent issues needing to be addressed, and summary of history gathered for each patient on schedule.

Clinical Visit Flow

- **Pre-visit huddle process**
  - Identify patient/family needs.
  - Specify who will go in and in what order or concurrently.
  - Provide warm handoff and communication if not in concurrent assessment.
  - Use trauma-informed approaches in all aspects of the visit (history taking, physical examination, treatment planning) and be alert for potential trauma triggers.
  - Provide joint treatment planning and shared decision-making with interdisciplinary team, patient, and caregivers.

Assessment and Plan

- **Patient/caregiver**
  - Develop a shared plan of care and provide to caregiver and child welfare (excepting confidential information).
  - Introduce care coordinator/family navigator as a resource to help with referrals, information.
  - Conduct follow-up visits early and often, especially if new placement setting or recent transition.
- **Clinical team debrief**
  - Clinical team debriefs may be conducted after each clinic, weekly, or monthly to review cases, troubleshoot issues, and celebrate successes.
  - Monitor for secondary traumatic stress symptoms in staff.
- **Child welfare colleagues:** Communicate plan of care after each visit and facilitate collaboration and coordination of child/family needs

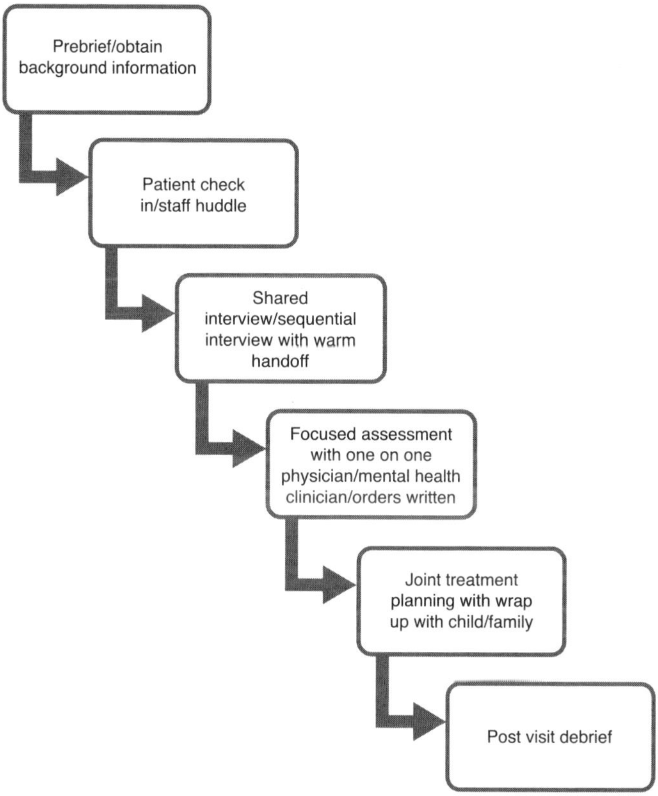

Figure 8–2. Sample of clinical visit flow in an integrated care model.

An example of a shared data system across sectors is IDENTITY, a software program that connects child welfare databases with the electronic medical record.[6]

Legal Rulings and Consent to Treat Regulations

Regulations vary from state to state and often from county to county. The Child Welfare Information Gateway has links to individual states to reference statutes regarding consent procedures.[14] Silos of care still exist despite efforts in many states to improve communication through legislative mandates and memoranda of understanding. A local breakdown of legislative efforts is available at www.childwelfare.gov.[14]

Release of information or memoranda of understanding with agencies involved may include but are not limited to

- Child welfare social workers and public health nurses
- Teachers, schools, and other education professionals
- Court Appointed Special Advocates
- Community health and mental health clinicians
- Early development regional centers
- Juvenile justice system

Considerations for Special Populations in Foster Care

It is important to consider the components of integrated care for specific subpopulations of children in foster care. For example, unaccompanied refugee minors in federal foster care may require interpreters as part of the visit. Prebriefing with the interpreter can help avoid retraumatization of the patient and secondary traumatic stress for the interpreter. Records are ideally obtained beforehand from the Office of Refugee Resettlement, and prior authorizations for the visit may need to be coordinated with the child-placing agency. For youth in juvenile detention, health visits may require coordination with both the youth's caseworker and staff at the juvenile detention center. There may be additional confidentiality or adolescent health–related concerns to consider. Other subpopulations of children in foster care requiring special consideration may include: infants born preterm, infants of parents with substance use disorders, children with medical complexity, children with significant developmental (such as autism spectrum disorder or intellectual disability) or mental health problems, and pregnant and parenting teens.

Monitoring of Outcomes

Measurement-Based Care

In addition to established and more commonly used pediatric screens for behavioral, developmental, and mental health (eg, PHQ-9, GAD-7, ASQ, PSC, as described in Chapter 12, Mental Health), a trauma-informed, integrated pediatric care practice for youth in child welfare should consider trauma symptom screens as part of their practice. The timing of screening may also be important. At entry to care, children are often in acute distress. One may consider deferring developmental and mental health screening to a follow-up visit while assessing for urgent issues such as suicidality, aggression, and potential harm to self or others. In integrated care settings, the trauma symptom and mental health screens may be reviewed by mental health clinicians and interpreted and discussed with pediatricians. The developmental screening tools may be reviewed by a clinician (eg, pediatrician or developmental specialist), and reviewed with the caregiver with recommendations for addressing more significant concerns. The key is communication within the team and family to address and support overall child and family health and well-being. Screens can also be used to monitor trauma symptoms and developmental progress over time.

Evaluation and Population-Based Outcome Measures to Consider in Integrated Models for Children in Foster Care

Integrated care models emphasize collaboration and communication among various disciplines; therefore, evaluation and outcome measures ideally include population-based or systems-based measures. Potential measures and outcomes to consider include continuity of care, placement stability (in a family-based setting), effective care coordination, and patient and caregiver satisfaction.

There are significant challenges to meaningfully measuring outcomes for integrated care models, including logistics of data gathering, tracking, and analysis to evaluate continuity of care, creating placement stability goals, identifying parameters for care coordination, and assessing patient and caregiver satisfaction. Thus, practices seeking to evaluate the effectiveness of their integrated care model must consider what to measure and which measures to use and may wish to partner with child welfare and a team of data or research experts. Developing a shared database among the various care agencies serving children in foster and kinship care could enable tracking of this highly mobile patient population and the use of claims data to potentially evaluate their physical and mental health and social outcomes.

Implementation and Sustainability of Integrated Care Models

Financial sustainability of integrated care models is dependent on funding sources. Most funding resources other than Medicaid will require outcomes data to commit to continued funding.[15] Other potential sources of funds are contracts with child welfare, county general health funds, and foundations. **Table 8-3** describes existing payment strategies to support integrated care models.

Table 8–3. Descriptions of Funding Sources to Sustain Integrated Care Model Clinics

Funding Source	Description
Federal/state/ county funding	Medicaid payment for care coordination models serving children in foster care may be an option in certain states.
Academic institutional support	Partnering with an academic institution to identify multidisciplinary partners, promote workforce development and build outcome databases can have immense benefits.
Philanthropic grant funds	Philanthropy and grants are often necessary to implement and sustain an integrated care medical home model.

Advocating to Sustain Integrated Care Models

Billing Considerations

The key to sustainability is finding continued funding sources. Integrated care models are typically not supported by current fee-for-service or Medicaid managed care payer structures. While insurance payment is essential, additional funding from philanthropic institutions and grants will be necessary. Academic institutions and children's hospitals can be excellent resources to identify multidisciplinary partners and find educational resources to promote workforce development. Scaling up will require changes to Medicaid payment structures to support collaborative care and care coordination. States will vary in their ability and willingness to allow for same-day billing for medical and behavioral health services, increase payment rates for evidence-based services in integrated care settings, and require managed care organizations to implement value-based payment strategies that support models achieving better outcomes for children in foster care. Researching county and state billing and reimbursement policies can open a discussion with funders about piloting different payment strategies.[16] Additionally, for information on coding for social drivers of health issues and services, visit https://downloads.aap.org/AAP/PDF/SDOH.pdf. Center for Medicare Services (CMS) also requires states to follow Early and Periodic Screening, Diagnostic, and Treatment (EPSDT) guidance, which includes covering services indicated as needed by a child upon screening and diagnosis.

Transitions

Children in foster care are often in transition among placements, or because of reunification or adoption, and may be lost to follow-up. No-show rates may still be high, and continuity of care may be limited. Child welfare can notify team members when placement changes occur and provide contact information to facilitate continuity of care. A discharge visit at the time of reunification is suggested to ensure the child has ongoing health care and to apprise the caregiver of the child's health status.

Variations in Family Needs

Longer visit times and more frequent follow-up are not always ideal for families. Clinicians must balance quality of care and time with patients and families against productivity and volume of patients served. Increase in utilization of telehealth services has expanded access to working caregivers and families in suburban or rural areas.

Staffing, Partnerships, and Sustaining a Healthy Team Environment

Integrated care settings are knowledgeable about trauma-informed care and can proactively create trauma-informed practices to recruit, train, and support staff, such as by facilitating teamwork, proactively addressing causes of burnout, and preventing or ameliorating secondary traumatic stress.

Key Takeaways

- Integrated care is an evidence-based, trauma informed approach that uses collaborative care among medical and behavioral health clinicians to address the multifaceted and complex health needs of children in foster and kinship care.
- Integrated care can occur through coordinated care, colocated care, or fully collaborative and integrated care. The extent of integration is dependent on a practice's ability to partner with behavioral health, available resources, and support (eg, personnel, space, funding).
- Lack of funding and outcomes data are threats to the sustainability of integrated care models.
- Fully integrated health care that is holistic, trauma informed, and culturally humble is considered the best practice for all children, including those involved with child welfare and other children with complex health needs. Pediatricians are on the front lines of this challenge to provide the best care and advocate for this integrated approach.

CHAPTER 9

Sexual and Reproductive Health Care

Channelle S. Carr, MD, MHS, FAAP
Camille A. Broussard, MD, MPH, FAAP

Understanding the Sexual and Reproductive Health Needs of Youth in Foster Care

Youth in foster care have a greater risk of acquiring sexually transmitted infections (STIs) and of teen and repeat teen pregnancy, as well as dating and sexual violence and/or exploitation, when compared with their peers without foster care experience. A large study found that youth with foster care experience engaged in sexual behaviors earlier, reported more sex partners, and were more likely to engage in casual sex and sex for money than were their peers without foster care experience.[1] Histories of trauma, placement instability, loss of relationships, and inadequate sexual and reproductive health (SRH) education and care all contribute to these disparate outcomes.[2]

Gap in SRH Knowledge Among Youth in Foster Care

Often, case workers, social workers, caregivers, and schools have not provided youth in foster care with SRH education or access to SRH services.[3–5] Youth with high placement instability are especially at risk because they may not have had a consistent trusted adult or school providing this education to them. This leaves a large gap in SRH knowledge for youth in foster care; these youth may reach out to peers and social media, which may provide inaccurate or incomplete information.[6,7] Furthermore, lesbian and bisexual girls in foster care have described receiving little inclusive SRH from trusted sources.[8] Thus, pediatric health professionals have an important role in providing SRH education and services to youth in foster care during medical visits.

Confidentiality and Consent Concerns

Youth in foster care have a right to the same confidentiality protections and ability to consent to SRH services as their peers in the general population. However, child welfare agencies may not have explicit policies that guarantee this confidentiality and consent, which can become confusing for all parties involved in care. Additionally, it can become challenging to keep SRH services completely confidential because youth often require assistance with transportation to appointments or with picking up prescriptions. Thus, pediatricians and other clinicians should only disclose the minimum information necessary as dictated by state law to ensure that youth can access SRH services (for example, request a group-home worker transport youth to a medical appointment but do not disclose what will occur at that appointment unless required by state law). Because confidentiality protections and the ability for minors to provide consent for SRH services themselves vary by state, it is critical for pediatricians and other clinicians to know their state law or consult their institution's legal team regarding these issues.

Importantly, clinicians should be mindful that many youth in foster care have had their private lives and histories disclosed without their consent in court or within multiple systems they have experienced and may not expect confidentiality from adults. Therefore, youth may not feel comfortable discussing their SRH concerns for fear of disclosure. Pediatricians and other clinicians should review confidentiality limitations at the beginning of the visit and ensure that discussions about SRH are conducted privately. Confidentiality may be broken when there are safety risks involved—for example, if youth express suicidal ideation, homicidal ideation, or abuse. Ideally, before any disclosure, clinicians should inform youth what information is about to be shared and with whom.

Access to SRH Care

There are numerous barriers to accessing SRH services for youth in foster care, including system-level, interpersonal-level, and individual-level factors within a socioecological model. See **Figure 9-1** for examples of these barriers. To overcome these challenges, pediatric health professionals play a critical role in expanding access to SRH services within their general practice. Becoming familiar and comfortable with providing SRH services as described in the following sections is essential to integrating SRH into primary care. Additionally, there are several resources that pediatric health professionals can use to provide their patients in the foster care system with SRH if additional or specialized care is needed. These resources include

- Clinics that provide Title X family planning (free or sliding-scale services)
- Local health department sexual health clinics
- Referral to adolescent medicine or obstetrics/gynecology specialists
- Planned Parenthood local sites

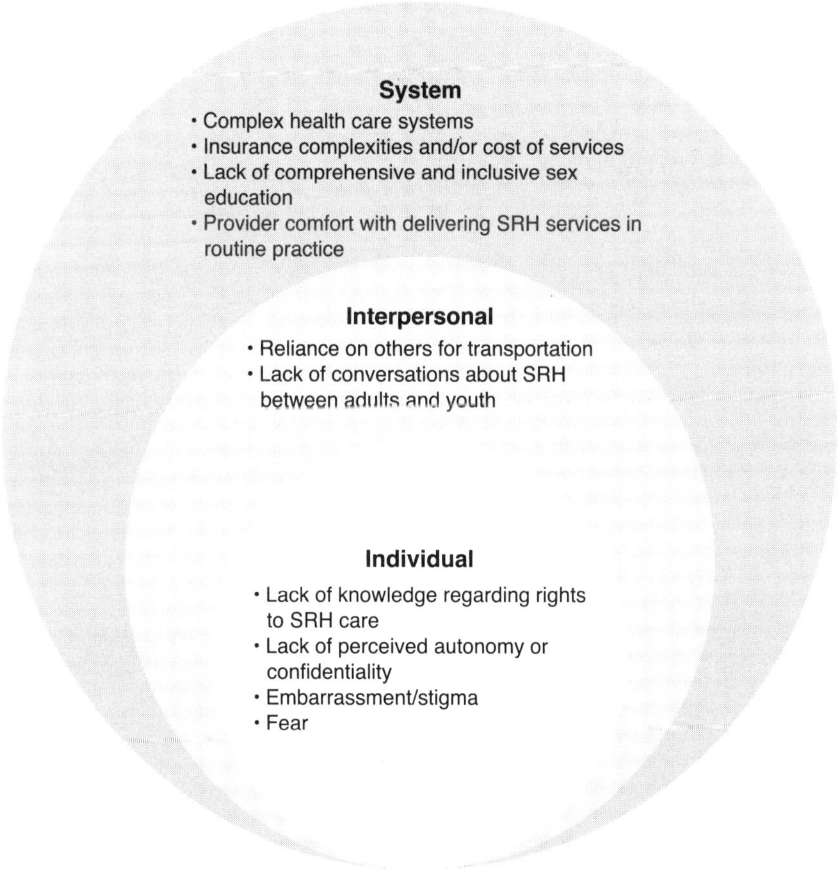

Abbreviation: SRH, sexual and reproductive health.

Figure 9–1. The social-ecological model reveals the multilevel factors within the individual, interpersonal, and system levels that affect access to sexual and reproductive health care for youth in foster care.

Providing Comprehensive SRH Care

It is the responsibility of the pediatrician to provide comprehensive SRH care, including taking an inclusive sexual history, STI screening, prevention education, diagnostic testing, screening for intimate partner violence, and family planning. Given the increased risk of pregnancy among youth in foster care, pediatricians and other clinicians should also provide preconception counseling and recommend prenatal vitamins to those youth of child-bearing age.

This discussion expands on the American Academy of Pediatrics (AAP) policy statements on Adolescent Sexual Health[9] and best practices for delivering SRH care to adolescents in clinical settings.[10] Furthermore, the Reproductive Health Equity Project for Foster Youth developed *The Foster Friendly Healthcare Toolkit: A Practitioner's Guide to Delivering Quality Sexual and Reproductive Health Care to Youth in Foster Care,* which provides detailed and tailored guidance on providing SRH services specifically to youth in foster care.[11]

History Taking During Medical Visits

Adopt the "5 Ps" approach to taking a sexual history: Partners, Practices, Protection from STIs, Past History of STIs, and Pregnancy Intention.[13] See **Box 9–1** for sample open-ended questions that comprise an inclusive sexual history.[12] Be aware that youth in foster care may be hesitant to share sensitive information with clinicians, given potential past histories of trauma, thus a trauma-informed approach to history taking is warranted.[8]

Obtain information on sexual and gender identity as a part of taking an inclusive sexual history. This can be important for affirming youth who may have experienced rejection by their family of origin due to their sexual and/or gender identity. Furthermore, some LGBTQ+ youth may have experienced discrimination within the health care system as well. See Chapter 27, Children and Youth Who identify as LGBTQ+, and Chapter 28, Additional Considerations for Transgender and Gender-Diverse Children and Youth, for more detailed information.

Gather information on what types of sex a youth engages in to appropriately screen for and counsel youth on STI and pregnancy risks based on sexual behaviors. Be mindful that sexual identity may not align with sexual behaviors.

Because youth in foster care are at increased risk of sex trafficking, the 6-item Short Screen for Child Sex Trafficking[14] and the 8-item Adult Human Trafficking Screening Tool[15] may be used in clinical practice as screening tools. See Chapter 23, Commercial Sexual Exploitation of Children, for more details.

Box 9-1

Sample Prompts/Questions in an Inclusive Sexual History

Sexual Identity

- Tell me who you are attracted to.

Gender Identity

- How do you see yourself in terms of gender?
- What name and pronouns should we use?
- When referring to your genitals, are there specific terms that you use?

Sexual Practices

- Some youth tell me that they have had anal, oral, or penile-vaginal sex. Do you know what those things are? Have you ever had those types of sex?
- Tell me about your sexual partners.
- Can you share with me the type of sex you are having? For example, some youth tell me they participate in anal, oral, vaginal-penile sex.
- Which body parts of yours touch which body parts of your partner(s)? (Alternatively: What body parts are involved in the type of sex you have?)

STIs

Screen for STIs based on Centers for Disease Control and Prevention (CDC) STI screening guidelines.[16] Youth in foster care are considered at higher risk for trichomoniasis (the most common curable nonviral STI) than are their peers[1] and thus should be screened for this in addition to chlamydia, gonorrhea, syphilis, and HIV. While this guidance is not a CDC recommendation, it is based on expert opinion and the recognition that these youth are at higher risk. Additionally, screening outside of CDC guidelines should be performed if requested by the patient.

STI screening collection sites should be dictated by the type of sex in which the youth engages (oropharynx, vagina, urethra, and rectum). Vaginal swabs for STI screening are considered the optimal sample type, compared with urine samples, for youth that have vaginas.[17] Self-collection of vaginal swab samples may be preferred by youth who have experienced trauma. However, urine samples are still adequate if properly collected (first catch of 5–20 mL with no urination in the previous hour). Clinicians may mark urine cups at the 20-mL level to limit the volume of urine provided and should ensure the urine sample is not too diluted. For men who have sex with men, the oropharynx, urethra (via urine sample), and rectum may be used as collection sites based on reported sexual activity.

Pediatricians can consult the current CDC STI treatment guidelines to find up-to-date guidance on treating patients who test positive for an STI, as well as guidance on providing partner treatment.[18] Many states allow for expedited partner therapy when pediatricians cannot ensure that the patient's sex partners from the previous 60 days will receive treatment. Providing expedited partner therapy, if allowed by local laws, can reduce the risk of reinfection. Patients should be counseled to abstain from sex for at least 7 days after they and their partner complete treatment.

Prevention of STIs is a critical conversation to include in the office visit. STI prevention includes[4]

- Condoms.
- Dental dams.
- Pre-exposure prophylaxis (PrEP; for further information on PrEP guidelines, refer to CDC guidelines[5]). Importantly, PrEP should be provided to anyone who requests it, however, there may be unique considerations regarding a youth's ability to consent based on local laws.
- Vaccination (human papillomavirus, hepatitis B).
- Counseling on reducing the number of sex partners as one method of harm reduction.
- Abstinence as a method of prevention.

Family Planning and Contraception

Youth in foster care should be provided with comprehensive and evidence-based family planning services. This includes contraceptive and pregnancy counseling on all available options, taking into account local laws. Counseling should be trauma informed and patient centered to allow for a shared decision-making approach. Specifically for contraceptive counseling, pediatricians should ask about past experiences with contraceptives, preferences for contraceptive method, and readiness to decide on a contraceptive method. Next, a discussion should occur to address the youth's priorities, concerns, and plan to execute the chosen method.[11]

Special considerations for youth in foster care regarding contraceptive counseling are detailed in **Table 9–1**.

Table 9–1. Advantages and Other Considerations for Contraceptive Methods for Youth in Foster Care

Contraceptive Method	Advantages for Youth in Foster Care	Other Considerations for Youth in Foster Care
Long-acting reversible contraceptives		
Subdermal progestin implant	• Little effort to maintain • Most effective form of contraception • Other than a small scar on arm, typically discreet • Reduces dysmenorrhea	• Requires an in-person visit for insertion and removal • Irregular bleeding is expected and can be a common reason for discontinuation
IUD	• Little effort to maintain • Discreet • Safe for nulliparous adolescents • Low discontinuation rates; patients are generally satisfied • Other than copper IUD, all other IUDs reduce dysmenorrhea	• Requires an in person visit for insertion, follow-up to check if IUD strings remain in place, and removal • For patients with a history of sexual trauma/abuse, insertion may precipitate retraumatization • Concern for pain with insertion may be reduced with topical or injectable (paracervical block) pain medication at the time of the procedure • Expulsion, although rare, may occur
Medium-acting contraceptives		
Depot medroxyprogesterone acetate injection	• Discreet • No daily effort needed • Reduces dysmenorrhea	• Requires injections every 11–15 weeks; patients will require transportation to appointments for intramuscular injections • Can precipitate medical trauma if there is any needle phobia • Known side effects are weight gain, decreased bone mineral density, and delayed return to fertility
Short-acting contraceptives		
Vaginal rings	• User-controlled method • Can be used in an extended cycle or continuous fashion • Reduces dysmenorrhea	• Patient needs to be comfortable with vaginal insertion • Consider if patient has sexual trauma history, as insertion can be triggering
Transdermal contraceptive patch	• User-controlled method • Reduces dysmenorrhea	• Lack of diverse skin complexions for patch color • Some patients may develop a skin reaction to the patch adhesive
Progestin-only pills	• User-controlled method • Reduces dysmenorrhea	• May require more stringent attention to exact daily timing than combined oral contraceptive pills
Combined oral contraceptive pills	• User-controlled method • Reduces dysmenorrhea • Can be used in an extended cycle or continuous fashion	• Requires daily adherence

(continues)

Table 9–1 *(continued)*

Contraceptive Method	Advantages for Youth in Foster Care	Other Considerations for Youth in Foster Care
	Barrier methods	
Condom	• Protects against STIs and HIV • Easy accessibility	• Must use for every sexual encounter • Requires partner acceptance for use
Internal condom (condom inserted into vagina)	• Protects against STIs and HIV • Can be inserted prior to sex	• Patient needs to be comfortable with vaginal insertion • Must insert for every sexual encounter • Can be harder to acquire
Diaphragm	• Can be ordered online after obtaining a prescription • Can be inserted prior to sex • Reusable up to 2 years	• Patient needs to be comfortable with insertion method • Must insert for every sexual encounter • Must use spermicide for effectiveness
	Emergency contraception	
Emergency contraception pills	• Over-the-counter option • Can be used up to 5 days after unprotected sex	• Requires effort from patient to either obtain a prescription or access the over-the-counter option
Copper IUD	• Can be used as subsequent contraception • Can last up to 10 years • Hormone-free option	• Requires an in-person procedure for insertion • For patients with a history of sexual trauma/abuse, insertion may precipitate retraumatization • Must insert within 5 days of unprotected sexual intercourse

Abbreviations: IUD, intrauterine device; STI, sexually transmitted infection.

Trauma-Informed SRH Care

Approach to SRH Medical Visits

A trauma-informed approach should be applied to SRH medical visits with youth in foster care.[11,20,21] Care should be taken during sensitive examination maneuvers (see **Table 9–2** for a trauma-sensitive approach to a physical examination), and patient dignity should be preserved by using adequate draping of the patient. Whenever possible, youth should be given choices on examination maneuvers and positions. Pediatricians should explain what to expect before and during the examination. Youth should be allowed to stop a sensitive examination at any time. Pelvic examinations can be especially traumatic for some youth. The provision of a mirror might be helpful to show and explain breast, genital/pelvic, or rectal anatomy to youth during the examination, if the youth consents. The youth can hold the mirror to be in control. A chaperone or another youth-identified safe person should be offered during examinations.

Table 9–2. Trauma-Sensitive Approach to a Physical Examination

The following resource provides approaches to a trauma-sensitive physical examination. The provider's goal should be to communicate respect and maintain/restore a sense of safety, autonomy and trust to avoid triggering feelings of fear, shame, vulnerability, and powerlessness.

<table>
<tr><th>DISCUSS</th><th>BEFORE EXAM</th><th>DURING EXAM</th><th>AFTER EXAM</th></tr>
<tr><td>While explaining the procedure, watch for signs of anxiety, fear, or discomfort</td><td>"Before we get started, I'm going to walk you through what we will be doing during the exam."
• What parts of the body will be examined
• What tools will be used
• How long it will take
"This is something I do whenever a patient has ______ (name symptoms)."
Normalize the exam</td><td>"First I'm going to _____."
Let youth know what you're doing prior to each step
Say - "First I will inspect the outside of the vaginal area"
NOT - "First I'm going to look at the outside of your vaginal area"
Say - "Allow your knees to fall toward the walls"
NOT - "Spread your legs"
Say - "Exam table"
NOT - "Bed"
Say - "Foot rests"
NOT - "Stirrups"
Say - "Take deep breaths"
NOT - "Relax"
Use simple, impersonal, nonclinical language</td><td>"I'm going to leave the room now so that you can get dressed. Once you're ready, I'll be back to share my findings and make a plan with you about what to do next."
*(share results and make treatment plan)</td></tr>
<tr><td>Provide adequately sized gowns/ drapes for modesty (cloth rather than paper, if possible)</td><td colspan="3">If youth need to remove clothing - "When needed, I will ask you to lift the left side of your shirt up to ______ so we can inspect ______."
Be specific
If using gown - "You'll wear this with the opening in the back."
If using drape - "You can use this as a sheet over your lap."
"I will step outside so you can change. When you're ready, let me know, and I'll come back in."
Knock & wait for permission before re-entering</td></tr>
<tr><td>ASK</td><td>"Any questions/ concerns before we get started?"<br>"Would you like to have someone else in the room during the exam for support?"
Offer to bring someone for support</td><td>"What words do you prefer to use when talking about your body?"
Ask youth's preferences
"Would it be alright if I placed my hand ___?"
Ask for permission before touching</td><td>"Any questions so far?"
Discuss findings and ask for questions
"How are you feeling about the plan?"<br>"How do you see this working best for you?"
Negotiate treatment plan</td></tr>
</table>

Reproduced with permission from Reproductive Health Equity Project for Foster Youth. *The Foster Friendly Healthcare Toolkit: A Practitioner's Guide to Delivering Quality Sexual and Reproductive Health Care to Youth in Foster Care.* 2022. Accessed December 2, 2024. https://fosterreprohealth.org/wp-content/uploads/2024/09/Foster-Friendly-Toolkit3-2024.pdf.

Reproductive Justice in Providing SRH Services

Youth in foster care often feel that they have no control. Using a reproductive justice lens in the clinical encounter, establishing that everyone has control over their own body and reproduction, encourages youth to engage in and control their own health care.

Be mindful of the possibility that a patient has experienced or is experiencing reproductive coercion by their partner or other clinicians. Use a patient-centered and shared decision-making approach for SRH services, especially contraceptive counseling, instead of leading always with a long-acting reversible contraception (LARC)-first approach. Young Black women in foster care have historically been subjected to reproductive coercion more frequently than other groups.[22] Thus, it is incredibly important for clinicians to be mindful of this to overcome biases and treatment preferences to support the patient. Youth in foster care may have been told that they would be unfit parents and should not become pregnant, which may further place the youth at risk for poor outcomes if they are judged or ignored. The PATH (Parenting/Pregnancy Attitudes, Timing, How Important) framework is one example of a person-centered approach (see **Table 9–3** for example prompts).

Table 9–3. PATH Framework for Asking about Reproductive Desires

PA	Parenting/Pregnancy Attitudes	"Do you think you might like to have (more) children at some point?"
T	Timing	"When do you think that might be?"
H	How Important?	"How important is it to you to prevent pregnancy (until then)?"

Adapted from PATH Framework. What Is PATH. Available at https://www.path-framework.com/whatispath. Accessed November 27, 2024.

Building Supportive Environments for Youth in Foster Care

Prevention, Educational, and Training Programs

To reduce disparate SRH outcomes for youth in foster care, more prevention programs and comprehensive sexual education are needed, specifically tailored to this population.[23] Training of foster parents and caregivers is critically needed, and some interventions have previously been piloted.[24–26] Importantly, youth in foster care need

- Age- and developmentally appropriate sexual education on puberty, anatomy, and reproductive processes. Advocates for Youth have developed digital content, called AMAZE, that youth can view and share with caregivers or other adults in their lives and that can be used by pediatricians to assist in these conversations and education (https://amaze.org; https://www.youtube.com/c/amazeorg).

- Education about consent and coercion regarding sexual behaviors. This is especially important in the context of potential past sexual abuse where the youth was denied the right of consent.
- Education on healthy relationships, including dating and sexual relationships.

Creating Safe Spaces and Fostering Open Communication in the Pediatric Office

Be mindful of the language, signage, office art, and materials available in the office to ensure an inclusive and welcoming space. Physicians can survey youth with lived experience regarding office space and consider their responses when designing welcoming spaces. Offer same-day SRH procedures, especially because youth in foster care may have more difficulty returning for appointments.

Key Takeaways

» Pediatricians have an important role in providing comprehensive, trauma-informed, and inclusive SRH education and services to youth in foster care during medical visits.

» Youth in foster care have a right to the same confidentiality protections and ability to consent for SRH services as their peers; however, there are barriers to maintaining this confidentiality that are unique to the foster care system.

» For pregnancy prevention and contraception counseling, a reproductive justice lens should be used to tailor SRH services in a person-centered and shared decision-making approach.

CHAPTER

10

Assessing Risk and Protective Factors

Miguel Nuñez, PhD
V. Faye Jones, MD, PhD, MSPH, FAAP

Children and adolescents in foster care face distinct disadvantages stemming from their challenging experiences before entering the foster care system and during their time within it. The very nature of the experiences that led children to their involvement with the foster care system are adverse (such as neglect or abuse). Furthermore, their foster care journey is often marked by additional challenges, such as placement instability, educational disruptions, and an absence of consistent support.[1,2] These adversities increase the likelihood of unfavorable outcomes. To help mitigate existing and future risk, clinicians can harness protective factors to bolster resilience. *Resilience* refers to the dynamic process by which individuals achieve successful adaptation (or maintain healthy functioning) following exposure to significant adversity.[3] Children may display resilience in the face of adversity, and clinicians have the opportunity to promote such ability.[4] It is important to differentiate between prevention, which involves building protective factors to mitigate the impact of future adverse outcomes, and treatment, which focuses on addressing the adverse effects that have already occurred. [5] While the risk and protective factors discussed in this chapter may also apply to children and adolescents in the general population, the assessment of these factors is particularly salient for youth in foster care. To effectively address the unique needs of this population, it is necessary to comprehensively assess risk and protective factors at individual, relational, and community levels. Such assessment should serve as a foundation for strategies aimed at enhancing youths' overall welfare. The chapter begins by outlining risk and protective factors to consider at different socioecological levels for children in foster care. Then, practical strategies for assessing risk and protective factors are discussed.

Risk Factors

Adversity can be present across different socioecological levels, including individual (eg, physical abuse) and interpersonal (eg, caregiver separation), community (eg, poverty), climate (eg, COVID-19), and cultural (eg, segregation).[6]

Individual Level

Nearly half of youth in foster care meet the criteria for a mental health disorder, a number nearly 4 times that of children and adolescents in the general population.[7] Children in foster care also have a high prevalence of complex trauma, further complicating their mental health presentations.[8] Yet not all youth who need mental health services receive them.[9] Implementing mental health screens in primary care settings can help identify youth who need additional mental and behavioral health care services. When appropriate, providing referrals to mental health clinicians and advocating for the youth to receive services are ways to limit the impact of mental and behavioral health disorders on affected youth.

Children in foster care are more likely than those in the general population to experience poor physical health.[10] There are estimates suggesting that 35% to 45% of children entering foster care have at least one chronic physical health condition.[11] The mortality rate is also higher among children in foster care than in the general population.[12] Continuity of care can play a vital role in managing physical health conditions. A trusted primary care clinician who is familiar with a youth's history and needs may offer opportunities to intervene and promote physical health. Continuity of care also provides the clinician with a better understanding of the patient's medical history and unique health care needs, enabling a higher quality of care through more informed decisions, a personalized approach, and detecting changes in the patient's health more effectively. A consistent primary care clinician can also serve as the point of coordination for different services needed by the child, including trauma-informed care, reducing the risk of fragmented or duplicated services. (See Chapter 17, Childhood Trauma and Resilience, and the American Academy of Pediatrics [AAP] policy statement "Trauma-Informed Care."[13])

The continuity of care may be particularly important for subsets of youth. Children with disabilities and those with physical health problems are at an increased risk of experiencing placement instability.[14–16] They are also more likely to have a longer length of stay in the system. Children with disabilities in foster care are estimated to have an average of 4 placement disruptions, compared to the mean of 2.37 placement disruptions among children without a disability. Furthermore, children with disabilities spend an average of 915 days in foster care, whereas children without a disability spend an average of 514 days in foster care.[15]

Risk factors at the individual level can compound and generate additional challenges. For example, adolescents with chronic illness are at increased risk of mental health conditions, including both internalizing and externalizing problems.[14] Given the high prevalence of physical and mental health conditions in this population, an integrated behavioral health approach may be beneficial in mitigating these types of risk. See Chapter 8, Integrated Models of Care, for additional discussion.

Children and adolescents who were or are currently involved with the foster care system should undergo screening for their social needs to ensure that gaps are identified and addressed. Research studies have revealed several areas where material hardships and risks exist, such as food insecurity, housing, employment, and transportation.[17] Poverty is a major player in identified social gaps, particularly in reports of food insecurity.[17–19] Using the US Census Bureau Supplemental Poverty Measure, Pac et al found poverty rates of 32% among children living with grandparents, compared with 20% for children living with foster parents and 17% for children living with parents.[20] A 2011 report by Murphey et al[18] stated that children who are in foster care and live with families that have incomes below the federal poverty line are 6 times more likely to experience food insecurity and 14 times more likely to experience severe food insecurity than children who live in households with incomes at 185% of the federal poverty line. Additionally, 1 in 4 kinship families report food insecurity.[19] A study of transition-age youth with foster care involvement by Park and associates[17] found that 30% of study participants were food insecure at ages 19, 21, and 23 years. By exploring and understanding these social gaps, the clinician can take steps to connect the family with social resources and other strategies to mitigate these challenges to youth well-being.

Relational Level

The top four circumstances associated with a child's removal from their family of origin are neglect, parental substance use, caregiver's inability to cope, and physical abuse.[21] These adverse childhood experiences (ACEs) reflect challenges in the child's primary caregiving relationships that may have a long-term impact on an individual's well-being. Children in foster care experience disproportionately more ACEs than youth in the general population, and even more than those from socioeconomically disadvantaged backgrounds (ie, children in families with income below the poverty line).[22] Adverse childhood experiences are documented to negatively affect well-being, including both physical and mental health outcomes, well into the adult years.[23] This may include chronic health conditions (such as asthma, obesity, sleep disturbance, diabetes) as well as developmental delays and mental health problems (such as anxiety, depression, and post-traumatic stress)[11,14,23] (see Chapter 12, Mental Health, and Chapter 17, Childhood Trauma and Resilience, for more in-depth information).

Even among children in foster care, those with a higher number of ACEs have a lower likelihood of reunification, and more placement instability, than those with fewer ACEs.[22,24,25] Clinicians working with children in foster care can lessen the impact of potential trauma secondary to ACEs by implementing mental health screening and referral as part of their routine care. Clinicians can use trauma-informed approaches and provide psychoeducation about the potential consequences of early childhood trauma on a child's health, mental health, and development. They can also offer guidance on trauma-informed positive parenting strategies to respond to existing symptoms.

There are challenges that should be considered if screening is implemented.[26] Among these is how to effectively utilize the information acquired. The AAP and the Centers for Disease Control and Prevention do not recommend screening specifically for ACEs based on the current science; instead, they recommend screening for trauma symptoms, which provides information that is more predictive at the individual level and can inform appropriate guidance and referrals. When indicated, referrals and coordination with mental health clinicians who provide evidence-based, trauma-informed treatment (or if unavailable, trauma-informed care focusing on organizational culture and practice) should be strongly considered (see Chapter 11, Screenings; Chapter 12, Mental Health; Chapter 17, Childhood Trauma and Resilience; and Chapter 38, Psychotropic Medication Oversight). The AAP provides information and guidance on the process of asking families about the impacts of adverse experiences.[27] Further, when clinical assessment or screening identifies a child with complex trauma, referral to a psychologist for a comprehensive mental health evaluation and evidence-based trauma treatment may be warranted. Occasionally, referral to a child and adolescent psychiatrist for potential psychotropic medication prescription and medication management may be indicated. (See Chapter 12, Mental Health, for additional discussion of screening for and responding to trauma symptoms.) Given the overlap of trauma symptoms with other mental health diagnoses, the primary treatment for children with complex trauma symptoms is comprehensive evaluation and evidence-based mental health treatment. In the past, there has been overprescription and overreliance by clinicians on psychotropic medication to address mental health and behavioral symptoms. Psychotropic medication is only indicated when comorbid conditions (eg, attention-deficit/hyperactivity disorder, anxiety, depression) have been identified after careful evaluation and institution of evidence-based therapy. It has been estimated that youth in foster care receive psychotropic drugs as much as 4.5 times more frequently than do their peers in the general population.[28] Such situations have resulted in civil lawsuits (for example, *M.B. v Tidball*). Specific steps that can help ensure that psychotropics are prescribed only when necessary include identifying mental health clinicians who are trauma informed, ensuring that a comprehensive trauma-informed mental health evaluation has been completed, ensuring treatment is specific to a comorbid mental health condition and the prescriber is following best practices for using lowest effective dose, monitoring for resolution of symptoms and potential side effects, and adhering to other safety guidelines for psychotropic medication use. It is reasonable to obtain a second opinion when a child has complex symptoms,[29] before beginning medication treatment. (See Chapter 38, Psychotropic Medication Oversight.)

Community/Systems Level

The amount of time that children spend in foster care, the type of placement, and the number of placements experienced are risk factors linked to poor outcomes. Spending more time in foster care, along with placement instability, has been linked with increased physical and mental health needs.[30] Children in family-based settings, particularly kinship care, appear to achieve more favorable outcomes and may have fewer placement disruptions than youth in non-family-based settings.[31,32] However, caution is warranted in interpreting results related to placement type, because youth in out-of-home care often experience multiple placements, including both family-based and non-family-based settings.[33]

Cultural dissimilarity between the foster family and the family of origin (eg, ethnicity, spoken language) may present challenges to cooperative parenting practices.[34] Further, cultural dissimilarity may interfere with positive ethnic identity formation and result in a child having fewer ethnically compatible social networks, which may lead to a lower sense of belonging and more social isolation.[35]

Youth who identify as lesbian, gay, bisexual, transgender, and questioning or queer (LGBTQ+) are overrepresented in the foster care system.[36] This population faces unique challenges when compared to their cisgender and heterosexual peers. In 2001, Feinstein and colleagues[37] reported on a study that found that 78% of LGBTQ+ foster youth in New York City were either removed from or fled their foster care placements due to unsupportive—or even hostile—environments regarding their sexual orientation or gender identity. One hundred percent of LGBTQ+ youth in the New York foster care system reported experiencing verbal harassment and 70% indicated being victims of physical violence because of their sexual identity while residing in congregate care. Nineteen years after the Feinstein and colleagues report, concerns regarding unsupportive and hostile foster care placements across the United States remained a concern.[36] Apart from further abuse, youth who are LGBTQ+ have a higher likelihood of congregate care placements and placement instability.[38] See Chapter 27, Children and Youth Who Identify as LGBTQ+, and Chapter 28, Additional Considerations for Transgender and Gender-Diverse Children and Youth, for information on caring for these youth.

Protective Factors

Protective factors are predictors of better adaptation in individuals who have experienced adversity.[39,40] In other words, they are things that help reduce the risk of developing problems in people who have undergone a difficult situation. Protective factors are not innate; rather, they develop over time.[39] As such, characteristics of the individual or the environment that are not malleable and amenable to intervention are not protective factors.[4]

Individual Level

Self-regulation, self-esteem, and interpersonal and academic skills are particularly salient protective factors for children in foster care.[41,42] Youth with more developed skills in these areas are better equipped to handle distressing or demanding situations that require cognitive, emotional, and behavioral control.

Self-regulation skills may help youth be less reactive, resist temptations, and engage in more thoughtful and constructive responses to challenging situations. Self-regulation is defined as the process by which the self changes its thoughts, feelings, and actions, including impulsive urges and task performance.[43] There is evidence to suggest that self-regulation may be improved with practice.[43] Realistic goal setting, and cognitive behavioral strategies, as well as psychoeducation on the relationship between nutrition, exercise, sleep hygiene, and self-regulation may help bolster these skills in youth who are in foster care. Self-esteem, or a youth's overall sense of their own worth, enhances their self-image and confidence, enabling youth to be more willing to take on challenges due to a stronger belief in their abilities to achieve their goals (ie, self-efficacy).

The presence of social support is a protective factor at the relational level; however, a youth's interpersonal skills may help them to develop healthy relationships. Children in foster care who possess effective communication, social awareness, and conflict resolution skills are more likely to build and maintain positive relationships with caregivers, teachers, peers, and others.

Lastly, school plays an integral part in children's lives. Youth who participate in extracurricular activities or have higher educational attainment show greater stability in their foster care placements.[42] In turn, greater stability may lead to higher future earnings in adulthood.[44]

Relational Level

The presence, type, and quality of the relationships established with children in foster care may act as protective factors. Children's development of skills that serve as protective factors depends on the guidance of, or teaching from, adults. The ability of adults to meet the needs of children determines the cultivation of such skills. Furthermore, peer relationships play an important role in children's development and behavior, particularly during adolescence. The literature indicates that children in foster care may benefit from regular contact with their biological parents,[41] living with a family member (kinship care),[32] and the presence of a caring adult.[45] Maintaining regular contact with biological parents can be direct (ie, visitations) or indirect (eg, phone calls, email). It is important to emphasize that contact with biological parents can also have negative consequences (eg, meeting with abusive parents can remind the youth of past trauma or generate new trauma).[46] As such, it is not only about contact with biological parents but the quality of that contact.[47] The contact must be properly planned, with appropriate support for the child, family members, and caregivers, to be successful and contribute to the assessment or rehabilitation in terms of a child's identified needs. Relatedly, the caregiver's skills in producing a warm and stable environment for the child with adequate supervision and discipline, and investment in nurturing the relationship with the child, are protective factors for youth in foster care.[41] For adolescents, in particular, the presence of a caring adult (such as a mentor or teacher) is linked to favorable outcomes as they age out of foster care.[45]

Community/Systems Level

As children in foster care learn to navigate their environment effectively, the community and systems to which the child belongs can either facilitate or inhibit the development of resilience. A positive school environment, a stable living situation, and support for independent living are salient protective factors.[42] Children in foster care may have experienced significant disruptions and changes in their living situation resulting in frequent school changes.

A positive school environment provides valuable stability and consistency, particularly during times of transition. Further, a positive school environment helps provide children in foster care with a sense of belonging and inclusion. Schools also often have access to resources and programs that may benefit children in foster care or may serve as advocates, identifying challenges early and connecting them to appropriate services.

A stable living situation may enhance academic outcomes by facilitating regular school attendance. Placement stability can also promote a secure attachment between the child and caregiver and enable children to form lasting relationships with peers, neighbors, and community members. Further, a stable living situation allows for continuity of care, as children can receive consistent physical and mental health care, which may be vital for monitoring and addressing their needs following removal from their family of origin. Notably, research suggests that children with disabilities in foster care are less likely to experience disruptions in placements with dual parenting, possibly because caregivers can provide support to each other and reduce the sense of parental burden.[15] This finding highlights the importance of supports for foster families with all types of parental compositions.

As youth near or begin their transition out of foster care, support for independent living plays a key role in promoting educational attainment, employment, adequate housing, and positive health outcomes. Depending on the state, this transition occurs when the youth reaches either 18 or 21 years of age.[48] To facilitate a successful transition, it is important for state policies to provide comprehensive support as youth adapt to the challenges of independent living and provide these young adults with the resources they need to thrive.[49]

While protective factors have been discussed here as distinct domains, it is important to reiterate that they are all interconnected. For example, youth with a stable placement (community/systems level) may be able to attend the same school regularly, allowing them to participate in after-school activities (individual level), which may facilitate friendships (relational level) and a sense of belonging at the school (community/systems level), promoting the development of their interpersonal skills (individual level), and nurturing a relationship with a caring adult such as a teacher (relational level).

Practical Application

The next step in assessing risk and protective factors is to gather data from the specific youth to determine the presence or lack of such factors. Data collection may occur through surveys, clinical interviews, observations, collateral records, and chart reviews. This section focuses on discussing survey options and suggestions for conducting the clinical interviews. At this time, there is no standardized measure that captures all the risk factors for the child welfare population. Clinicians could consider developing their own questions that target the risk factors (such as "How many placements have you had?") as part of their intake form or clinical interview. In settings utilizing an integrated behavioral health approach, the mental health specialist can assist to ensure a holistic screening. Clinicians may also opt to use screening instruments. See Chapter 11, Screenings, and Chapter 12, Mental Health, for further discussion about screening instruments.

Currently, there is no validated instrument that assesses all protective factors discussed with a sample of children in foster care. There are validated measures of resilience, such as the Child and Youth Resilience Measure–Revised.[50] Researchers previously suggested that measures of resilience should be integrated into clinical practice.[51] However, there is currently no agreed-upon method of assessing resilience.[52] Resilience is context specific, meaning that a one-size-fits-all measure of resilience is often not applicable across different groups, including children and adolescents in foster care.[40] Instead, resilience may be assessed through the presence of protective factors identified in the literature rather than general measures of resilience. For example, self-regulation could be assessed through the Adolescent Self-Regulatory Inventory (ASRI),[53] and self-esteem could be assessed through the Rosenberg Self-Esteem Scale (RSES).[54] The difficulty of applying this approach to children in foster care lies in the length of time that such a request may take if assessing each domain. For this reason, preparation prior to the visit could be helpful. Information from medical record review could help to identify which surveys may be used to fill in any information gaps and strengths that can serve as starting points to engage youth in discussions.

Of note, while resilience is often associated with a strength-based approach, it is crucial to carefully balance this perspective by considering the risk factors. Unfortunately, there are instances where resilience is inappropriately used to minimize systems' responsibilities in ensuring the safety of children, which can lead to actions that invalidate a child's experiences. Furthermore, this narrow focus on resilience may overlook other areas of a child's life that could be negatively affected and may influence the withholding of needed resources.[55]

A recent development in the literature is the examination of positive childhood experiences (PCEs), which serve as promotive factors for healthy outcomes.[56] The literature distinguishes promotive (associated with favorable outcomes even after accounting for childhood adversity) versus protective (moderating the effects of adversity) effects, suggesting more research support for PCEs as promotive factors. Further, PCEs appear semi-independent from ACEs, such that experiencing one does not preclude experiencing the other. The first study of PCEs looked at the links that these experiences have with adult outcomes.[57] However, subsequent research has shown a positive impact of PCEs on adolescents.[58] More research is needed to assess the role of PCEs with youth in foster care specifically. However, PCEs provide a framework that can be used to screen a youth's potential assets and resources. The 7 PCEs are the ability to talk with family about feelings, the sense that family is supportive during difficult times, the enjoyment of participation in community traditions, feeling a sense of belonging in school, feeling supported by friends, having at least 2 non-parent adults who genuinely care, and feeling safe and protected by an adult in the home.[57] Some, but not all, of the PCEs overlap with the protective factors mentioned earlier in this chapter that apply specifically to children in foster care. As with risk factors, other methods apart from surveys will likely be needed for a comprehensive assessment.

If the clinician prefers to assess risk and protective factors as part of a clinical interview, they should be mindful of the following:

- **The developmental age of the child.** Children's communication style varies by their developmental stage. Younger children may need to express themselves through play or nonverbal cues. Relatedly, cognitive abilities, such as attention span, memory, and abstract thinking, differ across the developmental spectrum and questions need to be tailored appropriately (eg, younger children with shorter attention spans benefit from concrete examples).
- **The impact of childhood trauma.** Clinicians should be aware of the range of behaviors that can be displayed as part of post-traumatic stress in children (eg, irritability). Further, clinicians should be mindful of the potential for eliciting a post-traumatic stress response during an interview and have appropriate contingencies in place to help the youth emotionally regulate.
- **Medical, mental health, and social history.** Preparing for an effective clinical interview includes a review of available records. Such review will provide guidance on ways to narrow the questions that need to be asked to complete the clinical picture. Further, it minimizes the reliance on the child's memory and the limited information that a foster caregiver would be able to provide for a child who has a history of multiple placement disruptions.
- **Individuals present in the examination room.** The people present in the room when the clinical interview takes place may influence the received responses. For example, a child may feel uncomfortable acknowledging certain experiences of trauma if their caregiver is present.

Regardless of the method used to assess risk and protective factors, the most important step is how the information gathered is used. Surveillance and/or screening for risk and protective factors as part of routine care is not the assessment in and of itself. A discussion of the results and collaboration on treatment planning with caregivers, the youth (when appropriate), and the child welfare social worker should follow at the conclusion of the assessment. Based on this discussion, identified ways of mitigating risk and enhancing protective factors should be implemented. By applying the information discussed in this chapter, clinicians can make important contributions to the well-being of youth in foster care by promoting resilience.

Key Takeaways

» The purpose of assessing for risk and protective factors is to promote resilience in an individual child; however, presence of protective factors does not negate treatment needs.

» The assessment of risk and protective factors should include a combination of different approaches, such as surveys, clinical interviews, observations, collateral records, and a chart review.

» Salient protective factors in this population include self-regulation, self-esteem, interpersonal and academic skills, social support, placement with a skilled caregiver, quality contact with the family of origin, a positive school environment, a stable living situation, and support for independent living.

» Salient risk factors in this population include poor mental and physical health, physical disabilities, ACEs, unmet social needs, unsupportive environments, a long length of time in foster care, non-family-based placements, a high number of placements, and cultural dissimilarity between the foster family and the family of origin.

» The most important part of the assessment is how the information acquired is being used in the service of the child.

CHAPTER 11

Screenings

Melissa Jimenez, MD
Elizabeth Wallis, MD, MSHP, FAAP

Introduction

In medicine, screenings are performed on asymptomatic populations to assess their likelihood of a particular disease.[1] Typically, screenings do not diagnose a disease. Rather, when positive, further diagnostic testing will be necessary.[1] Screenings may be laboratory based (such as a blood draw to test for anemia) or question based (such as a patient health questionnaire to screen for depression).

In recent years, research focusing on the physical and mental health of children in foster care has shown that this population has more complex medical and mental health needs than their counterparts in the general population. Given the high risk of physical, developmental, and mental health problems in these children, health screenings upon entering foster care are extremely important. Previously, standards for screenings during medical visits for children in foster care were unclear. In 2005, the American Academy of Pediatrics (AAP) first published guidelines for the medical examination of children in foster care.

Initial Health Screen

The initial comprehensive health assessment is discussed in detail in Chapter 2, Health Care Visits: Type and Periodicity.

Laboratory Screening

Due to the increased risk of physical health problems in children in foster care, as well as often few to no medical records being available to the physician, the AAP provides recommendations for laboratory screening in this population (see **Table 11–1**).[2] Given the variability in the prevalence of specific infectious diseases (eg, syphilis) among communities in the United States, the decision to include screening for a given infectious disease may best be made by understanding local data. Previous studies show a low prevalence of infectious diseases in children in foster care.[4] Further study is needed to determine whether changes to current recommendations are warranted. Presently, the following laboratory studies are recommended for infants, children, and adolescents entering foster care[2]:

- **Hemoglobin:** The AAP recommends universal screening for anemia at 1-year and 2-year-old health supervision visits. For children in foster care, hemoglobin should be screened at the initial visit for all children younger than 6 years as well as adolescent females. Consider an annual hemoglobin or complete blood count up to age 6 years and for postmenarchal females.
- **Hemoglobin electrophoresis:** Hemoglobin electrophoresis testing is recommended for children at risk for hemoglobinopathies.
- **Lead level:** Lead levels should be obtained at least once for all children between the ages of 6 months and 6 years, if records are not available. Lead levels may also be considered in children with pica.
- **Dipstick urinalysis:** Previously, the AAP recommended that all children undergo a dipstick urinalysis at the age of 5 years and adolescence if they were sexually active. However, multiple large-scale studies showed that the incidence of chronic kidney disease (CKD) in the general population was low, so the recommendations have been dropped. However, it is unclear whether youth in foster care have a higher rate of CKD; thus, further studies are needed to evaluate the recommendation for dipstick urinalysis at the initial medical examination for this population (toilet trained and older than 2 years).
- **Tuberculosis**: An interferon-gamma release assay (IGRA) or a tuberculin skin test may be used to screen for tuberculosis; however, according to AAP guidelines, IGRA is now the preferred screening method for children of all ages.[5] It is recommended that children in congregate care receive yearly screening for tuberculosis.
- **Hepatitis B**: Screening for hepatitis B surface antibody is strongly recommended for all children to ensure they have been vaccinated and to confirm that they have responded to the vaccine.
- **Hepatitis C**: Screening for hepatitis C is strongly recommended for children of all ages who are at increased risk. Individuals at increased risk for infection with hepatitis C include children with HIV, those born to mothers

with hepatitis C, and anyone who has a history of injecting drugs.

- **HIV**: Screening for HIV is strongly recommended for children at increased risk of infection, and if proper consents have been obtained. The strongest risk factor for children to develop HIV is being born to a mother with HIV infection. HIV screening is also recommended at least once between the ages of 13 to 17 years.
- **Syphilis**: Screening for syphilis using a rapid plasma reagin test is strongly recommended for all ages (except for neonates with adequate maternal testing).

Additional Screening for Adolescents

In addition to routine screening of all children entering foster care for anemia, lead, CKD, and infectious diseases, adolescent-specific screening recommendations exist. Further assessment is recommended by the AAP for adolescents in foster care, specifically to screen for drug, alcohol, and tobacco use; sexual activity; pregnancy; and sexually transmitted infections.[2] The Substance Abuse and Mental Health Services Administration recommends screening for drug, alcohol, and tobacco use through the use of a brief intervention and/or referral to treatment as part of routine health care (see Chapter 21, Substance Use).[6] In addition to the aforementioned initial screening laboratory studies, screening for gonorrhea, chlamydia, and trichomoniasis in sexually active adolescents is appropriate. A pregnancy test should be performed for adolescents who could be pregnant. See Chapter 9, Sexual and Reproductive Health Care, and Chapter 22, Pregnant and Parenting Teens, for further guidance.

Developmental, Educational, and Mental Health Screenings

More than 80% of children and adolescents in foster care have one or more developmental, educational, or mental health problems as a result of the early life adversity they have endured.[7] Children in foster care are more likely to be born preterm, lack prenatal care, have been exposed prenatally to drugs or alcohol, and have experienced trauma and neglect. All of these factors put children in foster care at high risk for significant developmental delays, educational problems, and mental health disorders. Comprehensive screenings for these conditions, performed by clinicians who can interpret findings in the context of early childhood trauma, are imperative for children in foster care and must occur soon after children enter foster care.

Table 11–1. Recommended Laboratory Screenings for Children in Foster Care[2]

Laboratory Screening	Method of Testing	Frequency
	Noninfectious Diseases	
Anemia	Point-of-care testing or venous sampling for CBC or hemoglobin/hematocrit	Initially,[a] then yearly up to age 6 years and for postmenarchal females
Lead poisoning	Venous sampling or point-of-care	Initially[a] for age 6 months to 6 years and for any child with risk
Chronic kidney disease	Dipstick or formal urinalysis	Initially[a]
Pregnancy	Point-of-care testing	Initially[a] for sexually active postmenarchal adolescents who could be pregnant, then as needed
	Infectious Diseases	
Hepatitis C[3]	Hepatitis C antibody test or NAT for HCV RNA	Initially[a] if at risk, including perinatally exposed infants (NAT for detection of HCV RNA at age 2 to 6 months and HCV antibody for age 18 months or older)
Hepatitis B	Hepatitis B surface antibody test	Initially[a] for all ages
HIV	Fourth-generation HIV antigen test and/or antibody screen	Initially[a] if at risk, at least once from age 13 to 17 years, and then annually for sexually active adolescents; may rescreen every 3 to 6 months for high-risk sexually active adolescents
Syphilis	Rapid plasma regain test	Initially[a] for all ages, then annually for sexually active adolescents; may rescreen every 3 to 6 months for high-risk sexually active adolescents
Gonorrhea and chlamydia	Urine DNA test	Initially[a] for sexually active adolescents, then yearly; also recommended routinely at least once starting at age 15 years; may rescreen every 3 to 6 months for high-risk sexually active adolescents
Trichomoniasis	RNA test	Initially[a] for sexually active adolescents, then assess local population prevalence and individual patient risk to determine need for yearly screening
Tuberculosis	IGRA preferred, may also use TST	Initially[a] and yearly if in congregate care

Abbreviations: CBC, complete blood cell count; HCV, hepatitis C virus; IGRA, interferon-gamma release assay; NAT, nucleic acid test; TST, tuberculin skin test.

[a] Initially upon entering foster care.

Developmental Screening

Screening for developmental delays should include a thorough evaluation of gross motor skills, fine motor skills, receptive and expressive language, social-emotional skills, cognitive development, and activities of daily living for children younger than 6 years.[8] Screening results should be discussed with the child's caregiver. The clinician can assess caregiver understanding of the child's developmental needs and offer developmentally appropriate guidance to help meet those needs. While there is no developmental screening tool specific to children in foster care, it is important that a standardized, validated tool be used and be administered by a clinician with experience in trauma and its sequelae in children.[8] **Table 11–2** outlines the timeline for developmental screenings as it correlates with periodic health supervision visits.[9]

Developmental screening is ideally accomplished within 30 days of entry into foster care; children with developmental delays should be referred for evaluation (see Chapter 13, Developmental and Educational Issues). For children younger than 36 months, Early Intervention services can conduct a full evaluation with consent of the child's legal guardian or educational surrogate. For children 36 months and older, full evaluation is done by the school district special education services. A child whose evaluation indicates need for services should receive an individualized treatment plan and initiation of appropriate Early Intervention services (<36 months of age) or special education services through the school district (>36 months of age). Periodic reviews should be completed to ensure progress is being made and that the child continues to receive the most appropriate services that meet their needs. As a child approaches school age, it is important that needs and services be reevaluated and transitioned into appropriate educational supports.

Screening for autism spectrum disorder (ASD) is a separate and very important part of a developmental evaluation. The diagnosis of ASD is often substantially delayed in children generally. Furthermore, the similarities in presentation that can exist between young children with an ASD and young children with a history of trauma and abuse or neglect are crucial to understand. At a minimum, ASD screening should occur at the 9-month, 18-month, and either 24- or 30-month health supervision visit and whenever there is a concern identified by the caregiver or clinician. Validated ASD screening tools should be employed; a variety of tools exist that are brief and relatively sensitive and specific. Some of the available screening tools are listed in **Table 11–2**.[10]

Table 11–2. Examples of Developmental Screening Tools for Youth in Foster Care

Developmental Screening	Screening for Autism Spectrum Disorder
Developmental Screening Tools • Survey of Well-Being of Young Children (SWYC) • Ages and Stages Questionnaire II (ASQ) • Bayley Scales of Infant Development (BSID, first, second, third editions) • Denver Developmental Screening Test (DDST) • Vineland Adaptive Behavior Scales II (VABS-II)	Autism Screening Tools • Modified Checklist for Autism in Toddlers (M-CHAT) • Developmental Behaviour Checklist-Early Screen (DBC-ES) (for children with developmental delays) • Screening Tool for Autism in Toddlers and Young Children (STAT) (not a first-tier screen)
Timing for Developmental Screening • Anytime clinician or caregiver has concern • Within 30 days of entry to foster care • At every health supervision visit, ideally 9-month, 18-month, and 24- or 30-month health supervision visits	Timing for Autism Screening • Anytime clinician or caregiver has concern • When a child enters foster care • 18- and 30-month health supervision visits

Educational Screening

Children in foster care have higher rates of virtually all educational problems compared with their peers not in foster care. About 45% of children in foster care qualify for special education services because of learning or behavioral challenges. More specifically, they have higher rates of special education placement, learning disabilities, intellectual disability, general achievement problems, and grade retention. It is also common to see significant discrepancies between IQ and achievement, resulting from academic deficits.

Pediatricians can ask about school placement, educational strengths and challenges, and whether a child has an individualized education program or 504 plan (see Chapter 13, Developmental and Educational Issues) and consider requesting an educational assessment to ensure they are placed in the appropriate educational setting and receiving the type and intensity of academic support needed. It is also important to keep in mind that the disruption of entering foster care, as well as any placement changes, may exacerbate educational deficits and necessitate additional screening and repeat evaluation, especially if there has also been a change in school. Best practice is to ask about educational concerns at the first encounter and monitor closely over the first several months in care so a timely referral for educational assessment can be made when indicated.

Mental Health Screening

The importance of mental health screening and ongoing reassessment cannot be overstated, as the prevalence of mental health disorders in children in foster care is high, and accessible treatments are often inadequate, disjointed, and not consistent with the evidence base.[11] (See Chapter 12, Mental Health.) Mental health screening for acute issues such as suicidality should occur at entry into foster care; a fuller mental health screening ideally occurs within 30 days. That said, it is important to remember that removal and entering care are themselves often traumatic and can affect a child's mental health, just as the time spent in foster care can change a child's mood and symptom presentation. These factors should be taken into account when considering mental health screening and subsequent evaluation.

First, a broad assessment of mental health symptoms and regulation of affect appropriate to a child's age and developmental stage should be completed. This includes screening for behaviors in different settings, gaining an understanding of a child's relationship to family members and caregivers, and inquiring about a child's interests, coping abilities, and areas of impairment. Screening for traumatic stress symptoms that may mimic mental health conditions is important, along with screening for specific mental health conditions including depression, anxiety, and attention-deficit/hyperactivity disorder. When concerns arise, screen for eating disorders and substance use disorders. Youth should be asked about symptoms of aggression, suicidality, impulsivity, self-injurious behaviors, and homicidal ideation. Recognizing the depth and overlap of traumatic stress symptoms and mental health disorders in children in foster care, screening for most urgent symptoms and ongoing reassessment of other symptoms is appropriate. Validated screening tools for individual mental health conditions should be used to further evaluate areas of concern that are identified. In particular, clinicians should have a very low threshold for the use of validated trauma symptom screening tools.

Using trauma-informed care skills, the pediatrician can frame asking questions about mental health as being important given what has happened to the child. Assessing traumatic stress symptoms is more important than direct inquiry about details of the child's trauma history, which can likely be obtained from child welfare. Understanding the reason for placement is important; this information can also be obtained from child welfare or the caregiver. While children will vary widely in how comfortable they are discussing their removal and placement, almost all children will respond to a focus on their strengths. The clinician can say that it is normal to feel angry, sad, confused, or even guilty and follow the child's cues (body language, facial affect, and words) about what they are comfortable discussing. An evaluation of a caregiver's understanding of the effects of trauma and loss and a child's symptoms can help them respond in a trauma-informed way to the child's behaviors and emotions. While the caregiver's ability to reassure the child they are safe and help the child regulate is key, their willingness to prioritize mental health care is also critically important. Mental health screening will likely occur at multiple points and not just when a child enters care. Many foster care medical homes screen at all health supervision visits unless the child is well established in treatment. Symptoms are likely to change, extinguish, amplify, or overlap, and a child's needs may also change. (See Chapter 17, Childhood Trauma and Resilience, for an in-depth discussion.)

Lastly, clinicians can collaborate with child welfare to develop a network of trauma-informed mental health services, including those that provide evidence-based treatment services, to meet children's needs.

Social Drivers of Health

Healthy People 2030 defines *social drivers of health* (SDOH) as the conditions in the environment in which a person is born, lives, works, learns, plays, worships, and ages that may affect a person's health, functioning, and quality of life.[12] The 5 broad domains of social drivers of health are (1) economic stability, (2) education access and quality, (3) health care access and quality, (4) neighborhood and built environment, and (5) community and social context.[12] SDOH are interconnected in many aspects of a person's life and contribute to inequity and health disparities. In screening, it is important to think about SDOH as they relate to a child's current environment as well as the environment surrounding their family of origin. These factors may change over time and should be regularly revisited. Even if a child is removed from their environment and placed in foster care, many of these SDOH continue to impact the child and their overall well-being.

Adverse childhood experience (ACE) screens are population survey tools designed to assess risk for poor outcomes in a population. Children in foster care are known to have, on average, higher ACE scores than other populations of children. Currently, the AAP does not recommend screening children in foster care for ACEs because these screens do not identify a specific, potentially treatable condition and are not predictive of outcomes at the individual level. Instead, the AAP recommends screening for traumatic stress symptoms and mental health, behavioral, and developmental problems that do have specific treatment. Identifying traumatic stress and mental health symptoms and disorders allows pediatricians to connect youth in foster care with evidence-based treatments.

Key Takeaways

- » Due to the increased risk of physical health problems in children in foster care, laboratory screening is recommended at the initial health screen.
- » Initial laboratory screening may include tests for hemoglobin, lead, tuberculosis, CKD, and bloodborne infections and STIs (HIV, syphilis, hepatitis B, hepatitis C, gonorrhea, chlamydia, and trichomoniasis).
- » Children in foster care should be screened for developmental delays and ASDs within 30 days of entering care, as well as with the same periodicity as children not in foster care.
- » Children in foster care have very high rates of mental health disorders and should have early screening as well as ongoing reassessment of symptoms.

CHAPTER 12

Mental Health

Brooks Keeshin, MD, FAAP

Mental health concerns are quite common among youth in foster care.[1] States either require or offer mental health assessments to ensure early identification of mental health concerns in this population, and although the systems and types of services vary,[2] there is an important opportunity for primary care to play an important role in the diagnosis and treatment of mental health issues among youth in foster care.[3] However, there are several things to consider that will require modifications or adaptations of the typical approach to the general pediatric population when responding to mental health needs among youth in foster care. This chapter will discuss what it means to take a trauma-informed approach to mental health care, screening, and diagnostic considerations, as well as mental health assessment and treatment options most commonly indicated among youth in foster care.

Trauma-Informed Care for Pediatric Mental Health

Trauma-informed care begins by recognizing and responding to the potentially traumatic experiences associated with foster care placement and realizing that those experiences likely exacerbate any observed mental health challenges identified by the youth, family, or system[4,5] (see Chapter 17, Childhood Trauma and Resilience, for more detailed information). Trauma and resultant traumatic stress mimic commonly observed mental health conditions that pediatricians routinely diagnose and treat. Youth may have symptoms indicative of depression, anxiety, and attention-deficit/hyperactivity disorder (ADHD), but those symptoms might be better explained by an underlying traumatic stress diagnosis where the symptoms of traumatic stress overlap with these common pediatric mental health conditions.[6]

Furthermore, secondary adversities that occur because of traumatic experiences can affect mood and behavior. Diagnosing any disorder is challenging in the context of a youth having been removed from their familiar environment and family supports, having to change schools or manage school disruptions, or experiencing changes in their social network. These adversities can understandably result in the development or exacerbation of symptoms that can be confused with disorders such as depression, anxiety, or ADHD. When the adverse situation is driving the symptoms, it is better to initially support the youth through the experience and their understandable responses rather than ascribing a particular nontrauma/nonadjustment diagnosis.

Of course, some youth in foster care have common mental health conditions that benefit from evidence-based approaches.[7] A trauma-informed approach appropriately acknowledges the great and varied impact that trauma and adversity can have on the development and persistence of symptoms and functional impairment, while not ignoring the potential that within the context of trauma and adversity reactions, common mental health conditions can exist.

Trauma-informed care must start well before the patient enters the door, with the clinician being thoughtful about which specific mental health screens to use and how those tools are interpreted. Furthermore, providers must feel comfortable engaging in the first steps of trauma-informed mental health care and be able to connect youth with specific evidence-based mental health treatments designed to address the trauma and nontrauma conditions found among youth in foster care.

A Trauma-Informed Mental Health Screening Approach for Youth in Foster Care

When entering foster care, mental health screening can highlight and prioritize mental health concerns in the context of other medical priorities. Furthermore, a combination of screens can specify the types of mental health challenges, essential for providing the youth, foster parents, and other professionals with the information necessary to care for the youth. Obtaining records or collaborating with prior and current mental health clinicians, as well as repeat screening over time, provides added information on an individual's response to treatment, which can inform treatment plan revisions.

This section outlines a trauma-informed mental health screening approach using self-report measures tailored to meet common concerns seen in older children and adolescents in foster care. In primary/outpatient pediatric care, the use of screens can decrease system and provider bias when evaluating mental health symptoms and provide an opportunity to begin a discussion that identifies the unique experiences of the patient. For younger children, caregiver report measures will need to be used; however, the younger the child and the less of a relationship that the respondent has with the child, the lower the reliability of mental health screening for these children. General mental health screens (such as the Strengths and Difficulties Questionnaire, commonly known as the SDQ[8]) may yield information to determine the appropriate next step in a younger child absent trauma-specific screens. With increasing age and increasing capacity to self-report, there is tremendous value in using screens with greater specificity for trauma and traumatic stress in older children and adolescents in foster care.

A critical component of addressing mental health in foster care is the use of a trauma screen.[9] It is important to note that trauma screens are different from adverse childhood experience screens that provide a score based on different types of adversity experienced in childhood. In contrast, an appropriate trauma screening tool will screen for both trauma exposures and trauma symptoms, which can assess for ongoing impact and guide treatment response. One example of such a tool is the Pediatric Traumatic Stress Screening Tool (PTSST), which is freely available through UtahPIPS.org/cpm.[10] This tool, adapted from the Brief University of California, Los Angeles (UCLA) posttraumatic stress disorder (PTSD) Reaction Index[11] and accompanying decision support, has open-ended trauma exposure questions that capture recent and remote experiences, as well as 12 symptom questions that stratify level of traumatic stress severity and guide the clinical team to a targeted clinical response, either as a stand-alone tool or integrated with information obtained from other mental health screens. Another trauma screen that briefly assesses for traumas and traumatic stress symptoms is the Child Trauma Screen (CTS).[12] The CTS asks 4 separate trauma-exposure questions (yes/no) and then asks 6 trauma-symptom questions using a 4-point Likert scale. Both the PTSST and the CTS have self- and caregiver-report options, are available in multiple languages, and use validated symptom-level cutoff scores that indicate a high risk of PTSD. The PTSST also offers a moderate risk category; 3 traumatic stress subscales around 1) sleep difficulties, 2) intrusion and hyperarousal, and 3) avoidance and negative mood; as well as clinical decision support to guide a trauma-informed response.

The value of understanding the presence or absence of trauma and traumatic stress when assessing other mental health concerns is twofold. First, in youth for whom there are concerns for other common conditions, the presence or absence of trauma and/or traumatic stress provides a context for the reported symptoms, informs differential diagnoses, and likely leads to a more evidence-based treatment plan for both traumatic stress–positive and traumatic stress–

negative conditions. Second, children and adolescents who experience trauma can have significant symptoms of traumatic stress without symptoms that are associated with other disorders, demonstrating that trauma screening cannot be limited to those who screen positive for mental health concerns.

For youth in foster care with depressive symptoms, the Patient Health Questionnaire A (PHQ-A), the most widely available depression-specific tool, is an appropriate screen. The American Academy of Pediatrics (AAP)-endorsed guidelines highlight how to stratify treatment based on self-report responses,[13] and the Guidelines for Adolescent Depression in Primary Care (commonly known as GLAD-PC) should be followed when no significant trauma symptoms are present. When trauma symptoms are present, consider an adaptation of the AAP depression guidance that leans toward addressing traumatic stress first, recognizing the significant syndromic overlap between depression and traumatic stress as well as the fact that trauma-focused psychosocial interventions provide significant relief to symptoms of depression when delivered to someone with traumatic stress.[6]

Instruments used to screen for anxiety in primary care include the Generalized Anxiety Disorder 7-item scale (GAD-7) and the 5-item Screen for Child Anxiety Related Emotional Disorders (SCARED).[14,15] A measure that focuses on generalized anxiety, such as the GAD-7, is a reasonable approach for older children and teens, in whom generalized anxiety disorder is common. However, the GAD-7 does not identify separation anxiety or social anxiety absent generalized anxiety symptoms, which tend to have an earlier age of onset, so when screening younger populations, the SCARED screen may be a better choice. In either case, anxiety disorder comorbidity is common, and having comfort using the full SCARED screen, with 41 items and pediatric anxiety subscales, is helpful for clarifying a diagnosis and treatment planning.

Suicidality should be routinely assessed in children and universally assessed among all children 12 years or older in foster care using approaches that have been validated and found to be safe for at-risk youth.[6,16,17] Several options commonly used in primary care include the Ask Suicide-Screening Questions (commonly known as the ASQ) and a stepped model that uses question 9 from the PHQ-A as the first screen, with a follow-up among positive screens using the short version of the Columbia-Suicide Severity Rating Scale (C-SSRS). The C-SSRS helps guide the appropriate level of suicide-prevention efforts by providing an initial stratification of low, moderate, or high-risk suicidality, focusing on the presence or absence of suicidal thinking and behaviors. Just like with any concern for suicide in children and adolescents, collateral information is critical to complement the direct assessment of the youth, and the adult caregivers in the child's life will be primarily responsible for any safety plan, including restricting access to lethal means, increasing access to urgent and crisis services, and appropriate follow-up with mental health clinicians. Therefore, within the limits of confidentiality, effective communication with the child welfare worker, the foster family, and ongoing mental health treatment providers will be critical during and after the assessment. Furthermore, among youth with a history of trauma, traumatic stress is highly associated with suicidal ideation,[18] reinforcing the need for effective trauma screening and responses when determining the most appropriate long-term care for youth who struggle with suicidal thoughts and behaviors.

Evidence-Based Assessment and Treatment for Youth in Foster Care

Assessments

A comprehensive mental health assessment for youth in foster care includes a combination of clinical interview, collateral information, and standardized measures to provide a complete picture of the youth's mental health strengths and challenges. Assessment by a mental health provider should include mental health symptoms, age of onset, exacerbating and ameliorating factors, and cognitive and developmental considerations, as well as relational and social capabilities. Standardized measures, including evidence-based trauma assessments, aid in the diagnostic process. A comprehensive trauma assessment should identify a wide array of trauma exposures and elicit a comprehensive understanding of trauma symptoms to help rule in or rule out conditions such as PTSD. One such example of a well-validated and widely available measure is the UCLA PTSD Reaction Index, which includes a comprehensive trauma history questionnaire, a timeline to document age of trauma exposures, and a validated 31-item trauma symptom measure that includes symptoms from all PTSD criteria as well as questions to identify the dissociative subtype of PTSD.[19]

Mental Health Treatment

Evidence-based interventions should be the first step in mental health treatment for several compelling reasons.[6] Youth are more likely to improve in a timely manner using a scientifically proven treatment, effectively addressing one of numerous challenges faced by youth in foster care. The risk of false attribution of challenges to a non-trauma-related childhood mental illness is high. Much of the complex treatment that youth receive in foster care does not start as complex but becomes complex over time due to a lack of initial treatment response to non-trauma-related diagnoses using treatments without a strong evidence base. Evidence-based treatments are not always successful; however, if a treatment fails, it is helpful to know that the treatment was appropriate and that the diagnosis and overall assessment may be worth revisiting rather than just recategorizing the disorder as treatment resistant. Notably, some families may not choose an evidence-based approach for various reasons, including personal beliefs, prior experience, or other preferences. For youth in foster care, when the county or state is the custodian and making decisions in the youth's best interest, evidence should be a strong factor in treatment planning. Furthermore, given the likelihood that youth may leave foster care over the course of treatment, when possible, it is best to involve the youth's family of origin in the assessment and treatment decision process, providing another opportunity to educate the family of origin on the importance of evidence-based care.

Trauma-Focused and Trauma-Informed Approaches

Widely available and evidence-based therapies for youth in foster care can be divided into trauma-focused and trauma-informed treatments. Trauma-focused treatments are designed to treat traumatic stress and co-occurring conditions. A highly evidence-based example of such a treatment is trauma-focused cognitive behavioral therapy (TF-CBT),[20,21] a manualized, modular approach for children and adolescents with traumatic stress and associated conditions. The first components of TF-CBT focus on improving the youth's capacity to understand trauma and begin to control symptoms through coping skills, enhanced symptom communication, and the introduction of the cognitive triangle (**Figure 12–1**) to connect thoughts, feelings, and behaviors. The second components of TF-CBT use a trauma narrative to facilitate gradual exposure and cognitive processing, decreasing the intensity and frequency of traumatic stress. The final components involve safety planning and child–caregiver relationship strengthening. It is important to note that although the caregiver's role is especially pivotal to this last component of the therapy, caregivers should be involved throughout TF-CBT. The caregiver in foster care does not have to be a member of the family of origin but rather can be any supportive, consistent adult in the youth's life whom the youth feels comfortable including in therapy.

TF-CBT is weekly, outpatient psychotherapy. Duration of treatment is generally 16 to 24 sessions, with longer durations for those with complex trauma. All youth in foster care are at increased risk for traumatic stress due to their history; therefore, it is reasonable for pediatricians and other clinicians to maintain a high index of suspicion for PTSD and other associated conditions for which TF-CBT might be the treatment of choice (such as traumatic stress with depression, anxiety, or behavioral challenges). However, it is incorrect to assume that simply because a child has entered the foster care system they would benefit from TF-CBT. TF-CBT is best used among youth who have one or more discrete traumatic experiences that are remembered and continue to affect the youth as measured by the presence of traumatic stress. However, outpatient TF-CBT is ideally suited for those youth who are attending school, maintaining placement in a home (foster or otherwise) setting, and stable enough for weekly psychotherapy.

When children lack clear evidence that their past experiences are directly leading to their symptoms or when dysfunction or severe emotional behavioral outbursts cannot be adequately managed by weekly outpatient therapy, a trauma-informed approach rather than a trauma-focused approach may be most helpful. For example, young children with significant externalizing behaviors will often benefit from trauma-informed behavioral management therapies such as parent–child interaction therapy (PCIT).[22] PCIT requires the child to have a certain level of consistency and connection with their caregiver. For teens who struggle with severe emotional and behavioral dysregulation, including self-harm and suicidality, dialectical behavioral therapy (DBT) is a good option to consider.[23] However, similarly to PCIT, DBT works best when there is a consistent and supportive caregiver who can participate in group sessions that include both caregivers and the adolescents. The youth's particular situation, including type of foster care placement, permanency, and existing supports, must be considered when determining the best treatment approach.

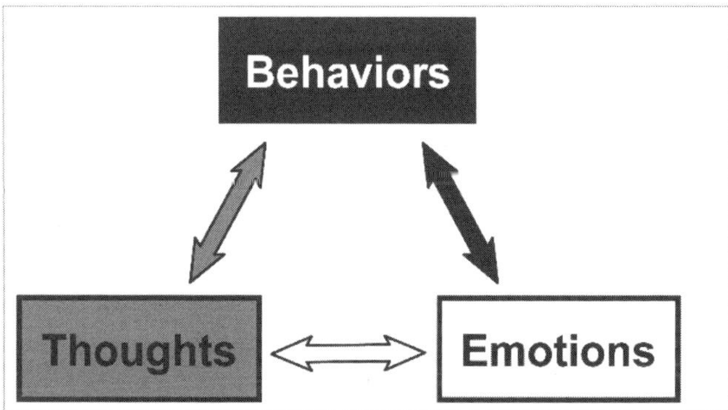

Figure 12–1. The cognitive triangle.

In-Office Interventions and Medication Management

Primary care pediatricians can introduce and reinforce many of the skills taught by therapists in trauma-focused therapy. Coping skills such as deep breathing, guided imagery, and progressive muscle relaxation, as well as approaches to mindfulness, can be quickly taught during clinical encounters. However, it is helpful to make concrete connections between the skill and the specific symptoms the skill addresses. This educates the patient and sets a reasonable expectation when the skill is used.[10]

A trauma-informed medication approach for youth in foster care is conservative and evidence based and addresses diagnoses that consolidate various symptoms, when possible, rather than favoring comorbidity.[6] Furthermore, a stepped-care approach, treating one potential pharmacological target to remission before reevaluating and addressing other targets, is preferred to avoid overly complex treatment regimens.

Sleep is a common challenge among youth in foster care and often dysfunctional in youth with traumatic stress, with or without co-occurring conditions, making it an appropriate initial consideration for intervention absent acute safety concerns.[6] Trauma-informed psychosocial strategies and basic sleep hygiene should be used first, such as implementing consistent bedtime routines, fostering connection between the caregivers at home and the youth, and encouraging calming evening activities before bed. It is also important to review and, when possible, reduce or eliminate any medications that may exacerbate sleep challenges. However, when traumatic stress challenges continue to affect sleep, short-term treatment with melatonin or prazosin can be considered.[6,24] It is important to follow up and ensure effective and sustained responses resulting in consistent sleep before reevaluating and considering other possible pharmacological interventions.

In addition to concerns about depression, anxiety, and ADHD, severe behavioral and emotional dysregulation is another common reason that youth in foster care receive psychotropic medication. All of these mental health concerns are more difficult to diagnose among youth in foster care who have a history of trauma and current evidence of traumatic stress, which could mimic common childhood mental health conditions. In general, trauma-informed interventions and addressing dysregulated sleep should be the first steps to address traumatic stress, followed by reassessment and then evidence-based treatment of remaining co-occurring conditions when indicated.[6] However, some youth in foster care may need a higher level of care, such as day treatment or in-home/wraparound supports for significant levels of dysfunction. When the severity of the mental health concerns or ongoing safety are the major considerations, consider psychiatric referral or consultation, possibly with a state-appointed oversight agency for youth in foster care if available (see Chapter 38, Psychotropic Medication Oversight).

Key Takeaways

- A trauma-informed approach to mental health balances the recognition of traumatic stress in all its varied forms with the understanding that youth in foster care can also experience non-trauma-related mental health conditions.
- Due to the risk of false attribution, it is critical that trauma be standardly assessed in pediatric and mental health settings and, when present, incorporated into the overall diagnosis and treatment planning, favoring a holistic understanding of the patient.
- Evidence-based measures and treatment modalities are preferred for youth in foster care with mental health challenges.

CHAPTER 13

Developmental and Educational Issues

A. Bird H. Gilmartin, MD, FAAP
Kristen Slaymaker, DO, FAAP

Background

Childhood and adolescence are foundational periods for healthy development, and loving relationships with responsive and nurturing adults are the cornerstone of healthy physical, mental, and social health outcomes. The first 5 years after birth encompass the most rapid period of brain development, but the brain continues to evolve in response to the environment throughout childhood and adolescence, fully maturing in the mid-twenties.[1–3]

Children in out-of home placement have a high likelihood of disruption in their developmental trajectories and educational performance because of ruptures in attachment relationships and the accumulation of adverse experiences and traumatic stress. Trauma that disrupts foundational brain structures is amplified as children mature, due to interference with the development of foundational circuits and structures, the consequences of which can resonate across the entire lifespan, from infancy through adulthood. Thus, the American Academy of Pediatrics (AAP) designates children and youth in out-of-home placement as children with special health care needs.

Nationally, children from birth to age 5 years comprise the largest portion (49%) of children entering out-of-home care, highlighting how critical the quality and stability of the foster care experience is during this crucial period. Attachment theory and resilience science both emphasize that healthy development depends on the continuous availability of safe, stable, nurturing caregiving and exposure to typical experiences and exposures.[4] (See Chapter 17, Childhood Trauma and Resilience.) Development, educational achievement, and mental and behavioral health trajectories are all at risk for children in out-of-home placement. Developmental delays (DDs) can be 3 to 4 times higher for children in foster care than for peers who have not experienced child welfare involvement.[5]

Effects on educational achievement are striking. Young adults in foster care are 3 to 4 times more likely to have been expelled from school and have lower high school graduation rates. Only a third of children in foster care meet state standards for reading attainment, a rate 2 to 3 times lower than the general population.[1,2,6–9]

Research suggests that children and youth in foster care use outpatient and inpatient mental health (MH) services at a rate 20 times higher than that of other children in poverty. MH and substance use disorders (SUD) are more common among youth in foster care (49.4% MH disorder; 3.3% SUD) than among those not in foster care (10.9% MH disorder, 0.6% SUD) across all ages.[10] In one study, they were almost 4 times more likely to have considered suicide and attempted suicide than peers never in foster care.[11]

Placement changes disrupt attachment relationships and are associated with compromised developmental trajectories, educational disruption, decreased academic performance (about 4 months loss with each change), and poor adult outcomes.[12–15]

Research shows that negative experiences, such as child abuse and neglect, exposure to violence, chaotic parenting, separation from parents, bullying, racism and felt discrimination, and environmental insults can also cause maladaptive structural changes in the developing brain. Positive experiences, such as responsive caregiving, stimulation and enrichment, opportunities for early education, and positive social interactions, promote healthy brain growth, learning, and healing after trauma has occurred.[1,2,5,6,16]

Children and youth in foster care often have a high trauma burden. Identifying this as a critical underlying factor for developmental and behavioral concerns helps pediatricians understand children in the context of what has happened to them, avoid misdiagnosis (eg, attention-deficit/hyperactivity disorder, oppositional defiant disorder, depression, anxiety), consider the presence of comorbid conditions, and initiate appropriate trauma-specific responses and therapies.[17] Moreover, positive developmental and educational experiences can mitigate the effects of abuse, neglect, family separation, and other challenges these youth may experience.[18]

The Intersection of Trauma, Culture, and Development

How an individual experiences a traumatic event is informed by their genetics, their prior experiences, their family's culture, and available supports, especially caregiving. There are complex historical and contemporary circumstances that contribute to the mental and behavioral health of children and youth in foster care, including interpersonal, historical, intergenerational, and cultural complex traumas.[19,20] Research shows that individual experiences with lifelong chronic marginalization and discrimination create a complicated interplay among genetic inheritance and gene expression and the responses of immunological, endocrinological, and neurological systems to trauma (see Chapter 17, Childhood Trauma and Resilience).[20–22]

Evidence shows that some children in foster care have parents who were also in foster care or suffer from their own trauma histories and resulting physical, mental, and behavioral health conditions. Trauma can be an intergenerational phenomenon and must be addressed at a family level, because children can only heal and recover in the context of safe, stable, nurturing caregiving.[23]

The Effects of Trauma on Development

Development is a dynamic and continuous process of adaptation to the environment. Children who grow up with significant adversity and inadequate buffering relationships adapt to that environment.[24,25] Trauma's developmental effects often present as delays in communication, cognition, social-emotional development, executive function, and self-regulation skills (often presenting as heightened sensitivity and reactivity to stress or perceived danger). Symptoms (see **Box 13–1**) can present as early as infancy and cascade forward across the age span unless identified and treated. Thus, it is essential that all professionals have a working knowledge of child development, the effects of trauma, and the biological necessity of providing safe, stable, nurturing caregiving and other positive childhood experiences.[26–28]

Caregiver's Role in Development and Education

Caregiving approaches that promote healthy development and resilience are crucial in caring for children who have experienced trauma, separation, and losses. Professionals involved with children in out-of-home placement can stress the importance of "time in," reassuring the child they are safe, predictable routines, and building self-regulation skills. Helpful family facing resources can be found at https://www.aap.org/en/patient-care/national-center-for-relational-health-and-trauma-informed-care/resources-for-families. They can stress early assessment and longitudinal monitoring of development and educational achievement by pediatricians who can connect caregivers to developmental and educational resources. Pediatricians can promote caregiver understanding of how prenatal exposures and postnatal trauma affect child

Box 13–1

Developmental Symptoms of Trauma by Age

Infancy/Early Childhood

- Developmental delays (most notably in communication, problem-solving and social-emotional skills)
- Difficulty regulating behavior and emotions (tantrums)
- Clinginess or fear of new situations
- Inconsolability, excessive crying

Preschool

- Loss of previously acquired developmental skills (loss of language, regression in toileting)
- Sleep difficulties (nightmares, night terrors, or fear of going to sleep)
- Separation anxiety
- Indiscriminate sociability (goes to anyone)
- Overreaction to minor events with tantrums, aggression
- Reenactment of trauma in play

School Age

- Concern over their own safety and the safety of others
- Retelling or playing out of the traumatic event
- Sleep disturbances
- Difficulty with attention, learning, memory
- Somatic symptoms (headache, stomach pain)
- Overreaction to minor events, withdrawal
- Challenges with peer relationships

Adolescence

- Shame or guilt; poor sense of self; hopelessness or helplessness
- Feelings of fear or vulnerability
- Difficulty identifying, expressing, and managing feelings; may be highly reactive or avoidant
- More frequent suspensions, expulsions, and time out of class
- Increased risk-taking/self-treatment behaviors (eg, self-injury, substance use, sexual activity)

development and behavior. Trauma-related behaviors and developmental issues can be challenging, and caregivers can benefit from appropriate guidance and support from pediatric and licensed mental health clinicians experienced and knowledgeable about the unique behavioral and emotional needs of traumatized children.

Children and families can benefit from referral to community-based home health services, Early Intervention (children under 3 years), and mental and behavioral health resources with expertise in evidence-based trauma-specific therapies (see Chapter 12, Mental Health). Pediatricians can refer preschool-age children (ages 3–4 years) to Child Find and help caregivers advocate with the public school special education team for an evaluation if there are learning, educational, or academic concerns to determine whether a child qualifies for special education services or Section 504 accommodations.[29] Pediatricians can encourage strength-based approaches and exposure to positive childhood experiences that promote healthy development even after trauma has occurred.

Child welfare staff are often involved in "dual planning" as they balance reunification goals and alternate timely permanency options. Allowing ample opportunities for families of origin to sustain their relationship with their child and achieve reunification is the best predictor of reunification. Families of origin need support and assistance in connecting to trauma-informed psychotherapy and substance use and mental health treatment for themselves. All families may need help with resources such as child care, respite, care coordination, peer support, employment, health care, transportation, stable housing, and food, as well as education about effective parenting strategies to help them develop the skills they need to provide a safe, nurturing environment for their child.

Pediatrician's Role in Child Development and Behavior: Surveillance and Screening

When evaluating children and adolescents in foster care for developmental, educational, and behavioral concerns, it is important to consider potential risk factors including historical and cultural trauma, genetic loading, prenatal exposures, and postnatal adversity and trauma. Every effort should be made to obtain as complete a record of the child's medical, mental, and behavioral health and social, developmental, and educational histories as possible. These histories can provide important information about prenatal substance exposure; neglect, abuse, and exposure to interpersonal violence; educational histories; mental and behavioral health histories; and functional impairments.[30] This essential information can assist in determining what assessments and care a child needs to achieve their optimal long-term developmental trajectory. This section focuses on the scope of issues children may present with and surveillance and screening considerations. Chapter 30, Neurodevelopmental Disorders: Identification and Intervention, details how to elicit a comprehensive medical history to assess prenatal, perinatal, and postnatal factors that can affect development.

Neglect, Abuse, and Exposure to Interpersonal Violence

Approximately 1 in 4 children experience some form of abuse or neglect.[31,32] Neglect is the most common reason for placement in foster care and often co-occurs with parental substance use disorder. It is important to remember that poverty can be conflated with neglect, especially when the investigator and family are from different cultural, racial, or ethnic backgrounds.[33] Neglect or living in dire poverty can lead to a paucity of typical childhood exposures, poor relational engagement, or inadequate schooling, housing, food, or health care. The overlap of intimate partner violence and child physical abuse (45%–70%) is significant.[34] Infants and children exposed to maltreatment and violence demonstrate significantly more internalizing behaviors (ie, anxiety, depression, withdrawal, and somatic complaints), externalizing behaviors (ie, attention problems, tantrums, aggression), poor academic performance, developmental delay, and an increased risk of chronic health problems.

Educational Histories

There is a high degree of educational neglect, school mobility, and inadequate follow-through with recommended educational accommodations (ie, individualized education program, Section 504) that can add to significant educational concerns for youth involved with child welfare.[35] Pediatricians should document the child's current school placement (school name, school district, current grade, history of grade retention) and services received in and outside of school.

Mental and Behavioral Health Histories

Historical information about mental and behavioral health conditions is often missing for this population. Children may have had poor access to needed services prior to care. Ideally, this history includes family medical and psychiatric histories, prenatal history and exposures, and postnatal traumas, including abuse and neglect. Obtaining a complete history of diagnoses, medications, levels of care, safety concerns (including self-harm and suicide), and interventions can clarify a child's mental and behavioral health needs.

Functional Impairments

Additional information regarding the child's functioning is helpful. Components to consider include regression or growth in development skills, nutrition and eating habits, toileting practices, sleep disturbances, attachment behaviors, externalizing and internalizing behaviors, and somatic complaints. Impairments may negatively affect engagement across different environments (ie, educational and therapeutic settings, child care, home, visitation, normalizing activities).

Developmental and Behavioral Screening

Developmental and behavioral screening can augment history, optimize risk detection, and provide opportunities to connect a child to helpful interventions. Screens should be corrected for gestational age up to age 2 years.[30] The high prevalence of development concerns, high-risk social factors, and ongoing stressors and uncertainties in this population led the AAP to recommend using a validated screening tool[36] and an enhanced screening schedule. The AAP recommends universal developmental and behavioral screening at the time of placement (to identify urgent issues), within 60 days after placement, and at all preventive health visits for children in out-of-home placements from birth to 66 months (see Chapter 11, Screenings). Any child with concerns should be referred to Early Intervention (<36 months) or the school district special education program (≥36 months). Any child with learning or behavior issues or a history of multiple school disruptions should be referred to special education. Increased screening frequency can identify children who are progressing, not progressing, or falling further behind over time.[10]

A table of acceptable measures can be found in the AAP clinical report "Promoting Optimal Development: Identifying Infants and Young Children with Developmental Disorders Through Developmental Surveillance and Screening."[37] Details on screening for mental health and traumatic stress symptoms can be found in Chapter 12, Mental Health.

Maintaining a Broad Differential Diagnosis

Pediatricians will ideally consider a broad differential for developmental, learning, emotional, and behavioral concerns since all are potential symptoms of cumulative childhood trauma, including abuse or neglect, prenatal substance exposures, fetal alcohol spectrum disorder (FASD), traumatic brain injury, autism spectrum disorder (ASD), and violence exposure. Genetic predisposition is another consideration. Maintaining a broad differential can reduce misdiagnosis, increase accuracy of treatment, and help pediatricians better educate caregivers.

Overview of IDEA, Educational Supports, and School Services for Children in the United States

Connection to early development and education supports makes a lasting positive impact in the general population.[38] Short-term benefits are seen in cognitive, language, social-emotional, adaptive, and motor skills development. Long-term outcomes include higher academic achievement and income and professional success.[39,40]

Navigating the complex terminology and services for children with learning and developmental problems can be very challenging. Numerous additional barriers reduce access to services for children in foster care, including difficulties obtaining consent, lack of care coordination across sectors, high turnover of child welfare professionals, and placement changes that can disrupt services. Understanding the regulations, terminology, and service sectors can help pediatricians educate families and advocate for individual patients and for systems changes to address barriers. This section focuses on the Individuals with Disabilities Education Act (IDEA), educational supports, and school services for children in the United States.

Table 13–1 contains a list of supports and services provided by Early Intervention (<3 years) and Child Find (3–18 years) for children covered by IDEA. The process for how and who is routinely assessed by Early Intervention and Child Find is highly variable across states.[9] The table lists useful information for clinicians, caregivers, and child welfare and other child-serving professionals. The reader may wish to pay particular attention to the topics of consent, type of service plan, and agencies responsible for services in the table.

In 2020 through 2021, 3.2% (360,000) of the resident population younger than 36 months in the United States received Early Intervention services and 6.2% (750,313) of the resident population ages 3 to 5 were served by Child Find. Over half of children served by Early Intervention services were eligible for Child Find after their third birthday.[42–45] Despite their higher prevalence of developmental delays and lower rates of academic achievement, children in out-of-home placement have lower rates of referral and connection to developmental/educational services than the general population, and the gap between need and services increases as children age. Children of color are screened and referred at lower rates, leading to delays in diagnosis and services compared with their white counterparts. Disparities are intensified by the variability and application of eligibility criteria from state to state.[10,16,19–21,42,43,46]

Table 13–1. IDEA/Educational Supports and School Services

	Early Intervention (EI), ages <36 months	Child Find (CF), ages 3–18 years
Responsible Federal Legislation	Individuals with Disabilities Education Act (IDEA), Part C	Individuals with Disabilities Education Act (IDEA), Part B
Child Abuse Prevention and Treatment Act (CAPTA) implications	All age eligible children in out-of-home placement are automatically eligible for an assessment with Early Intervention	All age eligible children in out-of-home placement are automatically eligible for an assessment with Child Find
Service classification	Educational	Educational
Who can consent	The caregiver who holds educational decision-making, most typically biological parents *Note: Early Intervention must document good faith efforts to contact biological parents. After 3 separate attempts, if unable to locate or reach the biological parent, EI is able to move on to the next responsible party. In the case of children in out-of-home placement, that would typically be the foster parent or kinship parent.*	The caregiver who holds educational decision-making, most-typically biological parents *Note: Child Find cannot move on to the next responsible party in the same way EI does*
Ages served	0–3 years of age	3–5 years of age
Program participation	Voluntary	Voluntary
Services	Services and therapies (occupational, speech and language, physical, social and emotional, developmental interventionists)	Appropriate public special education for children ages 3–5 years with identified developmental delays and disabilities that have an educational impact
Cost	Typically free; some states use a sliding scale; services cannot be denied based on a family's ability to pay	Typically free; some states use a sliding scale; services cannot be denied based on a family's ability to pay
Type of service plan used	Individualized Family Service Plan (IFSP)	Individualized Education Program (IEP)
Responsible agency	Variable: Health, Human Services, Education, Developmental Services, Family and Social Services, Rehabilitation Services, Public Health, Health and environment, Developmental Disabilities	Public school district of residence

(continues)

Table 13–1 *(continued)*

	Early Intervention (EI), ages <36 months	Child Find (CF), ages 3–18 years
Qualification for services	1. A child lives with a parent with a documented intellectual disability or developmental disability (state specific). 2.The child has a disability or developmental delay (states have different thresholds for the degree of delay required to qualify). 3. The child has a categorical or established condition (qualifying conditions vary from state to state).	1. All children enrolled in EI will be assessed to see if they still need ongoing services beyond their third birthday. If they continue to qualify for services, they will automatically qualify for Child Find. 2. States must follow IDEA, but they can have distinct guidelines on who qualifies for each disability type. 3. IDEA states that children who have one of 13 types of disabilities may qualify for special education and an IEP. To be eligible, the disability must adversely affect a child's educational performance.[41]

Eligibility for Educational Supports and School Services

IDEA is a federal law that covers Early Intervention and Child Find services and requires public school districts to provide special education and related services to children with disabilities. IDEA states that children who have one of 13 types of disabilities (**Box 13–2**) may qualify for an IEP. To be eligible, the disability must adversely affect a child's educational performance.[41]

States must follow IDEA, but they can have distinct guidelines regarding who qualifies for each disability type, resulting in some variation in service provisions among states and even individual school districts within states (**Box 13–3**). State laws may not contradict or provide less than federal requirements, although that can be challenging to assess.

The IEP document can be reviewed and revised at any time, but at least annually. By law, a copy of the IEP must be supplied to the family in their primary language of literacy, so they can read and understand their child's classification and what services they receive in school. A formal reevaluation with updated testing should occur every 3 years.[48]

After evaluation, a child may receive services under an IEP or a 504 plan. Special education services are one of the supports provided by IEPs, whereas 504 plans provide accommodations. Services are provided through their public school district. Key differences between the 2 plans are outlined in **Table 13–2**.

Box 13-2

Disability Classifications Accepted by IDEA

Thirteen Disability Classifications Include[41,47]:

- ▲ Intellectual disability
- ▲ Hearing impairment
- ▲ Deafness
- ▲ Speech or language impairment
- ▲ Visual impairment (including blindness)
- ▲ Serious emotional disturbance
- ▲ Orthopedic impairment
- ▲ Autism
- ▲ Traumatic brain injury
- ▲ Other health impairment
- ▲ Specific learning disability
- ▲ Deaf-blindness
- ▲ Multiple disabilities

Box 13-3

Essential Components of an IEP[41,47]

- ▲ Statement of child's present levels of performance
- ▲ Annual goals (intended measurement of progress)
- ▲ Special education
- ▲ Related services
- ▲ Supplementary services (including frequency and where services they will take place)
- ▲ Any modifications necessary for statewide assessments
- ▲ Transition goals/services (for age 16+)

Children in foster care experience school disruptions and learning issues for various reasons including the effects of prenatal substance exposure, neglect, and trauma on brain development; educational neglect in their birth homes; and multiple placement changes. Thirty percent to 50% of youth in foster care receive special education services through an IEP, yet these youth are still more likely to repeat a grade and have poor academic achievement, and

Table 13–2. Key Differences Between IEP and 504 Plan

Characteristic	Individualized Educational Program (IEP)	504 Plan
Law governing	Individuals With Disabilities Education Act, federal law governing provision of special education services to children with disabilities	Originates in anti-discrimination law; applies to children who do not qualify for special education
Eligibility	Determined by a comprehensive multidisciplinary evaluation based on specific disability categories (**Box 13-2**), at least one of which must affect a child's performance	No formal testing required; services available to a child with a physical or mental impairment that limits 1 or more life activities
Reevaluation	Can occur at any time; must occur at least annually with formal reevaluation (including testing) every 3 years	
Funding	Federal, state, and local	State and local

are 3 times more likely to drop out of high school, compared with their peers not in foster care.[49] Although children in foster care qualify for school services under both IDEA and Section 504 as previously noted, they do not consistently receive necessary educational accommodations because of lack of consent and school transitions that often accompany placement changes. A federal law, the Fostering Connections to Success and Increasing Adoptions Act 2008, P.L. 110–351, now requires that child welfare agencies develop an educational plan for each child in care and maintain them in their school of origin if in their best interest.[16,50] Children in foster care with a positive connection to their school (eg, positive teacher and peer relationships, a supportive environment) have been found to have better academic outcomes and school attendance than those without that important connection.[51,52]

Learning Disorders

The highest level of education an individual completes is highly dependent on academic proficiency in reading, writing, and mathematics. Academic proficiency is a strong predictor for health, well-being, and life expectancy.[22,53]

It is estimated that 1 in 5 children has a learning disorder that affects proficiency in these core areas.[54] Learning disorders are heritable, with a risk of recurrence of 50% to 60% in families with an affected first-degree family member, although psychosocial factors can affect clinical manifestations as well.[23] Learning challenges must be present for longer than 6 months despite academic interventions for consideration of this diagnosis.[37] Intellectual disability, lack of instruction, school absences, trauma, and attention challenges need to be ruled out when considering a learning disorder. Individual achievement testing uses a standardized assessment measure to assess performance in different subjects. This can be broad-based or specific to 1 subject.

There are 3 primary management approaches to address specific learning disorders in the educational setting.

1. **Remediation** may be offered to reduce performance gaps in basic academic skills, through provision of specialized instruction (eg, special education, speech therapy, tutoring).
2. **Accommodations** through a 504 plan may include extended time on assignments, paraprofessional support, and adaptive equipment (eg, text-to-speech/speech-to-text software, keyboarding).
3. **Modifications** may be considered to reduce the volume of work required.

Diagnostic Considerations

Children and youth in foster care are often diagnosed with ADHD, FASD, oppositional defiant disorder, bipolar disorder, adjustment disorder, depression, and/or anxiety. Several of these are discussed in more detail here because of their overlap with traumatic stress symptoms. Accurate diagnosis can be challenging because traumatized children may present with both trauma symptoms and 1 or more of the following comorbid conditions:

- The overlap between ADHD and trauma symptoms includes hyperactivity, impulsivity, and difficulty with concentrating and paying attention. Both conditions may also present with trouble listening, restlessness, sleep issues, and being disorganized.[55] Medications used to treat ADHD may be ineffective or have side effects when a child's symptoms are trauma related[56] (see Chapter 38, Psychotropic Medication Oversight).
- Fetal alcohol spectrum disorder is a consideration in children with developmental, learning, cognitive, or behavioral problems and is more common among children involved with child welfare.[57] In most diagnostic schema, documented prenatal alcohol exposure is necessary for a diagnosis, but this can be challenging to clarify.
- Fetal alcohol syndrome is a subset of FASD characterized by dysmorphic facial features, growth restriction, and neurologic involvement (structural or functional), but symptoms and signs vary across a broad spectrum.[58,59]
- Prenatal exposure to other substances, including opiates and methamphetamines, can result in neurobehavioral impairment. Polysubstance exposure

is common among children involved with child welfare, making it challenging to identify a single cause for functional differences.[60,61]

- Autism spectrum disorder also shares similarities with trauma symptoms (relational dysregulation, inattention, difficulty with transitions, language delay) and can cooccur with trauma symptoms. Concern for ASD should result in referral for full evaluation by an expert in this area.

Management Considerations

Management considerations of identified behavioral, emotional, and/or learning issues include:

- A pediatrician may refer to specialists for assessment (ie, developmental or mental health clinicians) and treatment.
- Multidisciplinary assessments are valuable and preferred.
- Assessments should be rooted in an understanding of trauma and its effects and include trauma treatment as part of the management plan.
- Learning and development should be assessed throughout childhood and adolescence.
- Developmental screening for children up to 66 months of age should continue in primary care settings according to AAP guidelines[37] for children in foster care to identify emerging issues.

Conclusion

The importance of understanding the profound effects that trauma can have on developmental, educational, and behavioral health trajectories across the life span (infancy into adulthood) cannot be overstated. Having a relationship with a safe, stable, nurturing caregiver is central to a child's recovery from trauma. If pediatricians are aware of important historical components and risk factors that children in out-of-home placement experience, they can help ensure timely screening and connection with necessary developmental, educational, and behavioral assessments and supports. Additionally, all professionals who have a role in ensuring the well-being of children and families must ground themselves in a trauma-informed care approach and understand the role of trauma in how a child presents to avoid potential harm through misdiagnosis and inappropriate responses and treatments. Identification of the root causes of developmental, behavioral, and educational concerns can favor correct diagnosis and connection to the most appropriate evidence-based treatments and interventions to support patients, families, and the clinicians who care for them. Applying a holistic, trauma-focused, culturally informed lens can help ensure the healthiest long-term trajectories possible for children and youth.

Acknowledgment

The authors wish to acknowledge the contribution of Adiaha Spinks-Franklin, MD, MPH, FAAP, to the early conceptualization of this chapter.

Key Takeaways

» The effects of trauma on child development are profound, with variable presentations by age.

» Children involved with child welfare are at high risk for developmental delays and educational achievement challenges.

» Caregivers and clinicians play a critical role in promotion of healthy development and resilience.

» Early referral to Early Intervention and/or Child Find is an important step that pediatricians can take to ensure optimal developmental trajectories for young infants and toddlers in out-of-home placement. Follow-up to ensure completion of assessment is critical.

» School-aged children may qualify for educational accommodations or supports through a 504 Plan or IEP.

» Consider traumatic stress in the differential when a child is having developmental, educational, or behavioral challenges.

CHAPTER

14

Oral Health

S. Thikkurissy, DDS, MS, MA
AnnMarie Matusak, DDS, MS

Overview of Dental Issues Among Children in Foster Care

Increased Prevalence of Oral Health Issues

Dental caries is the most common chronic noncommunicable disease of childhood. According to the American Academy of Pediatrics (AAP), the overall reported prevalence of dental caries is 45.8% among children age 2 to 19 years, with 23% of children age 2 to 5 years, 52% of children age 6 to 8 years, and 57% of children age 12 to 19 years having dental caries.[1] The prevalence of dental issues is higher among children in foster care compared with children who have not experienced foster care. A 2021 study from the University of Minnesota found that the prevalence of dental caries in foster populations was 12% higher compared with those with no experience in foster care (44% vs 32.2%).[2] Additional findings included that children with a history of foster care were nearly 20% less likely to see a dentist for both routine dental care and specific dental issues. Morón et al found that children in foster care were 1.6 times more likely to experience pulpitis (painful inflammation of the dental pulp, a result of untreated dental caries that has progressed), 5.8 times more likely to have a diagnosis of severe gingivitis (gingival inflammation that can lead to bleeding gums and, in medically compromised children, mucosal translocation of pathogenic bacteria into the bloodstream), and 1.3 times more likely to require dental extractions.[3]

Risk Factors for Dental Issues

Risk factors for dental issues include lack of access to culturally aware and pediatric-specific dental care; lack of access to fluoride and dental hygiene routines such as brushing, and the presence of special health care needs. The American Academy of Pediatric Dentistry (AAPD) cites transitory familial settings as an underlying reason for "high risk for caries."[4] Montano-DiLeone[5] described how transitory living situations impact dental care among children experiencing homelessness:

> Many children and adolescents who are homeless have no early or routine access to dental care. In addition, parents or caregivers often are unaware of the importance of dental care in early childhood. Children within this population do not receive adequate fluoride, regular professional care, or oral hygiene training.

Children with special health care needs are also a population at risk for dental caries.[4] Children in foster care may present with a complex overlay of risk factors for dental issues, including social instabilities and complex health care needs. This chapter will frame oral health in the context of the child or adolescent in the foster care system.

Assessing Dental Caries Risk in Children: AAP/AAPD Standards

Caries risk assessments are, in essence, a premanifest predictor of disease. Typically, screening instruments will account for biological, medical, and socioeconomic variables and attempt to fashion a risk for disease from these variables. The Oral Health Risk Assessment Tool developed by the AAP can be found in **Figure 14–1**. With this tool, certain elements may be weighted differently than others. For example, a child with asthma may not have as high a risk for caries as someone who has visible plaque on their teeth and does not use fluoride. Risk assessments balance pathological and protective factors to provide a clinical picture. This cumulative clinical impression is intended to further guide preventive regimen recommendations, such as use of higher-strength fluoride in adolescent patients, and professional visit periodicity.

Both the AAP and the AAPD recognize the singular importance of partnerships between dental and medical professionals. While oral health specifics are rarely taught to any great length in medical school, engagement with community pediatric dentists and dental training programs allows physician trainees to understand their role in caring for patients (and families) at higher risk for dental disease. While clinical examination of caries might be more challenging, understanding basic concepts such as "lift the lip" and assessing for frank cavitations, oral abscesses, and facial swelling allows physicians to provide fundamental oral health counseling as well as guidance to seek professional dental care. The AAP also has a Brush, Book, Bed program, which links oral health to a regular nighttime routine. Both the AAP and the AAPD recognize the value and importance of fluoride as an anticaries agent and a staple of risk-reducing strategies. The AAP Caries Risk Tool (AAP-CAT) created with Bright Futures is a straightforward and clinically applicable document to help physicians assess the oral cavity (**Figure 14–2**).

American Academy of Pediatrics Oral Health Risk Assessment Tool

The American Academy of Pediatrics (AAP) developed this tool to aid in the implementation of oral health risk assessment during health supervision visits. Since a validated caries risk assessment tool does not currently exist, this tool includes factors known to be related to childhood caries. The form provides a framework to assist the pediatric clinician to identify risk as well as modifiable behaviors to optimize patient oral health.

Instructions for Use

Use this form in conjunction with the **AAP Oral Health Intake Form**, to collect information from parents/caregivers on home care and habits that contribute to both protective and risk factors. That information will help inform the **Action Plan** and the family's **Self-Management Goals**.

The child is at high risk for caries if any of the risk factors below are reported or found in the physical exam. In the presence of multiple risk factors or severe clinical findings, the clinician may determine the child should be seen by a dentist as soon as possible.

Patient Name:________ Date of Birth:________ Date:________

Visit: ☐ 6 month ☐ 9 month ☐ 12 month ☐ 15 month ☐ 18 month ☐ 24 month ☐ 30 month ☐ 3 year ☐ 4 year ☐ 5 year ☐ 6 year ☐ Other

RISK FACTORS

Mother or primary caregiver had active decay in the past 12 months ☐ Yes ☐ No

Does not have an established dental home ☐ Yes ☐ No

Continual bottle/sippy cup use with beverage other than water ☐ Yes ☐ No

Does not drink fluoridated water or take fluoride supplements ☐ Yes ☐ No

Frequent snacking on sugary and/or sticky snacks ☐ Yes ☐ No

Has not received fluoride varnish in the last 6 months ☐ Yes ☐ No

Does not have teeth brushed twice daily ☐ Yes ☐ No

Does not use fluoride toothpaste ☐ Yes ☐ No

Medicaid eligible ☐ Yes ☐ No

Special health care needs ☐ Yes ☐ No

PHYSICAL FINDINGS

Obvious decay ☐ Yes ☐ No

Restorations present (Fillings or Silver Diamine Fluoride Present) ☐ Yes ☐ No

White spots or decalcifications ☐ Yes ☐ No

Swollen or bleeding gums (gingivitis) ☐ Yes ☐ No

Visible plaque ☐ Yes ☐ No

Oral Health Risk Determination: If YES to any of the above, this patient is considered HIGH risk for dental disease. Determine ☐ HIGH / ☐ LOW risk; follow **Action Plan** below.

ACTION PLAN

	High Risk	Low Risk
Apply fluoride varnish	☐ Every 3 months	☐ Every 6 months
Refer to a dental home	☐ Yes	☐ Yes
Set self-management goals with caregiver	☐ Yes	☐ Yes

SELF-MANAGEMENT GOALS

Reviewed

- ☐ Brush twice daily with fluoride toothpaste.
- ☐ Regular dental visits for child and caregiver(s).
- ☐ Wean off bottle and use only water in sippy cup
- ☐ Less/no juice. No soda.
- ☐ Drink fluoridated water.
- ☐ Less/no junk food or candy. Replace with healthy snacks.
- ☐ Have teeth treated with fluoride varnish every 3-6 months.

COMPLETED ACTIONS

	Yes	No
Oral health risk assessment	☐	☐
Visual exam of the mouth	☐	☐
Fluoride varnish application	☐	☐
Anticipatory guidance	☐	☐
Referral to a dentist	☐	☐

MANAGEMENT OF HIGH RISK CHILDREN

High-risk children should receive professionally applied fluoride varnish. Caregivers should be counseled to brush teeth twice daily with an age-appropriate amount of fluoridated toothpaste. Referral to a pediatric dentist or a dentist comfortable caring for children should be made with follow-up to ensure that the child is being cared for in the dental home.

American Academy of Pediatrics DEDICATED TO THE HEALTH OF ALL CHILDREN® Bright Futures NIIOH

Figure 14–1. Oral Health Risk Assessment Tool developed by the American Academy of Pediatrics.

Reproduced from American Academy of Pediatrics Oral Health Risk Assessment Tool. Available at https://downloads.aap.org/AAP/PDF/oralhealth_RiskAssessmentTool.pdf.

Physical Findings

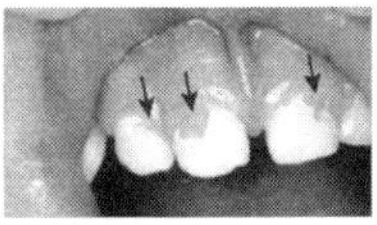

Obvious Decay

Tooth decay is the decomposition of the tooth structure due to acid caused by bacteria and can appear on any surface of the tooth. Decay can range in color from yellow to black. When obvious decay is present, the child should be considered high risk and referred for immediate dental care.

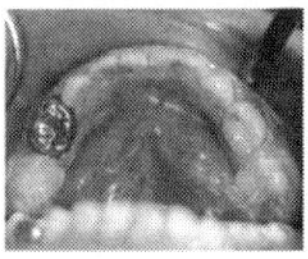

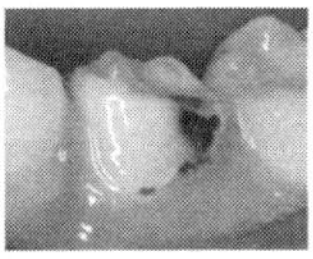

Restorations Present (Fillings or Silver Diamine Fluoride Present)

Restorations indicate that decay occurred and was treated. Restorations can present as materials such as silver diamine fluoride, metal, alloy, plastic, glass ionomer, or porcelain. A child who has been treated for decay is at continued risk and should be under the regular care and supervision of a dental professional.

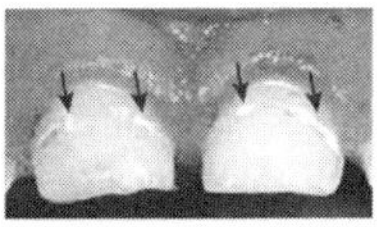

White Spots / Decalcifications

Decalcification is an early sign of tooth decay, takes the form of white spots on the teeth, and commonly presents along the gum line. Remineralization can be achieved with fluoride, in particular application of fluoride varnish. When calcifications are present, the child should be considered high risk and referred for immediate dental care.

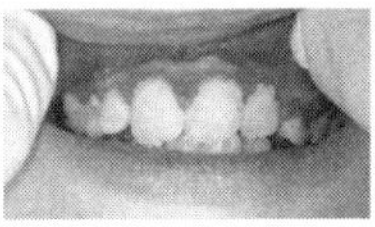

Swollen or Bleeding Gums (Gingivitis)

Gingivitis is the inflammation of the gums. Pediatricians can teach patients and their families good oral hygiene skills to reduce inflammation.

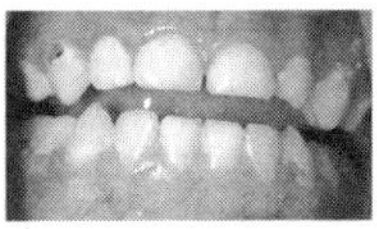

Visible Plaque

Plaque is the soft and sticky substance that accumulates on the teeth from food debris and bacteria. Pediatricians can teach parents to remove plaque from the child's teeth by brushing and flossing.

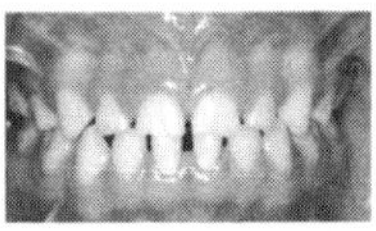

Healthy Teeth

Children with healthy teeth have no signs of early childhood caries and no other clinical findings. They are also experiencing normal tooth and mouth development and spacing. Apply fluoride varnish if child has not received treatment in prior six months.

For more information about the AAP's oral health activities and resources, email oralhealth@aap.org or visit www.aap.org/oralhealth.

American Academy of Pediatrics — Bright Futures — NIIOH

Figure 14–2. Clinical assessment in a pediatric oral health assessment.

Reproduced from American Academy of Pediatrics Oral Health Risk Assessment Tool. Available at https://downloads.aap.org/AAP/PDF/oralhealth_RiskAssessmentTool.pdf.

Potential Barriers to Dental Care Access

The Affordable Care Act (ACA) requires most insurers to cover a package of health care services known as essential health benefits, with pediatric dental care explicitly identified as a covered service. The benefit for children and adolescents provided by Medicaid is known as Early and Periodic Screening, Diagnostic and Treatment (EPSDT) services, which provides for a full array of prevention, diagnostic, and treatment services, including oral health and dental services, for infants, children, and adolescents younger than 21 years in families with low income.[6] However, the challenge of finding a dental home that accepts the specifics of Medicaid or ACA-approved insurers can negate these federal legislative advances. Children in families with low income, including those in the foster care system, are typically seen in safety-net clinics, which can include dental schools, children's hospitals, and regional health departments. Special health care needs in pediatric patients are a major challenge to dental care access. Very often, management of complex medical needs in conjunction with oral health needs requires additional training that goes beyond what is taught in the traditional dental school curriculum. Kerins et al[7] noted in 2011 that the US dental care system has "extremely limited capacity to care for children with special health care needs," with these children often requiring care in a children's hospital or by a pediatric-specific provider. As noted earlier, social factors, such as transitions in living situations that can occur with foster care placement, can lead to additional dental care access challenges. Obtaining consent may be another challenge when anesthesia or a procedure such as extraction is medically necessary.

Delivering Oral Health Care

Routine Care

According to the AAPD, all children should have their first dental visit by age 1 year or within 6 months of eruption of the first tooth. While actual dental caries prevalence is low in the 1-year age group, the purpose of this visit is to provide age-based and development-based anticipatory guidance, including the use of fluoride, toothbrushing, potential for dental trauma, and enrollment in a dental home. This includes the use of office-based fluoride therapy (varnish), which is a higher concentration than that found in toothpaste. The use of fluoride varnish as an office-based prevention strategy also extends to pediatricians, who, in many states, can apply fluoride varnish (as a reimbursable medical code). Most oral health recommendations are subsequently based on a 6-month periodicity. However, there are instances of high risk for dental caries in which increased periodicity to 3-month examinations may be beneficial. Insurance coverage of periodicity varies among states, and providers should review their state and insurance coverage details. In some cases, a letter of medical necessity may be authored by the treating physician or team to increase periodicity of examinations or fluoride varnish based on assessed risk.

Treating Oral Health Problems

The literature consistently demonstrates that pain (both visceral and perceived) alters a child's behavior. Trauma experiences can also affect behavior and tolerance of dental procedures. Pediatric dentists are specifically trained in the psychology of normal and abnormal child behavior development, including the management of children who have experienced early childhood trauma.

A key principle is reinforcing the establishment of a dental home as defined by the AAPD. The dental home is the "ongoing relationship between the dentist and the patient, inclusive of all aspects of oral health care delivered in a safe, culturally sensitive, individualized, comprehensive, continuous, accessible, coordinated, compassionate, and patient- and family-centered way regardless of race, ethnicity, religion, sexual or gender identity, medical status, family structure, or financial circumstances."[8] This definition intentionally includes groups with special needs, such as those in foster care, and children with special medical needs. Ideally, the dental home is continuously accessible and independent of foster placements.

The extent of dental work and child behaviors can affect the need for advanced behavior guidance in addition to communication and nonpharmacological approaches. Adjuncts, such as nitrous oxide, are key to the provision of individualized care. Pharmacological interventions often require interactions with large safety-net providers, such as regional children's health centers, health departments, and providers with access to pharmacological services (procedural sedation and operating room care, for example).

In areas where these interventions are not readily accessible, a provider may be required to use protective stabilization to safely manage high-acuity dental pain, using a trauma-informed approach. Further exploration of trauma-informed approaches within pediatric dentistry, including the training of dental students and development of new approaches to care, could improve access to trauma-informed dental care.

Future Directions to Improve Access

Strategies for improving access to care for this population in foster care are multipronged, including (1) collaboration between medical and dental providers, (2) an infrastructure that supports access to care, typically through adequate reimbursements, and (3) a means of tracking a patient's needs between foster care placements. These elements are essential in providing a dental home for children and adolescents in the foster care system.

Key Takeaways

» Children in foster care typically have a high risk of dental disease.

» Fluoride varnish applied at visits to a pediatrician or other physician is a supportive strategy for reducing the burden of dental disease in this population.

» Oral health may be deprioritized during foster care placements but can contribute to significant behavior and pain-associated issues.

CHAPTER

15

Measuring Health Care Outcomes

Tagrid M. Ruiz-Maldonado, MD, MS, FAAP
Kristine A. Campbell, MD, MSc, FAAP

Medical processes and interventions support health outcomes that pediatricians can identify, track, and measure. Measuring health outcomes is important for establishing best practices, revealing gaps in clinical performance, identifying program needs, improving patient and family satisfaction, and fostering accountability. By selecting outcomes relevant to their clinical population, pediatricians caring for children and adolescents in foster care can better evaluate the impact of their practice on their patients' health. Furthermore, outcome measurements can demonstrate the effectiveness of a clinic in meeting the needs of a selected population, providing clear, objective results that can help drive funding and support, and are a crucial part of ensuring longevity at the systems, clinic, and patient levels.

Much of the discussion regarding measuring health outcomes inherently overlaps with quality improvement processes and research, which are outside of the scope of this chapter (see Chapter 39, Improving Care, Expanding the Field). Instead, this chapter focuses on understanding, selecting, and measuring *patient-centered* and *process-based* outcomes that have meaning for youth in foster care and their caregivers, for the pediatrician and clinical staff caring for these patients, and for the child welfare system tasked with providing substitute care for this population. This chapter aims to (1) identify key domains relevant to youth in foster care, (2) introduce an approach to selecting health outcomes within these domains, (3) review the process of choosing measures for selected health outcomes, and (4) discuss the intersection of pediatric health outcome measures and local, state, and national objectives to improve the health and well-being of youth in foster care.

Health Domains for Foster Care Pediatric Practice

The World Health Organization has broadly defined *health* as a multidimensional construct composed of overlapping physical, mental, and social domains.[1] The identification and definition of health domains are integral to the comprehensive assessment of health, as they allow for an organized approach to selecting meaningful outcomes and measures.

The American Academy of Pediatrics (AAP) Periodicity Schedule[2,3] recommends age-specific screening across the domains of physical, mental, developmental, and behavioral child health, as well as the social and emotional environments in which a child is growing and developing. While the standard periodic screenings recommended by the AAP are necessary, they are not sufficient for youth in foster care. As detailed in Chapter 1, Core Components: A General Overview, and Chapter 2, Health Care Visits: Type and Periodicity, youth in foster care require more frequent and different types of visits. Given the unique aspects of providing care to youth in foster care, it is important to consider a systems health domain in addition to the domains previously mentioned.

Rather than specific outcomes and outcome measures, the systems health domain reflects key players and processes intrinsic to this population's health (**Table 15–1**). This can include tracking completion of health visits and health screening as recommended for youth in foster care by professional health organizations or as mandated by county or state child welfare policies. Identifying and documenting key players in supporting the health care needs of youth in foster care can aid in further evaluating clinic effectiveness. Processes considered routine for typical patients—consent for immunizations or medications, for example—can become complex for children and adolescents in foster care. Furthermore, a child's caregiving team—foster parent(s), caseworker, or care manager—may change without notice. These systems issues can be challenging in the routine clinical encounter; in an after-hours emergency context, they can become urgent. Correct and early documentation of these issues, and accessibility within the medical record, is critical to providing optimal care for a child or adolescent in foster care. Pediatricians must be aware that there are different models of health care coordination for children in foster care and should be familiar with the model(s) in their region or state. These may include specialized health records, assigned care managers, or home health nurses to provide on-site support. Developing relationships with people not directly "in the room" is important to successfully implement health care plans and ensure continuity of care over time.

Table 15–1. Systems Health Domain: Key Players and Processes to Include in the Medical Record of Youth in Foster Care

Key Players and Processes	Examples
Caregivers	Family of origin (unless rights are terminated) Foster, kin, or group home caregiver Current caseworker(s) and specific role(s)
Health care team	Primary care Subspecialists Physical, speech, or occupational therapists Mental health care clinicians Current nurse or other care manager Psychotropic oversight program manager and clinicians
Medical decision-making	Data-sharing system (eg, health passport, electronic health record) Proxy permissions (eg, family of origin, foster family, caseworker) Consents for information sharing with stakeholders Consents for immunization, medication, reproductive health care Consents or protocols for emergency medical decision-making Plans for after-hours contacts in case of emergent medical needs
Health visits	Initial screening examination within 72 hours Comprehensive health assessment within 30 days Follow-up health assessment within 60–90 days

Selecting Health Outcomes for Foster Care Pediatric Practice

Within each AAP-recommended health domain are specific outcomes of importance to patients, caregivers, clinics, and agencies. **Table 15–2** outlines examples of outcomes within each health domain that may help illustrate the comprehensive health status of youth in foster care. It is important to note that, in reality, some outcomes may fall into multiple domains, reflecting an underlying integrated care model.

Pediatricians may also consider the needs and priorities of local agency partners in developing a "toolbox" of health screens. Meeting with child welfare administrators or foster care agency leaders in the community may promote cross-sector collaboration related to critical health issues, such as substance use disorders, mental health and evidence-based trauma treatment, reproductive health, or suicidality and self-harm, which may be difficult to effectively manage without a pediatrician's support.

Finally, pediatricians should be cognizant of the best sources of information for their clinical setting. For example, focus groups and key stakeholder data may help identify specific needs and help establish priorities for screening and evaluation of youth in foster care in a particular community. Additionally, family and patient participation, by way of family advisory boards and lived-experience perspectives, may provide valuable input. Awareness of these

Table 15–2. Examples of Health Domains, Outcomes, and Measures to Document When Assessing and Tracking Health Status of Youth in Foster Care

Domain	Outcome	Measures
Physical Health	Ongoing health evaluation[a] and preventive care	Growth parameters (including BMI and OFC[b]) Immunizations (catch-up and scheduled) Oral health assessment and topical fluoride Dental referral (by age 12 months) Recommended screening labs such as blood lead levels Hearing screening Vision screening
	Chronic health care needs	Comprehensive problem list Current medications, dosing, and prescribers Medical equipment, settings, and suppliers Allergies and adverse reactions Schedule of care Hospitalizations
	Physical abuse and neglect concerns	Complete head-to-toe skin exam
Mental Health	Mental health history	Current diagnoses Current medications, dosing, and prescribers Current mental health therapies (eg, PCIT, TF-CBT) Inpatient or residential mental health care Substance or alcohol use disorder Suicide attempts or self-harm
	Mental health screening	Depression and anxiety (eg, PHQ-9, GAD-7, SCARED) Childhood traumatic stress (eg, CPM-PTSST, UCLA PTSD-RI Brief Form) Alcohol, tobacco, or other substance use (eg, CRAFFT, BSTAD) Suicidality and self-harm (eg, ASQ, C-SSRS)[b,c]
Developmental Health	Developmental history Developmental screening (at every health supervision visit)	Developmental risks and diagnoses Current developmental interventions General developmental screening (eg, Ages and Stages Questionnaire, SWYC) Autism screening (eg, M-CHAT, SWYC)
	Education history[b]	Schools attended Grades completed School performance School contacts Individualized education program Early childhood intervention plan

Table 15–2 *(continued)*

Domain	Outcome	Measures
Psychosocial Health	Environment	Type of placement (eg, congregate care vs family-based settings) Household members and relationships History of placement changes Activities and barriers to participation Employment and access to salary[b] Peer group Trusted adults
	Sexual history[b]	Pronouns Chosen name, if applicable Access to birth control (eg, condoms, LARC) Consider STI screening (joint decision with patient[b])

Abbreviations: ASQ, Ask Suicide-Screening Questions; BMI, body mass index; BSTAD, Brief Screener for Tobacco, Alcohol, and other Drugs; CPM-PTSST, Care Process Model Pediatric Traumatic Stress Screening Tool; CRAFFT, Car, Relax, Alone, Forget, Friends, Trouble; C-SSRS, Columbia-Suicide Severity Rating Scale; GAD-7, General Anxiety Disorder-7; LARC, long-acting reversible contraception; M-CHAT, Modified Checklist for Autism in Toddlers; OFC, occipitofrontal circumference; PCIT, parent-child interaction therapy; PHQ-9, Patient Health Questionnaire; TF-CBT, trauma-focused cognitive behavioral therapy; SCARED, Screen for Child Anxiety Related Disorders; STI, sexually transmitted infection; SWYC, Survey of Well-Being of Young Children; UCLA PTSD-RI, University of California at Los Angeles Post-Traumatic Stress Disorder Reaction Index

[a]Recommendations may vary by state.

[b]Age dependent

[c]At initial placement

sources and their overlap may promote opportunities for partnership to fill gaps in health care and improve the delivery of needed resources.

When selecting health outcomes, the following questions may serve as a useful guide:

- What outcomes are important for the clinician's particular clinical setting?
  - How will the outcomes be defined, selected, and measured?
  - Are the outcomes short-term, intermediate, or long-term?
  - Are there valid, efficient, and accessible instruments to measure the selected outcomes?
- What clinical resources will be required to measure and track the outcomes?
  - Are the data of interest already collected or stored in the health record?
  - Will an increased number of staff members be needed?
  - Will a computer program be needed?
  - Will staff members require special training?
  - How will a clinician respond to negative outcomes?
- How will an adequate response to a pediatric health screener be ensured?
  - Who will be made aware of screening results that require ongoing care or resources?

- How will identified concerns be tracked across placement changes and reunification?
- How will a clinician know that a particular goal has been achieved?

Clinical care and integrated care management should be carefully weighed when assessing health outcomes of youth in foster care. These broad, intersecting themes establish a conceptual framework around which the pediatrician can organize health outcome selection within each domain.

Measuring Health Outcomes for Foster Care Pediatric Practice

Once the outcomes of interest are selected, instruments to measure each outcome can be identified (see **Table 15-2**). Except in rare circumstances, pediatricians are encouraged to rely on tested, published instruments to ensure validity and improve comparability across clinical settings. For example, tracking the percentage of patients screened at the recommended time frame allows pediatricians to identify trends, such as whether the clinic is able to consistently provide appointments or if caseworkers and foster families are presenting to care and adhering to discussed health recommendations. Similarly, the use of established screeners for mental health, such as the Patient Health Questionnaire-9 (PHQ-9), and for child development, such as the Survey of Well-Being of Young Children (SWYC), helps improve early detection of emerging health and developmental concerns and supports comparison with broader populations of children in the community. The AAP Bright Futures Toolkit provides links to common tools recommended for well-child visits as well as screening and assessment tools that may be driven by specific patient, caregiver, or pediatrician concerns.[4]

Of note, programs and interventions vary across states; therefore, relevant outcome measures may vary. For example, while one clinic may find it important to track completion of health instruments to ensure adherence to recommended guidelines, another may focus on tracking the results of such instruments to identify trends and advocate for increased funding for resources and programs. Pediatricians and other clinicians caring for youth in foster care should be familiar with the resources, programs, interventions, and funding and oversight agencies that apply to their clinic and patients. Pediatricians are encouraged to work with key cross-system players to determine whether goals do or should overlap. Additionally, pediatricians may collaborate across systems to develop a shared language related to health risks and outcomes to improve the response to ongoing health care needs in this population.

Pediatricians could also identify diverse sources of feedback applicable to their clinic and practice through outreach to key stakeholders at the local and state levels. Recurring process and case reviews may provide opportunities for identifying trends in patient care that may be positively or negatively affecting patient outcomes. As with selecting important health outcomes, family input also carries crucial value and can be obtained by way of lived-experience evaluations, satisfaction surveys, and patient advisory councils.

Finally, pediatricians should recognize the potential for systematic tracking of health outcomes within a clinical practice to support continuous quality improvement efforts and identify opportunities to improve care. Resources related to quality improvement training from the AAP include the Bright Futures Quality Improvement page and the Education in Quality Improvement for Pediatric Practice program, also known as EQIPP.[5,6]

Using Clinical Health Measures in Local, State, and National Collaborations

In recent decades, policy efforts have mandated increased access to health care, mental health, and integrated services for children and adolescents in foster care.[7] The Families First Prevention Services Treatment Act mandated that the child welfare system take on increased responsibility to ensure youth in foster care receive adequate health care, particularly related to mental health.[8] These mandates were meant to help bolster the health care and child welfare partnership, promoting cross-system collaboration while increasing efforts to avoid fragmentation in patient care. Ideally, this collaboration will result in a shared responsibility to understand and address outcomes for youth in foster care.

While selection and implementation of child health measures in the pediatric clinic are primarily for detecting and responding to individual patient needs, a pediatrician caring for youth in foster care may find opportunities to work with colleagues in child welfare to achieve shared goals, with particular focus on increasing well-being within child welfare. The following shared goals may be considered during evaluations at the individual child or program level:

- Child evaluations
  - Identify health needs for individual children in foster care
  - Fill gaps in health history to ensure continuity of care
  - Monitor service referral and receipt
  - Support coordinated interdisciplinary care

- Program evaluations
  - Support efficient service delivery and implementation
  - Contribute to evaluating the effectiveness of services on child health

Just as it is important for clinicians to be aware of state-specific programs, interventions, and services related to youth in foster care when selecting and measuring outcomes, they should also be mindful of outcomes closely followed at a national level. The Child Welfare Outcomes Report (CWOR) is a congressionally mandated report published annually by the US Department of Health and Human Services.[9] The report addresses states' performance on nationally accepted objectives established in consultation with key state and local administrators, advocates, researchers, legislators, and other experts in the field of child welfare. These objectives correspond to the 3 goals of child welfare as established by the Adoption and Safe Families Act of 1997—permanency, safety, and well-being.[10] Data for these measures are obtained from the National Child Abuse and Neglect Data System and the Adoption and Foster Care Analysis and Reporting System.

The national outcomes covered in the CWOR[9] are as follows:

- Reduce the recurrence of child abuse and/or neglect
- Reduce the incidence of child abuse and/or neglect in foster care
- Increase permanency for children in foster care
- Reduce time in foster care to reunification without increasing reentry
- Reduce time in foster care to adoption
- Increase placement stability
- Reduce placement of young children in group homes or institutions

While the CWOR is designed to inform Congress, the state, and the public about state performance, clinicians should also recognize that health care outcomes may have significant downstream effects on national outcomes. It is therefore important that pediatricians and nonphysician clinicians, when discussing local outcome measures and integration of health care and child welfare services, do so understanding the underlying interests of the child welfare system while seeking collaboration and establishing common cross-system goals.

Conclusions

The needs of children and adolescents in foster care have been abundantly described, with recent attention focused on chronic illness and mental health. However, there is a paucity of guidance for monitoring and responding to these needs in the pediatric clinic working with the foster care community.[11] Pediatric programs can support implementation and expansion of evidence-based health care for youth in foster care by tracking meaningful outcome measures for children in these programs. Reliable and valid measures of health outcomes can be shared with key stakeholders and policymakers in order to justify maintenance, expansion, or modification of health care services for youth in foster care.

Measuring outcomes is important not only to understand the current program or clinic status, but also to help determine whether what is being done is "working." Measuring outcomes of youth entering, currently in, and exiting the foster care system requires close collaboration among numerous key players. Pediatricians have a responsibility to define and measure outcomes to help support an iterative process aimed at addressing prevention; bolstering quality, ongoing care; and improving the physical, mental, developmental, and psychosocial health of children and adolescents in foster care.

Key Takeaways

- Measuring health outcomes serves multiple purposes, including establishing best practices and identifying program and patient needs.
- Consistent measurement of health outcomes for children in foster care can improve both individual health and population-based systems of care for a population at risk for both short- and long-term physical and mental health challenges.
- For children in foster care, a unique "systems health domain" composed of key players and processes is critical for appropriate care and continuity in the health care system.
- Selecting and measuring meaningful outcomes for youth in foster care requires communication and collaboration between clinicians and the child welfare system to reflect shared values and priorities.

Part 2. Culture of Foster Care

CHAPTER

16

History of Child Welfare in the United States and Issues of Disproportionality, Inequity, and Injustice

Camille A. Broussard, MD, MPH, FAAP
LaToya Montgomery, MSW, LCSW-C

Importance of Reviewing the History

Understanding the history of the US child welfare system is of paramount importance for pediatricians. Historical knowledge aids in the understanding of policy shifts, challenges, inequities, and injustices that have shaped the current landscape as well as resulting racial disparities and racial disproportionality, such as the overrepresentation of Black and Indigenous children in the child welfare system (see **Box 16–1** for definitions).[1] Moreover, a retrospective view enables pediatricians to advocate for improved policies, services, and interventions, ultimately enhancing the care provided to children and families. Maya Angelou once stated, "Do the best you can until you know better, then when you know better, do better"; thus, once we gain knowledge of where we have been and currently are within the structure of the child welfare system, we should aim to do better and make the system better.

The history of child welfare in the United States traces a trajectory from early charitable efforts and orphanages to institutional reforms and the evolution of foster care and adoption, reflecting societal evolutions in attitudes regarding child and parental rights and the role of government in welfare and protection. However, structural racism, inequities, and injustices have also been embedded in the child welfare system, which makes understanding its whole history imperative for pediatricians caring for children and families in the system. While this chapter focuses on racial disproportionality, it also acknowledges the overrepresentation of other populations in the child welfare system, including lesbian, gay, bisexual, transgender, and questioning or queer (LGBTQ+) youth and children with disabilities, as discussed in Chapter 27, Children and

Youth Who Identify as LGBTQ+; Chapter 28, Additional Considerations for Transgender and Gender Diverse Children and Youth; Chapter 30, Neurodevelopmental Disorders: Identification and Intervention; and Chapter 31, Children With Medical Complexity.

Box 16–1

Racial Disparities Versus Racial Disproportionality in the Child Welfare System

- **Racial disparities:** inequitable differences in decision-making points and outcomes in the child welfare system experienced by racial or ethnic groups.
- **Racial disproportionality:** the proportion of a given racial or ethnic group in the child welfare system is either larger (overrepresented) or smaller (underrepresented) when compared to that group's proportion in the general population.

Brief History of Child Welfare in the United States

The United States has a complicated history as it relates to children and their welfare. It was common in the 19th and early 20th centuries for children to be sent to work without protection in industries such as agriculture, textile mills, mining, and factories. Orphanages, like those established by the Children's Aid Society in New York City and other charitable and religious organizations, provided the only social services to impoverished, orphaned, or homeless children. Charles Loring Brace, who founded the Children's Aid Society, believed that children would benefit from being placed in families rather than remaining impoverished, on the streets, or in institutions.[2] This led to the Orphan Train Movement from 1853 to 1929, which is generally recognized as the beginning of foster care as an alternative to overcrowded orphanages. Thus, more than 120,000 children (largely of Italian and Irish descent), transported by trains from eastern cities westward, were placed with foster families on farms. Because this occurred before federal involvement in child welfare and protection, the outcomes of these placements varied, with some children finding loving homes and others being maltreated or subjected to harsh labor conditions on the farms.

During this period of orphanages and early foster families, legislation for the protection of small animals was more common than legislation protecting children. In fact, Henry Bergh, who formed the American Society for the Prevention of Cruelty to Animals (ASPCA) in New York in 1866, was consulted in 1874 regarding the first case of child abuse and neglect in the United States to evoke widespread public concern (see **Box 16–2**). This case led to the formation of the New York Society for the Prevention of Cruelty to Children in 1875. However, federal involvement in child welfare and protection would not be formalized until 1912, when Congress created the federal Children's Bureau to investigate and report on the welfare of children in the United States.

Box 16-2

Case of Mary Ellen (1874)

Mary Ellen was a child left orphaned by the death of her father and destitution of her mother. She was sent to live with a couple in New York for what we now know to be foster care. During this era, *foster care* involved a couple taking in a child and reporting annually to a religious society about the child's life progress. Mary Ellen was severely physically abused and neglected in this home after the husband died. A neighbor overheard Mary Ellen being harmed and attempted to have a mission worker intervene. The mission worker, Etta Wheeler, was unable to intervene due to the lack of procedures and enforcement of laws to protect children. As such, Henry Bergh and an ASPCA lawyer, Elbridge Gerry, appealed to the New York State Supreme Court to hear the case of Mary Ellen and advocated for protections. A judge found the foster mother guilty of assault and removed Mary Ellen from her care. Mary Ellen subsequently was placed with Etta Wheeler's family, married at 24 years old, had children of her own, and lived to be 92 years old. Her case inspired the formation of the New York Society for the Prevention of Cruelty to Children, believed to be the first organized child protective agency.

The Evolution of the US Child Welfare System

Once the Children's Bureau was formed, federal legislation would lead to the evolution of the modern child welfare system (see **Table 16–1**).[3–5] This included establishment of the first federal funding for child welfare services via the Social Security Act (SSA) of 1935 and Aid to Families with Dependent Children (AFDC) benefits. However, eligibility for AFDC benefits included home suitability requirements. The Flemming Rule of 1961, which required states to provide services to make a home suitable or remove children from unsuitable homes, was a reaction to mass expulsions of needy children from AFDC entitlements by states due to the "suitable homes" clauses.[3] Subsequently, the Flemming Rule and the 1962 Public Welfare Amendments to the SSA triggered increased removal of children from what were deemed to be "unsuitable homes," which were largely homes with unwed mothers and other parents whose behavior was deemed immoral. Additionally, the Child Abuse Prevention and Treatment Act (CAPTA) of 1974, the first major federal legislation addressing child maltreatment, established systems of assessment and identification of child maltreatment, including mandatory reporting. All of these legislative acts expanded the foster care system and led to a rapid increase in the number of children entering out-of-home placements; today, there are about 400,000 children in foster care on any given day and over 200,000 children enter foster care each year in the United States.[6]

The Adoption Assistance and Child Welfare Act of 1980, the basis of the modern child welfare system, established the federal government's role in administration and oversight of child welfare services. It specified

- Federal rules governing child welfare case management, permanency planning, and foster care placement reviews
- The development of state plans on how child welfare services are delivered
- An emphasis on family preservation by making "reasonable efforts" to keep families together through (1) prevention of out-of-home placements by providing services or (2) family reunification as soon as possible
- The creation of Title IV-E Adoption Assistance program, which encouraged adoption of children from the foster care system[3,4]

The Adoption and Safe Families Act (ASFA) of 1997 made more significant changes to the child welfare system by emphasizing child safety when considering family preservation and promoting adoption as a permanency decision through earlier termination of parental rights if reunification was not accomplished within a reasonable time frame.[3] More recently, the Family First Prevention Services Act (FFPSA) of 2018 included historic child welfare reforms with the intention of preventing children from entering foster care by allowing children to remain at home through the increased use of evidence-based and evidence-informed prevention services for parents who can enhance parents' understanding of child development and behavior and promote safety and nurturing. In addition to supporting prevention services (eg, parental mental health services, parental substance use treatment services, and evidence-based parenting interventions), the FFPSA provides more support for kinship caregivers (kinship navigator programs, for example); establishes placement, quality, and oversight requirements for residential treatment programs for youth in care to reduce unnecessary use of congregate care; and allows states to increase the age of youth to remain in care up to age 23 years.

Table 16–1. Timeline of Major Legislation and Historical Events in the Evolution of the Modern Child Welfare System in the United States

Year	Legislation or Historical Event	Impact on Child Welfare
1912	Creation of Children's Bureau	Required to investigate and report on welfare of children; instrumental in reducing infant mortality and ending child labor
1935	Social Security Act (SSA)	Title V, Part 3: Established first federal grants for child welfare services to give states funding for protection and development of child welfare agencies with local programming and services, especially for rural areas Title IV: Established Aid to Dependent Children (ADC) for states to provide cash welfare payments for needy children who lived with a parent or close relative in a suitable home
1961	Flemming Rule	Established that states could not deny ADC benefits to needy children living in unsuitable homes; required states to either (1) provide services to make the home suitable or (2) remove the child from the home and place the child in a suitable placement while providing financial assistance
1962	Public Welfare Amendments	Expanded eligibility for federal foster care; provided that foster care payments could be made directly to foster families, child care institutions, or child placement agencies; formally defined *child welfare services*; renamed ADC to Aid to Families with Dependent Children (AFDC) to expand welfare payments to assist parents in addition to children
1965	Social Security Amendments	Established Medicaid and Medicare programs and included eligibility under Medicaid for children in foster care
1967	Social Security Amendments	Moved child welfare services into a new Title IV-B of the SSA
1974	Child Abuse Prevention and Treatment Act (CAPTA)	Required states to have a system for receiving and responding to child abuse and neglect allegations; established mandatory reporting
1978	Indian Child Welfare Act (ICWA)	Set minimum federal standards for the removal and placement of Native American children to reverse their systematic removal from families and tribes and subsequent placement in non-Native environments; delineated child welfare case jurisdiction between state and tribal governments
1980	Adoption Assistance and Child Welfare Act of 1980	Recognized as the foundation of the modern US child welfare system; foundational in reforming the foster care system by emphasizing family preservation, family reunification, and adoption assistance for those who cannot be reunified
1997	Adoption and Safe Families Act	Emphasized child safety and expedited permanency decisions with the intention of reducing the amount of time children spend in foster care, including allowing states to pursue earlier termination of parental rights to provide release for adoption
2018	Family First Prevention Services Act	Emphasized children remaining in the home to prevent children entering foster care through increasing prevention services delivered to the family

Historical Foundations of Racial Disproportionality and Inequities in the Child Welfare System

Throughout US history, children who are Black, Indigenous, and people of color (BIPOC) have experienced a disproportionate amount of separation from parents, family members, and communities, often due to federal and state policies. When discussing child welfare, it would be remiss to dismiss the history of Black children being taken from their parents and sold during the institution of slavery. Enslaved Black children were dehumanized, considered property of enslavers, and had no rights for child protection. In addition, the history of the people indigenous to the United States should be acknowledged, as they have also experienced significant injustices, including forced displacement, physical and cultural genocide, and parent-child separation, which is discussed further later in the chapter. See Chapter 26, American Indian and Alaska Native Youth, for a detailed discussion of the historical context and trauma regarding the disproportionate number of Indigenous children in the system.

Initially, Black children were excluded from child welfare and protection; however, as key policies were enacted, Black children became overrepresented.[7] During the early periods of exclusion, Black communities often would care for Black children needing support or kinship caregivers.[7] The Flemming Rule became a catalyst in this shift from underprotection to overrepresentation.[8] Despite attempting to correct abuses of the AFDC's home suitability requirements, the Flemming Rule shifted to a focus on neglect, with an emphasis on placing children whose families needed financial assistance into out-of-home care. Consequently, the Flemming Rule was systemically used to oppress and separate Black families experiencing financial difficulties.[8] Furthermore, the mandatory reporting requirements expanded by CAPTA in 1974 led to a system focused on reporting and investigation instead of supporting with service provision. Subsequently, BIPOC children were disproportionality reported to the newly created hotlines.[9] In ensuing years, the war on drugs, its associated stereotypical narratives, and its disproportionate impact on Black families led to further increases in removals and overrepresentation of Black children in the 1980s and 1990s. Additionally, arguments have been made that the AFSA of 1997 has led to disproportionately increased termination of parental rights for Black families instead of the provision of preventive services.[7]

Indigenous children have also experienced unjust and deliberate family unit and tribe separation, especially through placement in Indian boarding schools starting in the early 19th century and lasting until the late 1960s. Thousands of Indigenous children were forced to attend these off-reservation residential schools, which were run by governments and churches. Notably, the stated purpose of these schools was forced cultural assimilation to the European way of life by prohibition of native languages and requiring English to be the language used; prohibition of traditional religions, practices, and ceremonies while promoting Christianity; and prohibition of traditional clothing and hairstyles.[10,11] Additionally, the schools placed children of different tribes together to further force assimilation and destroy traditions. These schools targeted American Indian, Alaska Native, and Native Hawaiian communities. The conditions were harsh, including manual labor by children, and corporal punishment was often employed to enforce school rules.[11] Generations of Indigenous populations were subjected to these schools, which were an integral part of Federal policy to take over tribal territories, resulting in historical trauma and the destruction of Indigenous communities, the legacy of which remains today. Furthermore, studies have shown that childhood attendance at Indian boarding schools was associated with poor adult and future generational health.[12–14]

Indigenous families continued to be systemically separated through the Indian Adoption Project and the Adoption Resource Exchange of North America (ARENA) from 1958 to 1978, during a collaboration between the Bureau of Indian Affairs and the Child Welfare League of America. ARENA became the national program tasked with placing "different" and hard-to-place children, the largest proportion of whom were Indigenous children, followed by children who were Black, Mexican American, older than 2 years of age, or had disabilities.[15] These programs placed Indigenous children with white adoptive families often without understanding the importance of extended family and tribal members in the collective care of Indigenous children.[15,16] It was then recognized during a US Congressional hearing in 1978 that Indigenous children were disproportionally removed from their homes, often unwarranted, with many subsequently placed in non-Native homes. This led to the passage of the Indian Child Welfare Act (ICWA) (see Chapter 26, American Indian and Alaska Native Youth, for details). Briefly, the main components of ICWA include recognizing tribal sovereignty over child welfare proceedings, preservation of Indigenous families, and ensuring tribal connectedness through placement preferences if a child is removed.

In summary, from the beginning of Indian boarding schools through ARENA, US policies resulted in permanently severing numerous generations of Indigenous children from their families and tribes, while ICWA attempts to restore preservation of Indigenous families and tribes.

Contemporary Inequities and Factors Contributing to Racial Disproportionality and Disparities

While Black children make up 14% of the US child population, in 2022 they accounted for 22% of children in the foster care system, which is down from 39% in 2000.[6,17] Indigenous and Latinx children are also overrepresented in the foster care system as compared to their percentage in the general US child population.[6] In addition to historical factors outlined above, recent contributors to racial disproportionality and disparities include structural factors such as the disparate impact of policies, decision-making bias along the child welfare continuum, and inequity in service provision, as well as family-level factors such as poverty, parental incarceration associated with mass incarceration of BIPOC people, and substance use. Furthermore, familial separation is occurring at the US-Mexico border for a new generation of migrant families coming to the United States. A comprehensive framework of disproportionality and disparity affecting Black families in the child welfare system has been developed, which can also be applied to other BIPOC families (See **Figure 16–1**).[18] This framework details how the following factors contribute to disproportionality:

- Disproportionate need
- Human decision-making
- Agency-system factors
- Placement dynamics
- Policy impact[18]

Intersection of Poverty, Substance Use, and Race

The intersection of poverty and race is amplified within the child welfare system, as BIPOC children living in poverty are disproportionally removed from their homes, largely due to neglect reports.[1] Public benefit programs have provided financial support to these families, and states that spend more on these programs have seen reduced rates of child maltreatment and foster care placement.[19,20] However, social service exposure (such as financial assistance programs, food stamps, housing assistance programs, and home visiting programs) among families living in poverty can increase visibility to mandated reporters, leading to potential surveillance bias, which can contribute to the disproportionate numbers of children living in poverty who enter the child welfare system.[21,22]

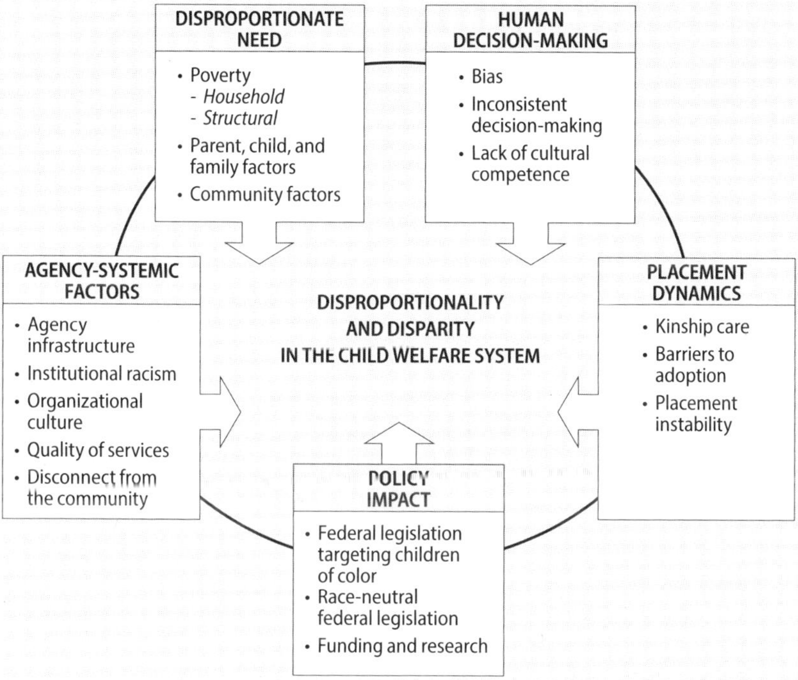

Figure 16–1. Conceptual framework of disproportionality and disparity in the child welfare system that considers disproportionate need, human decision-making, placement dynamics, policy impact, and agency-systemic factors.

Reproduced from Boyd R. African American disproportionality and disparity in child welfare: toward a comprehensive conceptual framework. *Child Youth Serv Rev.* 2014;37:15–27.

Concern about oversurveillance can be a barrier for low-income BIPOC families in applying for needed benefits.[21,23] Given that neglect and parental substance use are the most common reasons for removal (occurring in 63% and 36% of cases, respectively, in 2021[24]), it is important for society to review prevention efforts. If public benefit programs are not robust or equitably delivered, BIPOC children will continue to be disproportionately removed from their families. Comparing and contrasting the general response to the crack cocaine epidemic of the 1980s with the current opioid epidemic starting in the 2010s highlights the differential treatment experienced by Black mothers who have used crack cocaine compared with white mothers who have used opioids.[25] While some states have taken more punitive measures against prenatal opioid use, there is more of an emphasis on connecting mothers using opioids to treatment, and the dehumanization that was experienced by Black mothers who used crack cocaine largely has not existed for mothers using opioids.[25] As a society, we must continue to work toward connecting all pregnant mothers using substances to treatment to reduce the removal of children when appropriate.

Bias Along the Continuum of the Child Welfare Decisions

Bias extends along all decision points within the child welfare system. To understand this bias, one must become structurally competent[26] and assess upstream determinants of decision-making.[27] With this perspective in mind, one can envision how bias at the structural and interpersonal levels has a major role in persistent racial disparities and disproportionality (See **Figure 16–2**). Furthermore, those who make decisions along the continuum of the child welfare system are affected by both external policies and internal child welfare policies. These policies need to be examined within their historical context as well. Along the child welfare decision-making continuum, BIPOC families are more likely to

- Be reported for suspected abuse and/or neglect (oversurveillance, overreporting by clinicians, mandated reporting)
- Proceed to investigation once a report is made
- Have a formal evaluation or medical workup conducted for abuse concerns
- Have an allegation substantiated once an investigation is performed
- Have removal as an outcome of the substantiation determination rather than service provision (for example, substance use disorder treatment, mental health treatment, parenting classes, or support for poverty)[1,18,28,29]

Once in care, BIPOC children are less likely to be reunified with families, less likely to be adopted from foster care, more likely to spend more time in care, more likely to have placement instability, more likely to experience termination of parental rights, and more likely to exit foster care by "aging out" with no permanent caregiver.[1,18]

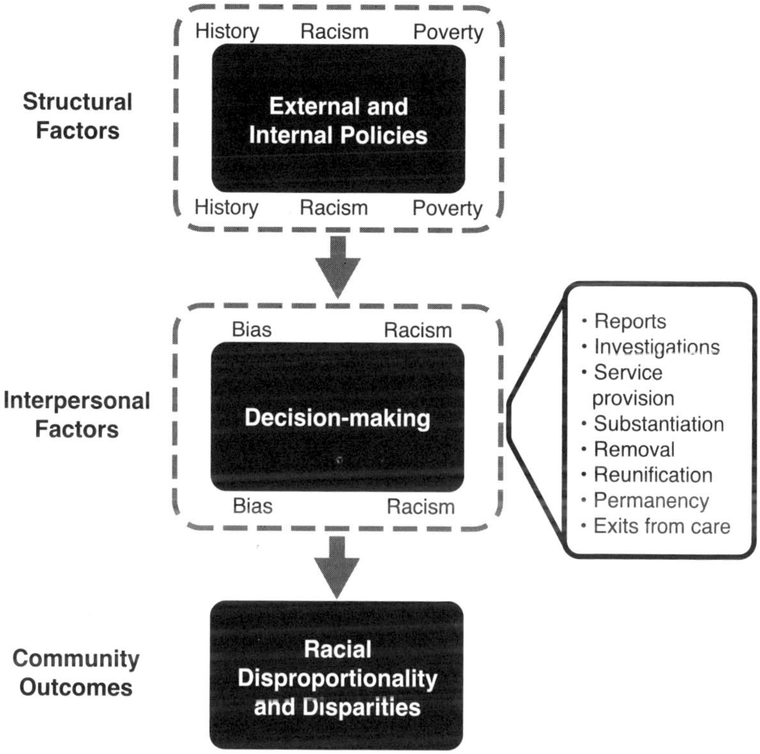

Figure 16–2. Structural and interpersonal factors affected by history, racism, poverty, and bias leading to racial disparities and disproportionality in the child welfare system.

Effect of Disproportionate Representation on Child Health and Well-Being

Disparities and disproportionate representation of BIPOC children in the child welfare system negatively affect children's health and well-being as well as those of their families and communities.[1,30] Disproportionate separation of BIPOC families continues the legacy of historical trauma and further propagates the loss of cultural and racial identity. This can lead to the perpetuation of intergenerational trauma, stress, and epigenetic changes affecting generations of BIPOC communities.[31,32] Furthermore, children describe loss and the harms of removal and placement in foster care.[33,34] Uncertainty and ambiguity dominate the conversations of these children. While the reported intention of the child welfare system is child protection, the experiences of children with lived experience continually demonstrate the failure of the system to protect children from lifelong poor outcomes in health and well-being.

The Need for Equitable Child Welfare Practices

Given this review of historical and contemporary inequities within the child welfare system, there is a critical need for advancing efforts for equitable child welfare practices, including researching and implementing culturally and racially responsive services. Community-based and tribal-based interventions with attention to creating authentic connections between agencies and communities could serve as gateways to providing such services. Additionally, turning attention to reforming policies that continue to perpetuate disparities and disproportionality is important. This involves examining biases that are still long held within the child welfare system and by individuals within that system. Centering the voices of those with lived experience in the child welfare system is paramount to understanding and reforming the system within an equity lens.[35] Without understanding and acknowledging these biases, the same inequities are likely to continue. All children deserve safe, stable, and nurturing relationships, ideally with their family of origin. Given the focus on these parent–child relationships, the importance of equitable prevention efforts, especially those related to families of historically minoritized racial and ethnic groups, impoverished families, and families affected by substance use, becomes more apparent in goals of family preservation. The American Academy of Pediatrics has provided recommendations for child welfare policy reform that promotes equity with a focus on correcting racial injustices:

- Build on the important prevention and family-strengthening goals of the FFPSA to further incentivize agencies to implement prevention programs and reduce child welfare involvement.
- Improve policies and practices related to reporting and investigating child maltreatment.
- Further strengthen federal policies to promote family-centered and family-based care for children and youth in foster care and ensure residential care is used only to meet clinical treatment needs.[36]

The Role of Pediatricians

Pediatricians take an oath to "do no harm." A famous web-throwing, blue and red Marvel character once said, "With great power, there must also come great responsibility." It seems appropriate to reference a superhero when thinking about pediatricians and their roles to serve and protect children. It is important for pediatricians to recognize their own potential bias when providing patient care. Are you more prone to want to involve child protective services if a family is experiencing poverty as opposed to when you have a perception that a family has access to more resources?

It is important to understand the responsibility that accompanies mandated reporting and acknowledge that intended and unintended consequences may occur in the process. A physician's testament of concern holds a great weight in the realm of child protection, with the utmost concern for a patient's safety and well-being. When making reports to child protective services, pediatricians should be transparent with families about concerns and the need to report. However, when a child's safety is not in imminent danger, pediatricians should use every resource available to avoid making a premature report and work with families to assess their needs and encourage parenting practices that promote safe, stable, and nurturing relationships that are culturally relevant. Recommendations have been made whereby pediatricians take an ethical and racially just approach to thoughtful reporting (see **Box 16–3**). These tasks will promote thoughtful reporting and equitable child protection efforts that are likely to reduce inequities in the child welfare system. Pediatricians, as prevention experts, can work to support and strengthen families of origin within their communities and help make child welfare more equitable.

Box 16–3

Thoughtful Mandated Reporting Using an Ethically and Racially Just Lens[37]

- Consider social/cultural context and alternative explanations when worried about child safety.
- Base concerns on evidence when possible.
- Avoid making assumptions and instead seek clarification from families about areas of concern.
- Reduce bias by ensuring internal consistency with reporting.
- Avoid conflating poverty with neglect, and recognize that lack of resources does not equate to not providing care.

Key Takeaways

- Understanding the history of the US child welfare system is important for pediatricians, because historical knowledge aids in the understanding of policy shifts, challenges, inequities, and injustices that have shaped the current landscape, including racial disparities and racial disproportionality, such as the overrepresentation of Black and Indigenous children in the system.
- This history traces a trajectory from early charitable efforts and orphanages to institutional reforms and the evolution of foster care and adoption.
- Contributors to continued disproportionality include structural factors, such as the disparate impact of polices, decision-making bias along the child welfare continuum (from reporting to exiting care), and inequity in service provision, and family-level factors, such as poverty, parental incarceration associated with mass incarceration of BIPOC people, and substance use.
- Pediatricians have a role in promoting more equitable child welfare practices, including taking an ethical, thoughtful, and racially just approach to mandated reporting. These efforts are likely to reduce inequities in the child welfare system and improve overall child health and well-being.

CHAPTER
17

Childhood Trauma and Resilience

Margaret Reynolds
Moira Szilagyi, MD, PhD, FAAP
Heather C. Forkey, MD, FAAP

Introduction

Trauma can be defined as stressful, dangerous, or frightening events either directly experienced or observed by individuals.[1] Whether it be separation from their family of origin or the events leading to separation, the traumas experienced by children in foster/kinship care affect them physically, emotionally, and developmentally.[2] This chapter aims to

- Explain the neurobiological and physiological responses to trauma and how those responses present clinically.
- Explain the role and physiology of the affiliate response in preventing the effects of and promoting recovery from stress.
- Outline what pediatricians can do to uniquely support children in foster/kinship care and their families.

Stress Response

Animals, including humans, evolved to have predictable stress responses enabling them to survive dangerous situations.

- In the freeze response, we become alert and stop moving to avoid detection.
- In the fight-or-flight response, we fight against or run away from threats.
- In the affiliate response, also called *tend and befriend*, we turn to other people for help when faced with threat.[3] The hormone oxytocin enhances our ability to interpret others' facial expressions, body language, and tone of voice, which enables us to determine if those we turn to will be likely to help us.[4] If we perceive safety, we gather others toward us and collectively

manage threat. If we feel threatened and are without affiliate support, we become more distressed, as we face the original threat alone.[5]

As children develop, the affiliate response is often the most effective way for them to manage stressful, new situations.[6–9]

Impact of Stress on Development

Understanding the various stress responses helps to explain why children can experience stress as positive, tolerable, or toxic.[10] Positive stress results from everyday challenges (academic tests, for example) that mildly stimulate stress responses in the context of caregiver support. With affiliate support, children learn to regulate and manage these stressors. Tolerable stress occurs with more significant life events (eg, divorce or the loss of a loved one) that could lead to physiological dysregulation but, when tempered by supportive affiliate relationships, become manageable experiences. Stress hormones take longer to return to homeostasis but eventually do because of caregiver support. Conversely, toxic stress occurs when children experience chronic or severe stressors (eg, abuse) without affiliate support.[10,11] When children without affiliate support face distressing events, their only options are fight, flight, and freeze. Repeated reliance on fight or flight can lead to dysregulation of the hypothalamic-pituitary-adrenal axis, and altered cortisol release may result in hyperarousal. Alternatively, children may freeze, manifesting as dissociation, inattention, or developmental delays.[9] These consequences are not random; they are predictable based on stress-response physiology.[12,13] Systemic and family factors potentially contribute to stress activation (eg, longer exposures to chaotic care, multiple disruptions from attachment figures) and modify gene expression.[6,14]

Clinical Manifestations of the Toxic Stress Response

Adaptation is the process of change over time for an organism to become better suited to its environment. Toxic stress results from alterations of physiology that can improve survival in threatening environments in the short term. Unfortunately, these changes have unfavorable long-term (potentially lifelong) consequences, including alterations in gene transcription, immune function, brain architecture, and connectivity.

Effects of Stress on the Immune System

In toxic stress, altered gene expression activates inflammatory pathways to respond to an injury while allocating fewer resources to fighting off infections.[15] Affected children may be more prone to infection and inflammatory conditions, such as asthma, obesity, metabolic syndrome, and eczema.[16] Children with chronic toxic stress are more likely to experience *sick syndrome*, or a feeling of unwellness precipitated by inflammatory mediators.[17–19] This can be evolutionarily advantageous, as people feeling sick will less frequently leave their homes and encounter predators. However, for children this can lead to problems with immune function, depression, and disruptions in school attendance and social networks.

Effects of Stress on the Brain

Neurodevelopment is highly reliant on the environment, including stressful, protective, and promotive experiences. Neuronal connections and structures developing earlier in life lay the foundation for subsequent development. Early changes thus cascade forward, having profound effects on future behavior.[20]

When children experience trauma without affiliate support, neurodevelopment adapts accordingly. For children in foster care specifically, adaptive changes that occur following traumatic experiences (hypervigilance to predict abusive behaviors, for example) may have maladaptive long-term consequences, such as misperception of neutral experiences as being threatening. Conversely, early supportive environments promote typical neurodevelopment and resilience despite later adversity.[6,11]

Certain behavioral health symptom clusters are commonly experienced by children with toxic stress reactions (see **Table 17–1**). Trauma presents on a spectrum from mild to pervasive (see **Figure 17–1**), based on the severity, frequency, and type of trauma, the child's age and stage of development when trauma occurs, and the presence or absence of promotive factors, such as protective relationships. While not all symptomatic children meet criteria for trauma diagnoses, those who provide medical care to this population should be familiar with the causes and symptoms of adjustment disorder, prolonged grief disorder, and posttraumatic stress disorder (PTSD). Developmental trauma disorder or complex PTSD results from repeated and severe interpersonal victimization without primary caregiver support, a situation more common to children in foster care. Toxic stress has been implicated in potentiating other mental health concerns, such as anxiety, depression, and psychosis. Children in foster care may be more likely to have a genetic risk for mental health concerns comorbid with trauma (eg, bipolar disorder, attention-deficit/hyperactivity disorder [ADHD], or depression).[9] Determining the cause of symptoms and specific diagnoses for children who have experienced significant adversity is challenging. Clinician biases can also lead to the misdiagnosis and underdiagnosis of chronic toxic stress in children, particularly children of color. Children in foster care, especially those from marginalized populations, are more likely to have symptoms ascribed to willful misbehavior rather than expected responses for a child who has experienced trauma.[24,25] Keeping trauma at the top of the differential diagnosis, knowing what to look for, prioritizing cultural humility, and having a toolbox of ways to respond facilitates high-quality care for children in foster care.

Table 17–1. Clinical Presentations Resulting From Toxic Stress[21–23]

Brain Structure	Normal Function	Physiological Change	Clinical Finding	Commonly Misidentified As
Reticular formation/ reticular activating system	Wakefulness	Overactivation	Short term: wakefulness to fight threat Long term: dysregulated sleep	Poor sleep hygiene
Ventromedial hypothalamic nucleus	Satiety	Inhibition	Short term: focus on fighting threat vs gathering/eating food Long term: overeating, food hoarding	Eating disorders; obesity-related eating behaviors
Amygdala	Emotional regulation	Hypertrophy	Short term: strong emotional response to threats to drive fight/flight behaviors; black-and-white thinking Long term: aggressive and impulsive behaviors	Oppositional defiant disorder; conduct disorder; bipolar disorder; ADHD
Hippocampus	Memory; accessing previously learned information	Limited function	Short term: amnesia surrounding the traumatic event Long term: learning difficulties	Academic challenges; learning disabilities; processing disorders
Prefrontal cortex	Executive function	Decreased connectivity with and regulation of other brain regions; delayed maturation	Short term: hypervigilance; black-and-white thinking Long term: impulsive behaviors; decreased inhibitory control; poor problem-solving	ADHD; oppositional defiant disorder; conduct disorder

Abbreviation: ADHD, attention-deficit/hyperactivity disorder.

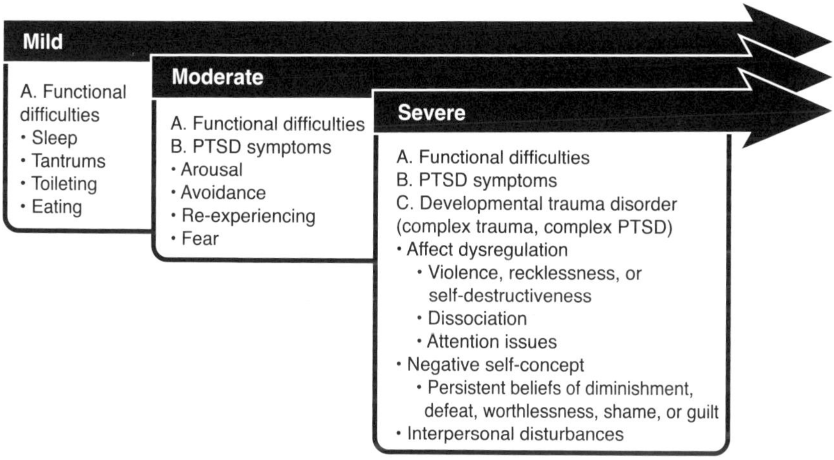

Figure 17–1. Spectrum of trauma symptoms.

Pediatric Clinical Response

Children heal from trauma via safe, stable, and nurturing caregiving relationships. The role of the pediatrician is to be a reliable resource for families and to nurture the caregiver–child relationship. As outlined in **Table 17–2**, the WITH mnemonic (Wonder, Investigate, Treat, Hope) provides the structure for this work, mapping onto the SOAP mnemonic (Subjective, Objective, Assessment, Plan) used in clinical practice. WITH begins by creating an environment in which children and families feel both physically and emotionally safe. Safety is the foundation of healing because one must feel safe to activate the affiliate structures of the brain.

Wonder

Children in foster care, along with caregivers, often present in a prolonged activated state of fight or flight. They may be physiologically unable to access higher brain processing and complex language. By remaining calm, attuned, and responsive, we can create the safety that enables families to move from fight or flight into thinking, learning, and better-regulated brain networks.

Wondering together with families builds trusting relationships in which they can feel safe and believe their clinician understands their perspective and the context of their lives. Just as caregivers can modulate children's stress responses with affiliate support, clinicians help patients and caregivers

Table 17–2. WITH Approach

Stage	Key Concepts	Concrete Action Items
Wonder	Engagement	Use verbal and nonverbal cues to signal safety, remembering that both nonverbal cues and language may vary across cultures.
		Ask open-ended questions to gain the perspective of the child and caregiver on the child's situation and symptoms.
		Share power.
Investigate	Surveillance and screening	Look for evidence that the child cannot access the affiliate response.
		Ask standard, open-ended questions about recent life changes.
		Use validated and population-specific screening tools to identify trauma-related symptoms and comorbid conditions.
		Be prepared to explain to families how and why screening tools are used as well as what results indicate and the corresponding indicated interventions.
Treat	Validation and normalizing of symptoms in context of trauma; providing indicated trauma-informed guidance and referrals	Synthesize all collected information to reach a diagnosis or diagnoses, and be familiar with trauma symptoms and diagnostic criteria for trauma disorders.
		Validate the child's and caregivers' emotions.
		Normalize the child's response to trauma (eg, "This is a normal response to an abnormal event—the trauma").
		Teach 3 Rs approach (reassurance, routines, and regulation).
		Provide recommendations for and warm handoffs to supports and referrals.
		Follow up regularly with patients and families to ensure they do not "fall through the cracks".
		Coordinate care.
Hope	Discussion and reassurance	Empower families by providing a diagnosis and/or language they can use to describe what is going on.
		Encourage families that things will get better and that there is hope for recovery, leveraging concepts like neuroplasticity.

modulate their stress. This can be especially critical for caregivers who carry the effects of their own experience of trauma, including intergenerational trauma. The idea of "angels" or "ghosts" in the nursery has been suggested in the literature, meaning that caregivers' responses to their children can often be derived from their own experience of being parented, for better or worse.[26,27] Regulating one's emotions may not come naturally to many caregivers, given their own past experiences, making this a challenging skill to model for the children in their care. However, it is important for clinicians to support caregivers in developing and modeling these skills to prevent the perpetuation of further trauma and harm. Reminding caregivers of their experiences of feeling safe and cared for (even if it was not with their own parents) and of experiences that they would not want to recreate with their own children can help parents mindfully approach their own work of parenting. To do this, we develop trust by using intentional linguistic, verbal, and nonverbal cues to communicate signals of safety, support, empathy, and curiosity.[28,29]

Intentional Language

For pediatricians, intentional language is familiar territory. We enter a patient's room by clearing our minds of the day's stressors and demands so we can be fully present. We greet the child, and subsequently greet the adults present, clarifying their roles. We introduce ourselves and anyone accompanying us. We ask about their concerns using sincere, open-ended questions, which provide insight into the child's situation and enable the family to control what information they share and how they share it. *Sharing power* means asking families about their priorities, what is most concerning to them, and what supports or interventions have or have not worked.[30]

We acknowledge and validate the emotions associated with concerns, while reinforcing the connection between trauma and symptoms, normalizing them. This delinks symptoms from intentionality or fault of the child. We validate that, even if the child is not to blame, these symptoms are still disruptive, concerning, or even frightening.

We must remain attuned to verbal and nonverbal cues that give insight into whether families feel comfortable or distressed—safe or unsafe. We can match our affect to the family's to empathize with their emotions without their intensity. For example, when a caregiver complains about the child's dysregulated sleep, matching the volume of their voice and gradually lowering to conversational pitch allows the parent to feel heard as we help them to regulate their emotions. Mirroring the family's wording reinforces that we hear them and demonstrates alignment between the clinician and family.[28,29,31]

We must also approach families with structural and cultural humility and seek to understand how systems, experiences, and culture affect their interpretation of what has happened and what might be helpful. Language interpreters and cultural brokers should be offered. Culture is not limited to one's race or ethnicity but extends to other sociodemographic identities, including religion, geography, socioeconomic status, immigrant status, and many others.

Verbal and Nonverbal Cues of Safety

In addition to *what* we say to patients, *how* we say it also promotes feelings of safety, which is fundamental to engagement and healing. *Neuroception* is the unconscious perception of threat or safety in our environment, and families with trauma histories may be particularly attuned to pick up on danger signals.[32]

Low-pitched sounds are perceived as being dangerous, while higher-pitched musical sounds and voices (such as "parentese") are soothing.[28] By maintaining a relaxed and slightly higher-pitched tone, clinicians appear less threatening to children who may be overwhelmed or scared in clinical settings. Children who have experienced trauma may misidentify fearful, anxious, or neutral facial expressions as anger or aggression. This extends to microexpressions, or smaller, subconscious facial expressions we make while listening or thinking. While unintentional, these can be perceived as lack of interest and may contribute to distrust. Closed body language (for example, crossed arms or turning away) can be interpreted as a lack of respect.[28,33] This reiterates the importance of being fully present when we enter an examination room. When culturally appropriate, maintaining eye contact, keeping an open posture, and leaning in communicate active listening and receptivity to what families are saying.

We must also watch for patient and caregiver interactions and reactions during the conversation. That information allows us to most appropriately engage in the context of the parent–child relationship. We should use simple, developmentally appropriate language, avoiding medical terminology. Traumatized children may be functionally younger than their chronological age because of how trauma affects brain development. However, youth, especially those of color, may experience adultification by caregivers and clinicians, when they are mischaracterized as being older than their chronological age and when others do not consider the effects of trauma on brain development. Similarly, if families appear frustrated or apprehensive, we may need to acknowledge their distress and explore options to ensure they retain a sense of control.

Investigate

In addition to gathering subjective information while wondering with the patient and family, collecting objective information about experiences, behaviors, and symptoms via screening, surveillance, examination, and diagnostic procedures is also important.

A Note About ACE Surveys

The Adverse Childhood Experience (ACE) questionnaire was designed for population research to determine the association between childhood adversities and adult health outcomes. ACE questionnaires are not validated clinical screening instruments and do not have predictive value at the individual level. There are no psychometric properties and clinical cutoff scores that help a clinician make clinical decisions for individual patients. Using ACE survey scores, especially in isolation, can result in missed opportunities to identify and address developmental, mental health, behavioral, educational, and functional symptoms resulting from early exposure.[34–40] Without adequate patient preparation, validation, and clinical utility, implementing ACE questionnaires clinically can be detrimental.[41–44]

Surveillance

Surveillance is "a flexible, continuous process whereby knowledgeable professionals [perform] skilled observations of children during the provision of health care."[9] This includes open-ended questions such as "Has anything scary happened to you or your child since the last visit?" or "Has anyone come or gone from the household lately?"[9,45] These create opportunities to discuss traumatic or relevant experiences. Questions about caregivers' concerns around behavior, sleep, eating, mood, and developmental milestones provide insight into how trauma is affecting their child's functioning. It is important to understand the child's functioning across usual childhood environments: home, child care, school, and with peers.

Screening

Screening is "the use of a standardized, validated tool to identify risk and determine the need for further evaluation."[46] Validated screening instruments are used to identify patients' risk of developing conditions or requiring services (eg, evidence-based trauma therapy). Atypical or concerning results on commonly used validated screeners for mental health and development should raise trauma as a diagnostic possibility. For children in foster care, screening with validated PTSD or trauma symptoms screening tools that include questions about experiences and symptoms is considered standard of care. (See Chapter 11, Screenings, and Chapter 12, Mental Health.)

Promoting Safety

Pediatricians must be intentional and establish safety when conducting surveillance and screening (see the earlier discussion in the section on "Wonder"). Having protocols for conducting screening ensures that families and staff understand how and why screening is being done.[47] Pediatricians should be prepared to review results with families and offer support in response to positive findings. Pediatricians should use screening instruments developed for the age, primary language, and risk level of their patient. Tools should have psychometric properties and be predictive at an individual level. When screening for childhood trauma in children in foster care, screening instruments ideally assess a child's strengths, symptoms, risk level, and current functioning.[47] Chapter 12, Mental Health, provides more details about the validated screening tools for PTSD and traumatic stress symptoms in the pediatric population and how to use these tools in clinical practice.

Trauma in children and adolescents may manifest as developmental, learning, behavioral, and mental health problems. Traumatic stress may not only result in PTSD or developmental trauma disorder but can also mimic or be comorbid with other behavioral health disorders, like attention-deficit/hyperactivity disorder, depression, and anxiety. Behavioral and mental health screening tools commonly used in many pediatric settings (eg, Vanderbilt ADHD Diagnostic Rating Scale, Screen for Child Anxiety Related Disorders, commonly known as SCARED) and developmental screening tools can be used in concert with the trauma-symptom screening tools to determine whether further diagnostic testing is needed to discriminate among these diagnoses and better direct management.[33]

Although physical health is affected by toxic stress, there are no biomarkers routinely recommended or clinically available. Pediatricians should consider whether physical symptoms and medical diagnoses are stress related, since families may prevent and manage flares of illnesses (eg, eczema, asthma) if they understand how stress affects their symptoms. Considerable research efforts are underway, and there is hope that biomarkers will be available soon.[48]

Treat

Treat maps onto the Assessment and Plan components of SOAP. Treating begins with using the information from Wondering and Investigating to name how trauma is affecting the child. By validating the patient's experience and normalizing their symptoms, we demonstrate affiliate support. Only then can we discuss a plan, including advice and tools provided in-office and treatments or services accessed by referral. Early response and treatment can lead to better long-term outcomes by building life skills and positively affecting cascading neurodevelopment.

Validate

After a patient identifies a history of trauma, it is important to pause and validate what we have been told before moving on. By using phrases like "I'm sorry that this happened to you" or "This is never supposed to happen to a child," we communicate empathy and begin to address what can be the "elephant in the room"—the trauma that has occurred. Using the phrase "I can understand" or "I understand" is not validating and often seen as not empathic, given that we cannot truly understand the unique circumstances that our patients have or are going through.

Psychoeducation and Normalizing

Pediatricians should directly name the trauma (if it is known to the child and caregivers) and its significance in relation to their symptoms. Verbalizing these effects reduces the stigma, guilt, and shame associated with discussing traumatic experiences. Pediatricians can normalize these responses with reassurance that the behavioral or health concerns are not uncommon after trauma. These are normal physiological responses to things that *happened to* the child or teen and do not mean that something is *wrong with* them.[33]

Many children in foster care are cared for by kin (actual or fictive), including aunts, uncles, grandparents, and family friends; additional time may be necessary to process and normalize the feelings of kin caregivers. Many may feel guilty that their loved one harmed or neglected the children or that they did not know or intervene sooner, or they may be distressed that child welfare is interfering in familial relationships. They may feel burdened by being cast in the role of caregiver or experience grief over the change in their life plans.[2,49–51] We can help kin caregivers by validating their feelings and normalizing their responses as reasonable.[52]

Trauma-Informed Guidance

During office visits, pediatricians can describe ways the caregiver can make a child feel safe, enabling them to escape the immediate negative consequences of the stress response. The "3 Rs" approach (reassurance, routines, and regulation) outlines this process.[9]

Caregivers can reassure children that they are safe through verbal messages of safety, such as "You are safe here." They can offer developmentally appropriate and trauma-informed comforting touch, such as hugs or rocking them in their arms.[31] For toddlers and older children, caregivers can use a heavy blanket or tent in the child's room to create a safe place. Reading with the child and using resources that address safety, safe spaces, and managing emotions (Sesame Street in Communities, for example) can promote safety.

Routines create predictability, an important part of safety for children who have lived in chaotic environments. We can recommend building predictability for meals, sleep, and playtime to minimize stressful surprises. Any changes in routine should be communicated to the child in advance so they can mentally prepare for the event. Caregivers must also prepare children for upcoming visits with parents and have a reentry routine that matches their temperament, such as time to be quiet or run off energy. Creating predictable environments builds trust between caregivers and children.[29,31]

Regulation is the process of gaining mastery over emotions and behaviors so individuals can engage in goal-directed activities. Regulation develops as children learn to identify, understand, control, and modulate emotions. The idea of changing their feelings may be new to children.[31] Pediatricians should model age-appropriate techniques for children in the office if they feel overwhelmed (focused breathing, muscle relaxation, and calming movements, for example) and teach these to caregivers to model and reinforce at home.[53] Children can only discuss their feelings if they can accurately identify and name them. Children take cues from caregivers, so caregivers remaining calm is crucial to regulation, as is looking at behaviors from the child's perspective, with the caregiver being a "feelings detective." Reading and watching shows with children provide opportunities to discuss what characters are feeling and how they manage their emotions. Children can practice their emotions through imaginative play and talk about emotions when they are calm.

Time-in is an opportunity for the child to pick an activity and the caregiver to pick a time they can focus on the child exclusively. Setting a timer for just 5 or 10 minutes, the caregiver and child have an opportunity to play or engage in a shared activity. Time-in can be prescribed and reviewed. Often the child is well regulated during time-in but may worsen in the hours after, suggesting that the child has gotten at least some of the support they need to regulate. Touching base with the caregiver to explain that behavioral response, and to find ways to extend time-in, will help.

Because children in foster care have experienced significant trauma, they often require a unique management approach. The AAP now recommends trauma-informed care as the universal approach to pediatric care.[33] The affiliate-centered approach (SHARE [Safety, Hurry, Attachment, Regulation, Efficiency]) is best suited for caring for children in foster care because it ensures collaboration between the clinician, caregiver, and patient, and grounds all interventions in keeping the child out of a fight or flight state (see **Table 17–3**).

Table 17–3. Trauma-Informed Approach to Managing Children in Foster Care[9]

Trauma-Informed Approach (SHARE)	
Safety	Start by emphasizing that the child will need to feel safe; describe caregiver responses to shut down stress response (eg, reassurance, routines, regulation [especially relaxation skills]).
Hurry	Identify immediate priorities vs those interventions that can wait a few days/weeks for referral to outside agencies. For example, a child who is self-harming or suicidal requires an immediate response, while a child with significant tantrums but who is otherwise safe may be able to wait for outpatient care.
Attachment	Recognize that the child may not yet have developed a trusting relationship with their new caregiver, even when that person is responsive, nurturing, and caring. The relationship may be short-term (not stable). Some therapeutic modalities require stability before therapy can begin as the continuity over time is crucial to supporting the attachment relationship. Discuss ways the caregiver can promote safety and nurture the child by holding the child's emotions, remaining available to the child physically and psychologically, being an attuned listener, and considering the child's perspective in day-to-day situations (see Regulation).
Regulation	A child who is dysregulated can lead to a disrupted placement. It can help to teach the caregiver ways to calm the child's stress responses (3 Rs, attuned listening, remaining calm, considering the child's perspective). Validate the caregiver's concerns, offer education about supporting the child, and build regulation skills.
Efficacy	Children in foster care and their caregivers often feel that courts, child welfare, and birth parents have more say than they do—that events happen to them and they have little or no agency. Support the caregiver's and child's coping abilities, their capacity to manage their emotions in response to events, and their ability to have some influence over their environment (in developmentally appropriate ways). Open communication and close follow-up can create opportunities for the family to check in with us for guidance and other help.

Abbreviation: 3 R's, Reassurance, Routines, and Regulation.

Referral Options

When referring patients to outside clinicians or integrated supports from mental health or social work, providing a warm handoff maximizes follow-up.[54] Describing the referral and introducing the family to the care partner directly removes the stress associated with meeting new clinicians. Families take cues from us just as children do from parents: if they feel safe in our settings, they can extend those feelings to new resources. We can also connect families to online and community mental health resources. For children needing evidence-based therapy, we can explain what the treatment offers and refer to clinicians who can help children process their trauma.[33] Communication with child welfare is necessary, may help facilitate the referral, and can streamline communication and collaboration among clinicians.

Pediatricians must consider multiple factors when directing children toward treatments for trauma. The interventions a child receives are often influenced by availability and accessibility. Intentionality is important when selecting interventions, even when choices are limited by local resource constraints. **Table 17–4** provides an overview of some services that may be appropriate for specific children in foster care and their caregivers. See Chapter 12, Mental Health, for information about evidence-based trauma therapies. Pediatricians can list evidence-based treatments available in their communities and work with child welfare and resource providers to develop systems for referral and communication.

Table 17–4. Spectrum of Services[31,55–62]

Type of Service	Example Service(s)	Goal(s) of Service
PTSD prevention treatment (after exposure, before symptoms)	Child and Family Traumatic Stress Intervention (CFTSI)	Prevention of PTSD after child has experienced a trauma through family
Foster parent-specific trainings	Resource Parent Curriculum (RPC); Attachment, Regulation, and Competency (ARC) Grow	Training and support for foster parents to promote understanding and response to traumatic reactions in children
Occupational therapy	Sessions focused on play, activities of daily living	Kids struggling with lower brain effects
Behavioral modification-specific treatment	Dialectical Behavior Therapy (DBT); Collaborative Problem Solving	Behavior modification, calming of dysregulation
Attunement therapies focused on building supportive relationships	Parent–Child Interaction Therapy (PCIT), Child–Parent Psychotherapy (CPP)	Promotes caregiver coregulation of child
Cognitive behavioral therapies	Eye Movement Desensitization and Reprocessing (EMDR) therapy; Trauma-Focused Cognitive Behavioral Therapy (TF-CBT)	Allows child to take trauma out of the lower brain, process in higher brain so it loses its ability to continue to harm the child
Complex trauma therapy	ARC; Neurosequential Model	Addresses the multiple ways that complex trauma affects children by first addressing lower brain concerns (safety, attachment, regulation) and later higher brain processes (processing experience, developing competency)

Abbreviation: PTSD, posttraumatic stress disorder

Follow-up and Care Coordination

Pediatricians should regularly follow up with patients, even after providing referrals. Creating care management lists that generate reminders to check in by phone or telehealth between visits can identify failed referrals, new symptoms, changes in caregivers, visitation, or education settings that can derail care and worsen symptoms. Foster care is laden with transitions and unpredictability; children easily fall through the cracks. Proactive follow-up and care coordination are essential to ensuring children and caregivers get the services they need in a timely manner and to minimizing fragmentation in care.

Hope

Ultimately, children in foster care and their families hope for healing and a positive future. At the end of each visit, families should feel optimistic. That said, hope is not the final step in the WITH paradigm; rather, it is an integral part of each step. Providing the family with words for what is happening, even without a specific diagnosis, can alleviate fear and offer hope. The affiliate stress response is grounded in physiology and provides the hope for healing. The physical, developmental, emotional, and behavioral consequences of trauma can be confusing and worrisome if not framed in the context of the physiological responses to stress. As we move to treatment, we are providing hope by giving clear reassurance that there are interventions and supports available to help the child process and recover from their trauma.

Children's developing brains can be shaped by toxic stress, but the converse is also true. Neuroplasticity explains how children overcome challenges with help from their caregivers and other adults (such as educators, child care, and mental health professionals). Plasticity is present throughout childhood and adolescence and into adulthood, providing hope for improvement with healing relationships and interventions. Since puberty is the second most active period of brain development and the brain only fully matures in the mid-20s, it is never too late to support a child. For medical professionals, caring for children in foster care is essentially fostering the hope of recovery through buffering relationships that leverage the healing of the affiliate response and the plasticity of children's brains. This prepares them to return to a safer, more stable home setting or find belonging in a kinship or adoptive home.

Key Takeaways

- » The affiliate response is a biological stress response that can be leveraged through safe, stable, nurturing caregiving to promote healing after trauma.
- » The effects of trauma on the brain and the body that cascade from the lack of safe, nurturing caregiving manifest as predictable behavioral, developmental, learning, physical, and mental health symptoms in children.
- » These toxic stress symptoms result from underlying physiological injury.
- » Pediatricians have a crucial role in recognizing and responding to trauma, including working "WITH" families to identify and manage the downstream sequelae of children's trauma and connecting families to services to promote healing.
- » Children in foster care are disproportionately vulnerable to toxic stress, as they have experienced inconsistent and unpredictable caregiving and the disruption of their primary attachment relationships. This is compounded by the increased likelihood of experiencing unstable placement while in foster care. Stability in the care of a safe, responsive caregiver is fundamental to healing. Pediatricians have the knowledge and skills to educate and support caregivers in dampening the child's stress responses and nurturing their affiliate response. High-quality caregiving and evidence-based interventions can leverage neuroplasticity to help change the negative behavioral, developmental, and health outcomes of trauma in children.

CHAPTER

18

Out-of-Home Placements

Lindsay Terrell, MD, FAAP
Katherine A. Ariano, MSN, RN, CCM, SANE-A, SANE-P
Sabrina Darwiche, MD, MPH

Introduction

There are different types of out-of-home placements (OHPs), with the most common forms being kinship care and licensed foster care; children may also be placed in therapeutic homes, group homes, or residential treatment facilities. Each form of OHP is associated with a unique set of strengths and weaknesses to address the medical, mental, and developmental health needs of children during the pursuit of permanency. Visitation with the family of origin during a child's time in OHP is another important consideration. Through thoughtful assessment and planning, physicians caring for children in foster care can assist all types of placement providers with the child's care and therefore assist with placement stability.

Overview of Legislation Related to Placement Types

The goal for all youth involved in the child welfare system is a safe, permanent home. In recent decades, this goal has expanded to include family preservation, leading to a greater emphasis on kinship care. This shift was facilitated by legislation such as the 1997 Adoption and Safe Families Act, which required states to give preference to family when considering OHP.[1] Despite this preference, adult relatives were often unaware that a child had been removed from a home, prompting the passage of the 2008 Fostering Connections to Success and Increasing Adoptions Act, which requires child welfare agencies to notify and explain all placement possibilities to all adult relatives within 30 days of a child's removal.[2] The emphasis on family preservation was taken even further with the 2018 Family First Prevention Services Act, which shifted funding from foster care to prevention services, including mental health services, substance use treatment, and in-home parenting training—all in an effort to reduce the rates of entry into OHP.[3] Presently, placement is mandated to be in the least restrictive environment to meet the child's needs, with 44% of children residing in nonrelative foster care and 35% residing in kinship foster care.[4] Chapter 42, Advocacy and Public Policy, includes further information on OHP legislation.

Placement Types

Placement type is an important factor in health and overall outcomes. In this section, kinship care, foster care, therapeutic homes, and residential care are outlined, followed by a discussion of outcomes across placement types.

Kinship Care

Kinship care refers to when a child resides with adult kin instead of their parent; it is the most common form of OHP, with approximately 4.3 million children in kinship care according to 2022 census data.[5] Each state defines *kin* differently, but typically it refers to a relative or an adult known to the family. While this community approach to child rearing has occurred for millennia, its more recent intersection with the child welfare system necessitates further categorization into 3 subgroups: private kinship care, informal kinship care, and formal kinship care.

Private kinship care is the removal of a child from their home and placement with adult kin without the involvement of the child welfare system. This is theorized to be the most common form of kinship care, but data are limited given the lack of involvement with a formal surveillance system. In comparison, placement in informal kinship care (sometimes referred to as *diversion kinship care*) occurs after an investigation by the child welfare system but without the child being placed in child welfare custody. This is in contrast to the 130,000 children in formal kinship care, in which a child welfare agency takes formal custody of a child.[4] Kin involved in formal kinship care may or may not be licensed foster parents. Assessments by child welfare agencies to ensure appropriateness of placement vary across jurisdictions. Qualifications can include passing a home assessment and the absence of a prior personal criminal or child welfare history. In some jurisdictions, informal kinship placements are associated with a lower level of screening.[6] Training requirements vary by type of kinship care and jurisdiction. In some instances, kinship caregivers may not receive any specific training before the child enters their home.

While there is significant state-by-state variation in the implementation of kinship care, the legislative emphasis on family preservation has led to a nationwide push toward kinship care as the goal OHP, as reflected in the increasing proportion of foster care placements that are with kin.[4,7] This stems from the belief that kinship care "enables children to live with persons whom they know and trust, reduces the trauma children may experience when they are placed with persons who are initially unknown to them, and reinforces children's sense of identity and self-esteem, which flows from their history and culture."[8] Despite these perceived benefits, it is important to note that kinship caregivers typically are older, have poorer health, have lower levels of educational attainment, have a lower income, and are more likely to live in an underserved or marginalized neighborhood.[9–11] Additionally, compared with nonrelative foster care, kinship caregivers receive less formal supervision, training, support services, and financial assistance.[11,12] So, while kinship care is generally believed to be the preferred OHP, the inequitable support received by kinship caregivers has significant implications for a child's health and permanency outcomes. However, the Administration for Children and Families announced in 2023 an attempt to address this inequity in the form of new regulations that would allow kinship caregivers to adhere to different foster care licensing standards, thereby increasing access to financial resources equivalent to those for nonkin placements.[13]

Licensed Foster Care

Licensed foster care refers to placement of a child in child welfare custody with a licensed or certified foster parent (also known as resource parents). Given the legislative push toward kinship care, nonrelative foster care is typically pursued only if no appropriate kinship caregiver is available. Approximately 44% of children in child welfare custody live with a licensed foster parent.[4] **Table 18-1** provides an overview of the strengths and challenges of each OHP type.

Foster parents complete specific training before receiving a license from their state to provide care for children in foster care. This training, usually 30 to 40 hours, is designed to equip prospective foster parents with the knowledge, skills, and tools necessary to provide quality care to traumatized children and adolescents. Topics covered can include child development, trauma-informed care, communication techniques, discipline strategies, cultural sensitivity, and legal aspects of child welfare. Additionally, licensing requirements may include a background check, a home fire inspection, and home visits with a social worker.

Table 18–1. Strengths and Challenges by Out-of-Home Placement Type

	Kinship (Nonlicensed)	Licensed Foster
Strengths	• Known to child; familiarity • Cultural identity promoted • Medicaid • Child care assistance	• Training and ongoing education support • Monthly stipend per child • Medicaid • Child care assistance
Challenges	• Typically no monthly stipend per child • Lack of training and ongoing education support	• Cultural identity of child may differ from foster family • Unknown to child; lack of familiarity

The foster care licensing process varies by location and agency. For example, some counties may train and license local foster families themselves while other counties may rely on private agencies. Regardless of how a foster parent is licensed, the process typically emphasizes the importance of providing a safe, stable, and nurturing environment that promotes the overall well-being and development of children in foster care, as well as encouraging the importance of reunification and co-parenting when possible.

Due to this extensive onboarding process, foster parents may have access to more extensive support services and resources compared with unlicensed kinship caregivers. For example, foster parents may receive more training on the effects of trauma and need for mental health therapy or local resources for children with developmental delay. Foster parents receive a monthly, age-based stipend per child: the older the child, the higher the stipend. Typically, this stipend comes as a monthly check that the foster parents can use at their discretion (eg, for school supplies, clothing, recreational outings, or child care). Many foster parents state that without this assistance, providing care for a child could cause a significant financial strain. Kinship providers can become licensed foster parents and have access to the same level of support.

Therapeutic Homes

Therapeutic homes, also known as treatment or medical foster homes, are a type of foster care placement geared toward serving children with greater medical, developmental, or mental health needs, while allowing those children to remain in a family environment rather than an institutional setting. Examples of children who may be placed in a therapeutic home include those with medical conditions requiring equipment (such as a gastrostomy tube) and children with autism spectrum disorder who need supports to complete activities of daily living. Determination of therapeutic foster home placement is guided by social service assessments, which may include professional input from licensed mental health and medical clinicians. Foster parents for therapeutic homes must complete several additional hours of training to be considered appropriately equipped to care for these children. Given the increased needs of this subset of children in foster care, therapeutic foster homes can obtain a higher monthly stipend compared with nontherapeutic foster homes. Therapeutic foster homes are generally available, via private agencies, to children in foster care; however, this varies among states.

Group Homes and Residential Treatment Facilities

Placement outside of a home environment may be described by a variety of terms. *Group home* and *residential treatment center* differentiate the 2 main types of congregate or institutional care. All of these terms refer to a placement type in which "professional caregivers are entrusted to look after the daily care and welfare" of children in OHP; this type of setting is generally considered more restrictive and intensive than in-home placements.[14,15]

A meta-analysis comparing children in non-kinship foster care placements with those in residential treatment found that placement in a home environment may facilitate better outcomes for children than placement in residential treatment.[16] However, there are potentially subsets of children for whom residential treatment or group care is the best option at a specific point in time because they may benefit from being in a nonfamily setting. Children who are in acute and severe distress, as well as those who are not coping well in a family environment (due to their previous experiences, for example) may benefit from residential care, such as group homes.[16] There are also group homes that exist for specific populations in foster care (eg, pregnant or parenting teens, those involved with the criminal justice system) and can assist with care tailored toward their particular situation. While every child deserves a home, some studies have found that children placed in group care do have good outcomes if there is positive caregiving and a holistic organizational structure.[16]

The 2018 Family First Prevention Services Act aimed to strike a balance between minimizing the number of non-family OHPs and meeting a child's potential placement needs by creating several categories of allowable nonfamily placement settings.[17] These include placements for pregnant or parenting youth, placements for youth involved with sex trafficking, and a model known as Qualified Residential Treatment Programs (QRTPs). QRTPs are accredited placements that must meet certain standards of care to ensure the placement is appropriate, is time-limited, and meets the child's treatment needs.[17]

Impact of Placement Characteristics on Health Outcomes

Data on medical, mental health, behavioral, and educational outcomes by placement type are summarized in the following sections. Regardless of placement type, placement stability is an important factor in health outcomes. By being proactive and thoughtful in terms of resource and referral connections, the physician caring for children in OHPs may help reduce placement disruption, thereby helping to ensure the health and well-being of this vulnerable population.

Medical

Comparing medical needs and outcomes across placement types is challenging. Studies show mixed findings, and it appears that both kinship and foster care show similar medical outcomes.[18] Children in foster care have high rates of undiagnosed or untreated medical conditions and face many barriers to receiving high-quality, timely, comprehensive health care. One study found that the number of placement changes a child experiences is significantly associated with more health care use, both planned and unplanned.[19] Additionally, children who experience multiple placement changes, are placed out of county, or are placed in underserved OHPs may struggle to access timely and consistent health supervision and subspecialty visits.

Clinicians should pay close attention to previously missed routine screenings (such as lead and hemoglobin), prescribed medications, past medical histories, possible undiagnosed diseases, and sexually transmitted infection testing in all children in OHPs. In addition, physicians can decrease the burden on families by offering a flexible visit schedule, assisting with mental health referrals, and providing a thorough after-visit summary.

Mental Health

Mental health outcomes are an important consideration, especially in the context of the traumas experienced by children in foster care, 80% of whom are estimated to have a mental health need of some kind.[20] Research comparing mental health outcomes across placement types has been limited by a lack of standardized measures. Nevertheless, a 2009 meta-analysis suggested that children in kinship care were twice as likely to experience positive emotional health as those in nonrelative foster care, while children in nonrelative foster care were twice as likely to experience mental illness.[21] Of note, while children in group homes or residential placements represent a minority of OHPs, these placements are designed and predominantly care for adolescents with significant mental illness.[22]

The seemingly protective effect of kinship care on mental health has been attributed to the stability and familiarity of a relative caregiver. However, studies also suggest that the perceived difference is reflective of a selection bias. Kinship caregivers may know the child through previous contacts and therefore may be less likely to provide OHP for children with severe mental illness and instead provide care only to children whom they can manage.[23,24] Furthermore, most children in kinship care are in private kinship care and therefore not system involved, potentially excluding them from surveillance of mental health outcomes. This is supported by research demonstrating that children in kinship care have lower utilization rates of mental health services related to access issues.[25]

Regardless of placement type, children who experience placement volatility have higher rates of externalizing and internalizing behavioral problems. Conversely, "behavioral problems [are] the highest risk factor associated with placement moves."[15] This suggests that poor mental health is both a cause and a consequence of placement disruption, further illustrating the need for permanency.[26]

Behavioral Health

Behavioral health is an important area for clinicians to assess. Children placed in kinship homes tend to have fewer behavioral issues, while their counterparts placed in foster homes tend to have greater behavioral and mental health needs.[15] A 2004 study found that placement disruptions of children in foster care increase as the number of problematic behaviors a child exhibits increases.[27] The study found a 17% hazard of disruption "for every child problem behavior reported," and this percentage increased when children were placed in nonrelative homes.[27] There is a threshold of behaviors that caregivers are able and willing to tolerate. Importantly, the likelihood of placement disruption was correlated with the number of children in the home—in other words, the threshold of problematic child behaviors may be lowered when a caregiver (kinship or nonkinship) has multiple children in the home.[27]

Assessment and management of impacts of trauma and behavioral health concerns are discussed in Chapter 12, Mental Health, and Chapter 17, Childhood Trauma and Resilience. It is important to note that behavioral health issues are a risk factor for placement disruptions. By being proactive in addressing behavioral problems in the context of childhood trauma, the clinician can be an asset in reducing disruption of foster placements.

Developmental Health

The presence of a developmental disability, among other things (eg, poverty, intellectual disability, mental illness, substance use disorders), increases the risk of a negative placement outcome.[28] "Children with developmental disabilities placed in foster care due to abuse and/or neglect are more likely to be placed in institutional care and less likely to achieve successful permanency placement with families."[28]

Educational Health

Chapter 13, Developmental and Educational Issues, discusses the important topic of education. Pediatricians should be aware of the potential protective factor of school stability for children in OHP, as well as potential risk factors for school instability, including placement changes. Placement instability has the potential to result in school instability for this population, and "when a change in child welfare placement is associated with a school move, youth are faced with the difficult challenge of simultaneously adjusting to a new living situation and a new school."[29]

Visitation

Given the emphasis on reunification in the child welfare system, visitation with biological family is typically a cornerstone of OHP and "is considered the primary intervention for maintaining the parent–child relationship."[30] Visitation represents a time when the child and biological family can spend time together despite the child being in OHP. This visitation may be supervised or unsupervised and occur in a multitude of settings, including the biological parent's home, a public site such as a park, child welfare offices, or, rarely, a well-designed visitation center. If supervised visitation is in place, supervision can be provided by kinship caregivers, child welfare workers, or another agreed-upon third party. There are also models of visitation where supervisors are trained in child development, parenting, and childhood trauma, and/or where parent supports such as parent-child interaction therapy are available. Child welfare agencies—based on their assessments of the family—will make recommendations to the court about visitation types and frequency. Physicians should understand that frequent and consistent visitation with biological parents may have a beneficial "impact on the levels of depression and externalizing problems of children in foster care."[30]

For physicians, it is important to encourage healthy relationships, not only between the child and their caregivers (biological, kinship, or foster), but also between biological parents and placement providers. When adults in a child's life can consistently model healthy interpersonal relationships and boundaries, the child benefits. Foster and kinship caregivers should be aware that visits with biological parents can be challenging for children, especially when a parent has significant mental health issues. Children may display internalizing and externalizing behaviors associated with visitation, which can be related to conflict in adult relationships, reexperiencing intrusive memories of trauma, or the trauma of separation. Ideally, caregivers are patient, prepare children for visits, and have a reentry period suited to the child's temperament after visits.

Permanency

When OHP is necessary to ensure a child's safety and child welfare and the courts are involved (all OHPs except private kinship care) it becomes the responsibility of the child welfare agency to identify a permanent home in a timely manner. A child achieves permanency when discharged from OHP by the courts into one of the following arrangements: reunification with parents, living with other relatives, guardianship, or adoption.

Unfortunately, children in OHP are vulnerable to placement instability, which can affect their ability to attain permanency. Approximately 40% of children experience a placement change within 6 months of entering OHP.[31] Children at highest risk of placement instability include those who are older; have a chronic physical, mental, or behavioral health condition; or have a delinquency history.[31] When comparing OHP types, children in kinship care are statistically less likely to experience placement disruption, leading to fewer mean placements compared with children in foster care.[21] In comparison, children in foster care have 2.6 times the odds of experiencing 3 or more placement settings compared with children in kinship care.[21] In addition to placement instability, children in OHP are at risk for prolonged placement. National data revealed that the median length of stay in OHP ranged from 6.1 months to 30.9 months, with only 11 states reporting a median length of stay less than 12 months.[20] Data comparing length of stay by placement type have been inconclusive.[21]

Nearly 90% of children who exited OHP in 2019 were discharged to a permanent home.[32] The remaining youth were unable to find permanency and exited care as they aged out, with a discharge reason of emancipation. While tens of thousands of youth were unable find a permanent home, the rate of emancipation has decreased by 5.7% since 2015.[32] Once again, children unable to achieve permanency tended to be older or have a disability.[32] When comparing permanency outcomes by placement type, data are mixed: children in foster care are more likely to be adopted, while those in kinship care are more likely to have a relative assume legal custody.[21] Neither placement type appears to increase the likelihood of reunification with parent.[21] Regardless of placement type, lack of permanency puts youth at risk of becoming unemployed, incarcerated, or unhoused; having mental illness; and having lower levels of educational achievement.[31,33]

Needs for Improvement and Future Research

Pediatric health professionals play a unique role in caring for children in OHP. It is important for pediatricians to understand the needs of these children in order to facilitate the practice of patient-centered, trauma-informed care and promote access to routine health care, mental health care, and subspecialty visits. These needs include, but are not limited to the following:

- All OHPs should emphasize and promote cultural identity. This is particularly important for OHPs that have racial, ethnic, or cultural identity discordance.
- Clinicians can play a key role in advocating for the least restrictive environment for the child.
- Clinicians should support the licensing of kinship caregivers to increase access to caregiver resources.
- OHP, regardless of placement type, can result in a disruption of medical records. Clinicians can advocate for collaboration with local child welfare agencies regarding standardized practices to obtain and pass forward comprehensive health information.
- Children with placement disruptions and high mental health needs are at risk of high rates of psychotropic medication use and should be referred to a pediatric psychiatrist for appropriate medication management. (See Chapter 38, Psychotropic Medication Oversight, for additional discussion.)
- Common challenges faced by foster and kinship homes include the need for ongoing training and support to address the needs of the children placed with them. The training and type of support necessary may look different for each family. Important aspects of training include training for the child's specific needs (eg, how to care for a gastrostomy tube), positive parenting strategies, child development, effects of childhood trauma, and how to respond using trauma-informed approaches.
- Access to resources such as mental health services, educational support, and respite care is crucial for all OHP caregivers, including kinship and foster caregivers, to ensure the overall well-being and development of the children they care for.
- Children at highest risk of placement instability include those who have a chronic physical, mental, or behavioral health condition. In addition,

higher numbers of placement changes and higher levels of care are typically associated with worse health and permanency outcomes.

Key Takeaways

- There are different types of OHPs, with the most common forms being kinship care and licensed foster care; children may also be placed in therapeutic homes, group homes, or residential treatment facilities.
- The goal for youth involved in the child welfare system is a safe, permanent home in the least restrictive environment possible. Consequently, recent legislation prioritizes placing children with kinship caregivers when feasible.
- Children removed from their home have increased medical, mental, and developmental health needs regardless of OHP type, requiring close follow-up and care coordination by a medical home.
- Most children in OHP eventually attain a permanent placement; however, this is frequently complicated by placement disruptions, and data are mixed on how OHP type affects permanency. Regardless, lack of permanency is a significant long-term social and medical risk factor.

CHAPTER 19

Factors Associated With Placement Stability and Permanency Outcomes

Lisa Nalven, MD, MA, FAAP

Introduction

Many children and youth who enter the child welfare system continue to struggle with issues of permanency and placement instability throughout their time within the system and upon exiting the system. Other chapters have discussed the reasons for the removal of a child from their family of origin, as well as associations that may exist related to a child's age, gender, race/ethnicity, and developmental/behavioral/medical history (see **Table 19–1**).[1] Once placed in a foster home, there are multiple protective and risk factors that affect a child's placement stability while in care and their resilience when exiting the child welfare system. Placement stability in the child welfare system considers duration and maintenance of placements, number of placements, moves, and placement breakdowns.[2] One way that the child welfare system attempts to reduce placement instability is through permanency planning, which creates a process of identifying and developing a long-term living situation with permanent relationships.

Placement stability, youth well-being, and outcomes when transitioning out of care are affected by individual, family, community, and structural factors and their interplay with the child welfare system. As discussed in detail in Chapter 16, History of Child Welfare in the United States and Issues of Disproportionality, Inequity, and Injustice, research indicates that there is disproportionality related to race/ethnicity for the number of youth who enter the foster care system, which continues throughout their experience in foster care and affects outcomes for permanency and transitioning out of foster care.

When a child is placed in out-of-home care, placement stability is critical to providing consistency and the opportunity to attach to a caring adult, which supports well-being and the chance to thrive. Placement instability leads to more compounding trauma for the child and disrupts connections to their family of origin, community, and foster family, which negatively affects behavior, mental health, educational outcomes, and ultimately permanency (adoption, reunification with family of origin, or legal guardianship).

Table 19–1. Profile of Children in Foster Care in 2022[a]

Race/Ethnicity	Percentage of Youth in Care
American Indian/Alaska Native	2%
Asian	1%
Black or African American	23%
Hispanic (of any race)	22%
Native Hawaiian or other Pacific Islander	<1%
White	43%
Two or more races	8%
Unknown/Unable to determine	2%
Age of Youth	**Percentage of Youth in Care**
Younger than 1 year	7%
1–5 years	33%
6–10 years	22%
11–15 years	22%
16–18 years	12%
19–20 years	2%
Placement Type	**Percentage of Youth in Care**
Foster family (nonrelative)	44%
Foster family (relative)	34%
Group home or institution	9%
Preadoptive home	5%
Trial home visit	4%
Supervised independent living	2%
Runaway	1%
Permanency Plan	**Percentage of Youth in Care**
Reunification with family of origin	52%
Adoption	28%
Aging out	5%
Legal guardianship	4%
Live with other relatives	4%
Long-term foster care	2%
Plan not yet established	5%

Table 19–1 *(continued)*

Time in Care[b]	Percentage of Youth in Care
Less than 1 year	40%
1–3 years	39%
3–4 years	13%
5 or more years	7%

[a] N ~ 370,000.

[b] Median time in care 15.5 months; mean time in care 22.6 months.

Data from Adoption and Foster Care Analysis and Reporting System (AFCARS) REPORT #30 – Preliminary FY 2022 Estimates (2023). https://www.acf.hhs.gov/cb/report/afcars-report-30. Accessed October 13, 2024.

This chapter reviews factors that affect the experience of youth in foster care from the time of placement until their exit from the system, as well as permanency outcomes, with attention to disproportionality and disparity across different racial and ethnic groups.

Overview of Stability of Children in Care

A literature review by Vanderwill et al[3] regarding stability and permanency provides an overview of placement statistics within in the foster care system and the factors involved. In 2017, approximately 240,000 children exited foster care. Of these, half were reunified with their family of origin and a quarter were adopted. Ten percent of youth acquired legal guardians, and the remainder joined relatives, aged out, or transferred to another agency. (Adoption and Foster Care Analysis and Reporting System [AFCARS] data for 2022 are similar to those from 2017). However, reentry into the foster care system was common: 10% after reunification and 10% to 25% resulting from adoption disruptions. National data indicate that children in care for less than 1 year are likely to have 1 to 2 placements, while 59% of those in care for more than 2 years will have 3 or more placements.[4] The number of placements increases with the time spent in care and varies by state. Furthermore, Black youth bear a disproportionate burden of placement instability compared with other groups, especially when they enter foster care at an older age, have an initial placement setting other than kinship care, display more externalizing behaviors, and are not in a racially matched placement, all while spending a disproportionately longer time in care compared with other groups.[5,6] Those who are in care longer also have less chance of reunification: reunification occurs for 54% of youth in care for less than 1 year and decreases to 26% of youth in care over 2 years.[7]

It is well established that placement stability is important to a youth's social, emotional, and behavioral well-being because it provides an environment that supports child development and attachment. Youth in foster care experience trauma a result of maltreatment, loss, and separation and are more likely to engage in externalizing behaviors that can negatively affect their relationship with a foster parent or cause them to experience discrimination, experience school instability, and require special education services—all of which negatively affect stability. In the face of these challenges, the foster parent requires appropriate training, ongoing support, and tangible resources to meet the needs of these youth.[3]

Multiple studies utilize the National Youth Transition Database (NYTD) and AFCARS data from different years to review factors associated with placement stability or instability and outcomes (**Box 19–1**).

Box 19–1

Placement and Stability[2,7–9]

Factors associated with increased placement stability

- Placement with kin
- Placement with sibling
- Cooperation between foster caregiver and family of origin
- Parenting skills of foster family
- Support systems and attentiveness to caregiver/child relationships

Factors associated with decreased placement stability

- Medically complex child
- Placement involving 3 or more children
- Placement in care as a result of parent substance use, sexual abuse, or physical abuse (vs neglect)
- Trauma, complex trauma, or high cumulative impact of adverse childhood experiences
- Externalizing behaviors
- Longer time in care
- Older age at initial placement (259% increase in instability seen for youth age 10 years or older versus those younger than 6 years[8])
- Unsuccessful reunification or adoption

Race and Ethnicity

Boyd[10] proposed a conceptual framework for Black disproportionality (representing 23% of those in care versus 13% of the general population) and disparity in the child welfare system that helps elucidate issues of racial/ethnic disproportionality with permanency and stability (see Figure 16-1 in Chapter 16, History of Child Welfare in the United States and Issues of Disproportionality, Inequity, and Injustice). Evidence strongly supports concerns that bias and inequities lead to disproportionately increased time in care for children who are Black, Indigenous, and people of color (BIPOC), and these concerns persist throughout the time a child is in care. Black children and families, both prior to removal of the child from their home and while engaged with the foster care system, receive fewer and lower quality services and fewer foster parent support services, have fewer caseworker contacts, and have less access to mental health and substance use services compared with other racial and ethnic groups. As a result, Black children are more likely to be referred for out-of-home placement (versus receiving in-home supportive services), experience more placement instability, spend more time in foster care, and historically are less likely to be reunited with their families of origin. [11]

Although this model was initially used to describe disproportionality and disparity as related to the Black population, other racial and ethnic groups are similarly affected. Black, American Indian, and Alaska Native youth are overrepresented in the child welfare system, with Hispanic youth being overrepresented in some states. Bias continues to exist in the reporting of child maltreatment and decision-making regarding investigation and placements of children of color.

Disproportionality in child welfare is thought to be related to other inequalities in larger society. Black families are reported to have higher rates of child maltreatment, infant mortality, and low-birth-weight infants compared with white families. Higher rates of out-of-home placement can be an outgrowth of living in a resource-poor community. Remaining in the system longer occurs because it is harder for a family to receive services needed for reunification. Black youth are more likely to be placed with kin rather than a licensed foster family and therefore receive fewer resources and services. Hence, the largest effect on disproportionality can be achieved through addressing socioeconomic disadvantages for people of color.[12]

Type of Placement

In contrast to child-specific factors, the type of placement (for example, foster-to-adoption families, kinship, foster family, group homes, and residential settings) can also affect stability. The highest rates of stability and permanency are with foster-to-adoption families, and these tend to involve children who are placed at younger ages. Kinship placements also tend to start at younger ages and are more commonly seen in Black families. This type of placement can help to preserve family relationships, culture, and community ties. Increased stability may also be related to children in kinship placements having fewer baseline behavioral and developmental concerns. Although kinship placements are associated with increased stability, these children are less likely to achieve permanency through adoption (that is, kin are less likely to adopt) and are more likely to enter guardianship upon leaving foster care. Although kinship placements may provide more stability, these families tend to receive less support and fewer resources from the child welfare system. Some studies suggest that after the first few years, stability in kinship care is no greater than placement in nonkinship families. More commonly, children are placed in nonrelative foster families, which have the lowest stability of the 3 placements discussed. Nonrelative foster placements are more likely to include children who are male, are older, and have developmental or behavioral issues, all of which are associated with less stability in a placement.[2] Youth placed in group homes or residential settings experience the highest number of changes in placement. It is not clear if this is related to characteristics of the youth, the environment, or both.[9] Of note, however, it is not a goal for a child to achieve long-term stability in a congregate care setting; rather, the goal is to move to a lower and hopefully more stable level of care when the group setting is no longer needed.

Children With Disabilities

In a study using data from AFCARS 2017,[13] Platt and Gephart[14] reported that 22% of children in foster care had a medical need or disability requiring specialized care; these children are more likely to change placements. (Of note, the National Survey of Children's Health for 2016 indicated that 44% of children in foster care were identified as having a specific mental health or developmental condition.[15]) A foster family requires appropriate experience, training, and resources to care for a child with disabilities or medical complexity. Without these, the challenges can result in disruption of a placement and decrease the chances of permanency. Placement in a new geographic location that is physically distant from the foster family can lead to health care disruption, which can affect a child's overall well-being and increase the stress or burden on a foster family. If appropriate care (educational, medical, mental health) is not available, a new placement is required. Children with disabilities have almost double the disruptions while in foster care (mean of 4 versus 2.37 for children without disabilities), and the occurrence of disruption increases with the number of disabilities and if the child is Black or Native American.

Moreover, a child with disabilities is more likely to spend a longer time in foster care and more likely than nondisabled youth to be in preadoptive homes, group homes, or institutions. Increased instability may be associated with an increase in externalizing behaviors of the child but also insufficient support and resources for the foster family. Out-of-state placements for the purpose of accessing appropriate supports and older and married foster parents predict stability for these children.[14]

Placement With Siblings

Placement with siblings has been demonstrated to improve placement stability and is associated with fewer placement changes due to problems or negative experiences in a foster family. Placement with siblings does not add to the relational loss experienced when a child is removed from parental care, and older children are less likely to run away if placed with siblings. If a child remains in foster care for a long period of time in a family of a different race, ethnicity, or culture, being placed with a sibling can be a positive factor. It is not necessary for siblings to be in the same home for the entire time in foster care or for all siblings to be together to have a positive impact. Despite these benefits, siblings may not be placed together for a variety of reasons: challenging sibling dynamics, inability to place siblings together, or placement of only part of a sibling group in care. Increased instability is seen in children who are Black and separated from siblings.

The economic, time, and energy demands on the foster parent in caring for a sibling group can increase stress and reduce quality of care (dilution of foster parent resources). This can result in sibling groups being moved more often than those placed without siblings. However, the benefit of sibling placement makes it imperative that resources be provided to support sibling relationships. If siblings are separated, efforts should be made to encourage sibling visitation to promote child well-being. In addition, recruiting a well-matched family is important; and having 2 parents, with 1 parent having flexible hours, may help to reduce the impact of dilution of resources over more than 1 child.[16]

Reunification

Nationally, only about 50% of youth leaving foster care are reunified with their family, despite legislation designed to provide resources to support reunification as a primary permanency goal.[13] In the birth to 5-year age group, rates of reunification vary greatly by state (8% to 31%). Infants and young children, especially those who were placed due to parental substance use, are less likely to be reunified than older children. In a 2021 study, LaBrenz et al[17] found no difference in the general rates of reunification among white, Black, and multiracial populations. Compared with white children, Native American children had lower odds of reunification, while Hispanic, Asian, and Native Hawaiian/Pacific Islander children had higher odds of reunification. Although there is a disproportionate number of Black and Hispanic children in the child welfare system, this did not seem to negatively affect their rates of reunification.[17] Disproportionality for reunification varies by state. Reunification is associated with older age, shorter length of stay in care, and statewide variables (such as lower poverty rates, higher reunification budget, lower teen birth rate, and greater drug rehabilitation resources for the population).

Parental substance use in BIPOC families has a significant effect on reunification and may be related to greater legal consequences and service inequities for substance use in this population compared with the white population. States without the Medicaid expansion have higher concentrations of Black families and more individuals in the Medicaid gap, resulting in less access to mental health services. This contributes to disparity in reunification because parents do not have access to the resources needed to treat their mental health issues and improve their ability to parent their children. Family factors that have a negative association with reunification include parental incarceration, single-parent household, parental substance use, and inability to handle the parental role.[17]

Transitioning Out of Care

Over the years, policymakers have sought to improve outcomes for children and youth in and transitioning out of foster care by increasing services. The Fostering Connections to Success and Increasing Adoption Act (2008) included incentives to support kinship care and adoption and allow youth who met certain criteria to remain in foster care after the age of 18 years in order to promote stability, education, and employment. Placement instability during time in care is associated with an increased likelihood of homelessness at transition, and homelessness is associated with lower rates of postsecondary education and higher rates of unemployment. Lower rates of postsecondary education lead to lower earning potential.

Resilience

Shpiegel et al[18] used the AFCARS and NYTD data beginning 2014 and followed youth longitudinally at 17, 19, and 21 years of age to describe "transition resilience." In this study population, two-thirds of youth demonstrated moderate to high resilience based on outcomes related to achievement in education and employment and the absence of early parenthood, substance use, homelessness, and criminal activity. Resilience can be viewed as the result of the interplay between risk and protective factors (**Box 19–2**).

Using combined indicators, 59% of transitioning youth demonstrated resilience at age 19 years and 55% by age 21 years.[18] Forty-two percent sustained resilience, but women fared better than men (46% vs 38%, respectively). At 24%, Native American/Alaska Native children had the lowest rates of resilience, in contrast with Asian and Native Hawaiian/Pacific Islander children, who experienced the highest rates of sustained resilience. Possible factors affecting the disparities included systemic bias as well as persistent poverty and the lack of employment opportunities in the community. Differences were not significant among white, Black, and Hispanic youth (42% to 44%) However, there are structural barriers to employment for young men of color.[18]

Box 19–2

Transition Resilience

Protective Factors

- ▲ Engaged in school or employment
- ▲ Absence of homelessness or housing instability
- ▲ No substance use referrals in the past 2 years
- ▲ No incarceration in the past 2 years
- ▲ Presence of supportive adult (eg, biological parent, foster parent, adult relative) by age 19 years
- ▲ Living in preadoptive home or with relatives at 17 years
- ▲ Longer placement stability at time of transition

Risk Factors

- ▲ Mental health issues by age 17 years
- ▲ Running away by 17 years
- ▲ Early parenthood
- ▲ Placement instability
- ▲ Discharge from foster care by age 19 years

Changing the Trajectory

Outcomes for youth in any setting are the result of the interplay between personal characteristics (such as personality and genetics) and the environmental experience (foster family, culture, society, and structures, for example). In the "social ecology" in which these youth exist, there are risk and protective factors that affect the child's resilience within and upon exiting the child welfare system.[18,19] The more supports a child has while in care, in addition to support and preparation for transitioning out of care, the greater the likelihood of a positive outcome (resilience).

At the policy and systems levels, more supports need to be provided to those adults caring for youth in care. Foster families (including kin) should be provided with the evidence-based training, resources, and supports required to care for and nurture youth. Intensive resources should be provided to youth and caregivers to address and reduce emotional and behavioral issues, which positively affects stability, a key factor in later outcomes. Foster families should be responsive to and, if possible, reflective of, a child's culture, language, and religion and consider other characteristics of the child and foster family. These families should not be chosen solely based on a family's willingness to care for a particular child. When possible and appropriate, improving bonding with the family of origin is important to a child's well-being. The provision of supports to the family of origin can also shorten time in care and promote reunification.[19]

One of the main outcomes of childhood trauma can be "social thinning," or loss of relational resources. Thus, as youth enter their teen years, and well in advance of transitioning out of care, those involved with the child should help them with developing a social network (social capital). This network must provide meaningful resources and opportunities to the youth. When a youth leaves care at 18 to 21 years of age, they are expected to live independently, yet they have lost the institutional support network (foster family and social worker). Moreover, many have not yet developed the skills to be successful on their own and need to develop skills for life, including relational. Skill development can be derived from a variety of resources: extracurricular activities, a structured program to support educational success and employment skills (specialized training can improve employment and income), and adult role models who may become long-term mentors. As previously discussed, stability in placement has a positive impact on education: remaining in the same school supports educational success (graduating high school and seeking postsecondary education). In turn, achieving a higher educational level enhances earning potential. Housing assistance is important so that youth can have a stable place to live after leaving foster care, which allows them to focus on advancing their education or maintaining stable employment. The guidance of a trusted adult or mentor may be required for youth to engage with these resources and to understand that these resources are meaningful for their future success.

Access to resources varies based on geographic location, which partly explains the disparities in outcomes. For example, a state legislative tuition waiver is associated with the attainment of a high school or general equivalency diploma, higher rates of enrollment in postsecondary education, and lower rates of incarceration. Extended foster care (remaining in foster care beyond 18 years of age) is associated with lower rates of homelessness and higher rates of enrollment in postsecondary education. Improving outcomes requires systemwide policies that not only provide needed resources and support for children, biological families, foster families, and kin but also address biases and inequities in the system.[12]

Conclusion

The pediatrician's most obvious role in the lives of children in the child welfare system is to provide appropriate medical care; however, pediatricians can provide much more. They can be part of the social capital that these youth need. The pediatrician may be the most stable adult in the life of a youth who has been in out-of-home care. It is also important for pediatricians to understand how many placements a child has had when providing care, as high placement instability can inform many risk factors for poorer outcomes. Knowledge and expertise in what supports a youth's comprehensive well-being as they transition into early adulthood provide a guide to the broader role that the pediatrician can fulfill. The pediatrician can leverage their role as a knowledgeable professional to not only advocate for the resources youth need in care and as they transition out of care but to also serve as a stable, reliable adult and mentor.

Key Takeaways

Pediatricians can support youth in care by doing the following:

- Mentor youth, and let them know that you are available between regularly scheduled medical visits to answer questions and provide support for needs that they express. Talk with them about their current concerns, any needs that they may not be aware of, and planning for their future.
- Assess the youth's relationships with current caregivers, and provide support to caregivers as needed.
- Advocate for youth and foster families when interacting with the larger system (this requires that medical records document the need for stability while in care, in addition to recommendations for mental health resources, community resources, and transition resources).
- Partner with case managers from child welfare to ensure appropriate resources are available to the youth, family of origin, and foster family while the youth is in care and during the transition to adulthood.
- Ensure that evidence-based interventions are used to support the youth, family of origin, and foster family.
- Ensure that the medical clinic has knowledge of and relationships with appropriate community resources that can support the youth while in care and during the transition to adulthood. Engage with social workers and other community professionals that can assist in making these connections.
- Have printed materials and links to digital material available for youth and foster families that provide information about what possible needs they may not have fully identified and resources that are available while in care and during the transition to adulthood.
- Educate youth about how they can care for themselves and what they need to have in place during the transition to adulthood (one educational resource from the American Academy of Pediatrics is available at https://downloads.aap.org/AAP/PDF/Foster%20Care/AgingOut%20FINAL.pdf).
- Learn ways that a primary care physician can support youth in foster care from those with lived experience. (An informative talk on the topic can be found at https://youtu.be/cCx2geBowiM?si=9BRdFtPRf-c6yYN8v)

Part 3. Adolescent-Specific Issues

CHAPTER 20

Transition-Age Youth

Colleen C. Katz, PhD, LCSW
Michelle R. Munson, PhD, LMSW
Amy Dworsky, PhD, MSW
Kym Ahrens, MD, MPH

Introduction

Approximately 20,000 young people "age out" of foster care each year.[1] This generally occurs between the ages of 18 and 22 years, depending on the state in which they live. Once they age out, youth are largely expected to support themselves and function as independent adults, which is incongruent with developmental neuroscience. Research has consistently demonstrated that transition-age youth face a constellation of challenges in the years after they leave care and tend to experience worse outcomes in a variety of key domains than their same-age peers who were not in foster care.[2] Several factors likely contribute to the challenges faced by transition-age youth, including adverse experiences they had before entering and while in care (eg, maltreatment, trauma, and placement instability), as well as the stress of an accelerated ascent into adulthood without adequate social, emotional, or economic support.[3–5] This chapter summarizes research on the experiences of transition-age youth related to five key outcomes: physical health, mental health, education, housing instability, and preparation for independent living. While the latter three of these domains lie beyond the walls of a physician's office, these are incredibly impactful social drivers that influence physical and mental health of transition-age youth in foster care. This summary aims to highlight issues physicians should consider when assessing the health of these youth in foster care and when providing them with health care services tailored to their unique needs.

Physical Health

Youth in foster care have higher rates of acute and chronic health problems compared with their peers not in foster care, and these differences are apparent upon entry into foster care.[6,7] Less is known about the physical health of youth transitioning out of foster care. Although some studies have found that these youth report generally good health, other research suggests they are at increased risk for several health conditions, including asthma, obesity, hypertension, and possibly diabetes.[8–10] Transition-age youth also have higher rates of disability[8] and unintentional injuries[11] and may display higher rates of eating disorder–associated behaviors, such as pica and food hoarding.[8,12]

Several factors are likely contributing to the increased health risks experienced among transition-age youth. These include high rates of adverse childhood experiences[13,14]; hypothalamic pituitary adrenal axis changes, increased inflammation, and other effects resulting from cumulative stress[15]; loss of continuity of care due to frequent placement changes,[16,17] especially if youth have been in foster care for an extended time; and overuse of urgent or emergent health care settings.[17–19] Not having a consistent pediatrician or other physician can decrease access to prevention and early intervention, both of which are critical to reducing adult disease burden.

Conversely, policy changes implemented in recent years have the potential to improve physical health outcomes for transition-age youth, including increased access to extended foster care, extension of eligibility for Medicaid until age 26,[20] and local, state, and federal policies to promote healthcare continuity and create medical homes for youth in foster care.[21] Other measures, such as decreasing placement instability, reducing homelessness, improving educational outcomes, and increasing access to mental health treatment would also be likely to have a positive impact on the physical health of transition-age youth.

Mental Health

Youth transitioning out of foster care are significantly more likely than their same-age peers to experience psychiatric and alcohol or substance use disorders (SUDs).[22–24] The recent CalYOUTH study found that approximately one-third of 19-year-olds with involvement in the child welfare system had at least one behavioral health disorder,[25] with the most common being major depression (9.6%), psychosis (9%), anorexia nervosa (6.5%), antisocial personality disorder (5.8%), substance use disorder (5.6%), social phobia (4.8%), and alcohol use disorder (4.6%). Other studies have found that posttraumatic stress disorder (PTSD)[26] and conduct disorder[27,28] are commonly diagnosed in transition-age youth. Past maltreatment[29,30] and foster care experiences, such as placement instability,[31] contribute to mental health problems among transition-age youth. Notably, the literature points to the misdiagnosis of mental health conditions, especially in youth of color as these youth may be labeled negatively due to behavioral manifestations of trauma instead of identifying needs or other more appropriate diagnoses.[32]

Studies have repeatedly shown that youth with child welfare experience are more likely than their peers to engage in suicidal ideation and attempt suicide.[33,34] Katz and colleagues[35] found that specific groups of transition-age youth were at increased risk for suicidal behaviors: (1) female youth, (2) youth with mental illnesses such as depression, anxiety, and PTSD, (3) youth with past experiences of maltreatment (especially neglect or sexual abuse) and (4) youth who identified as sexual minorities. Lesbian, gay, bisexual, transgender, and questioning or queer (LGBTQ+) youth with psychiatric and behavioral health issues appear to engage in alarmingly high rates of suicidal behavior, with over 95% reporting suicidal ideation.[35]

The child welfare system may help some young people access mental health services, including psychiatric assessment, psychotherapy, and psychotropic medication, when there may have been barriers previously.[36–38] However, as is the case with physical health, access to mental health treatment may be compromised when youth age out of foster care, and receipt of mental health services may decline as a result.[37,39] Teaching these youth to manage their own psychiatric and behavioral health care while they are still in foster care is critical if they are to feel adequately prepared to manage it by themselves after they have exited the child welfare system.

Education

The educational challenges faced by transition-age youth are well documented. These youth are less likely to have a high school diploma or general equivalency diploma (GED) than their peers.[2,40,41] Several factors likely contribute to this difference in high school completion, including enrollment in underfunded and low-performing schools, frequent school changes due to placement instability, and high rates of grade retention, suspension, and expulsion.[40,42–45]

Although these youth report similar aspirations for postsecondary education as their peers outside of the child welfare system,[42,43,46] they enroll in college at lower rates[47] and are less likely to complete their first year when they do enroll.[44,48–50] Consequently, they are less likely than their peers to graduate with a college degree.[2,44,51] Only 2% to 10% of transition-age youth earn a 2- or 4-year college degree by their mid-20s,[47] compared with nearly half of 25- to 29-year-olds in the general population.[52]

Many transition-age youth who enroll in college report feeling unprepared, reporting academic, social, and financial challenges.[45,53] Social support, both formal and informal, has been repeatedly identified as promoting postsecondary educational success among transition-age youth,[54–58] especially for those with marginalized identities.[59,60] Remaining in foster care beyond 18 years of age is associated with increased rates of college enrollment,[61,62] and participating in campus support programs is associated with increased rates of college persistence.[63] Also, receipt of educational and training vouchers is associated with increased rates of college persistence and graduation.[63,64]

The lack of postsecondary educational attainment among transition-age youth directly affects their ability to secure and maintain gainful employment.[65] Transition-age youth who have completed at least some college are more likely be employed and have higher earnings than those who have only a high school diploma or GED.[66] This is important, because numerous studies have shown that transition-age youth have a hard time earning enough money to lift themselves out of poverty.[67,68]

Housing Instability

One of the biggest challenges transition-age youth face is maintaining stable housing. Research suggests that between one-quarter and one-third of these young people will experience homelessness after they age out of foster care.[69–72] Although the experiences of these young people vary widely,[73] the potential adverse consequences of being unhoused are clear.

Research indicates that young people experiencing homelessness are at high risk for a range of negative outcomes related to their physical, mental, and behavioral health.[74,75] Youth experiencing homelessness have high rates of pregnancy and sexually transmitted infections.[75,76] This may be due, at least in part, to the fact that these youth are often forced to engage in survival sex, defined as trading sex for money, food, drugs, or shelter.[77,78] Youth experiencing homelessness also have high rates of psychiatric health disorders such as depression, anxiety, PTSD,[74,75,79,80] and SUDs.[75] What is less clear from the research is the temporal ordering (ie, which circumstance occurred first). Psychiatric health and SUDs can be both a cause or a consequence of homelessness, and homelessness can exacerbate preexisting psychiatric health or

SUDs.[74] Finally, youth experiencing homelessness have a much higher mortality rate than the general youth population.[81]

Several factors likely contribute to the poor health of unhoused youth. Practicing good personal hygiene can be a challenge for young people experiencing homelessness. Many also suffer from poor nutrition and lack of sleep. Additionally, living on the streets or in congregate settings increases the risk of skin, respiratory, and infectious diseases.[74,82] Last, but certainly not least, many youth experiencing homelessness do not have access to basic health care services due to a lack of health insurance and difficulty navigating the health care system.[74,83] Given this increased risk of homelessness, it is critical to ask transition-age youth in foster care what their plans are for housing before they age out of care. After aging out, it is critical for physicians to continue to ask at medical visits about this population's housing situation because the physician may discover a youth is couch surfing with friends or relatives, is living in a shelter, has moved back in with their family of origin, or has become homeless.

Preparation for Independent Living or Extended Care

Preparation is essential for youth aspiring to have healthy and fulfilling adult lives.[84] Preparing for adulthood requires resources, opportunities to make mistakes, and adult support and guidance. Inequities in these areas, coupled with the deleterious consequences of removal from their home (eg, trauma, grief, loss, shame) contribute to some of the adverse outcomes experienced by transition-age youth.[85]

For decades, youth in care have reported a lack of planning and preparation for their transition to adulthood.[86,87] Although the Foster Care Independence Act of 1999 doubled the amount of federal funding allocated to states for independent-living services and subsequent legislation has expanded the number of young people eligible for those services, a recently published systematic review of independent living programs suggests the impact of these programs is limited.[88] Additionally, these programs have been criticized for focusing too much on "hard skills" and not enough on how to develop and maintain healthy relationships and how to access and engage in health care and other needed services,[88] both of which are key to all aspects of health in adulthood.

Since 2010, states have had the option to extend federally funded foster care to age 21 years, and nearly all states currently allow at least some young people to remain in care beyond their 18th birthday. Evidence suggests that extended foster care is associated with better youth outcomes, such as higher levels of educational attainment and social support, higher rates of employment, increased savings, and lower rates of homelessness, justice system involvement, and early parenting.[69,89]

Pediatricians can help prepare older youth in foster care for the adult health care system by supporting them in making their own health care decisions so they can learn while they still have a safety net. They can also engage transition-age youth in health education, including psychoeducation, while also helping them build the self-advocacy, problem-solving, and decision-making skills that they will need as they embark on adult life.

Conclusion

Transition-age youth face numerous health challenges, many of which are a consequence of factors outside of their control. Pediatricians and other medical professionals can make a significant impact on the lives of these youth by educating themselves about the factors that influence the health of transition-age youth; by connecting them to support services in education, employment, and housing domains; and, importantly, by partnering with these youth to plan for their increased independence in managing their health care. Specifically, pediatricians and other medical professionals can partner with transition-age youth in the management of their health by routinely allowing time for questions during medical visits, providing youth with a "health summary sheet" so they can easily access all of their health information, educating them about their chronic health conditions and associated medications, providing education about medical insurance options, and supporting the identification of a new adult medical provider as they transition out of pediatric care. Finally, pediatricians can practice trauma-informed relational care by assisting transition-age youth in identifying supportive adults that can help guide them in young adulthood.

Key Takeaways

Pediatricians and other medical professionals can make a significant impact on the lives of transition-age youth by

- Partnering with them to plan for their increased independence in managing all aspects of their physical and mental health care
- Supporting the establishment of the self-advocacy, problem-solving, and decision-making skills that youth will need in the management of this health care
- Routinely allowing time for questions at the end of visits
- Providing them with a "health summary sheet" so they can easily access all of their health information
- Supporting the identification of new primary care clinicians when they are preparing to move

CHAPTER 21

Substance Use

Megan Radenhausen, PhD
Camille A. Broussard, MD, MPH, FAAP
Sarah J. Beal, PhD

While adolescence is an important period of growth and development, often contributing to resilience across the lifespan,[1] it is also a period of risk for substance use, with alcohol, marijuana, and nicotine being the substances young people most commonly report using.[2] Additionally, the number of overdoses and overdose deaths, largely attributed to fentanyl, continue to increase in young people.[3] Rates of substance use are estimated to rise as high as 49% for youth in foster care,[4–6] which is higher than for their peers in the general population of the United States.[7]

Several factors may contribute to the increased risk of substance use among young people in foster care. Maltreatment,[8] social adversity,[9] and parental substance use[10] are common exposures for young people in foster care,[11–13] all of which increase the risk of adolescent substance use. Additionally, youth in foster care have higher rates of mental health concerns[14] and may use substances to self-medicate, particularly when there is limited access to behavioral health services.[15,16] Use of substances exacerbates mental health symptoms.[17] As a result, it is not surprising that there are higher rates of substance use and substance use disorder (SUD) among young people in foster care compared with their peers in the general population.[4]

Recent strengths-based approaches to understanding adolescent substance use[18] highlight adolescence as an important period for preventing SUD, primarily through delaying the initiation of substance use to reduce the risk for SUD in adulthood.[19] Adolescents in foster care may experience more pronounced consequences of substance use and SUD as a result of school and social disruptions, an increased risk of juvenile justice involvement due to substance use,[20] and health risks[21] that are potentially exacerbated by substance use. Finally, there are subgroups of young people in foster care who face additional discrimination, including lesbian, gay, bisexual, transgender, and questioning or queer youth, which may further increase their risk for SUD and exacerbate the effects of substance use.[22,23] For these reasons, every young person in foster care should be screened for substance use during their health care encounters in a manner that is without bias and ensures confidentiality.

Screening, Brief Intervention, and Referral to Treatment

Screening, Brief Intervention, and Referral to Treatment (SBIRT) is the gold standard for brief interventions that address substance use. It was designed to be used in a variety of settings including schools, primary care, and emergency departments. The 3 main components of SBIRT are illustrated in **Figure 21–1**.

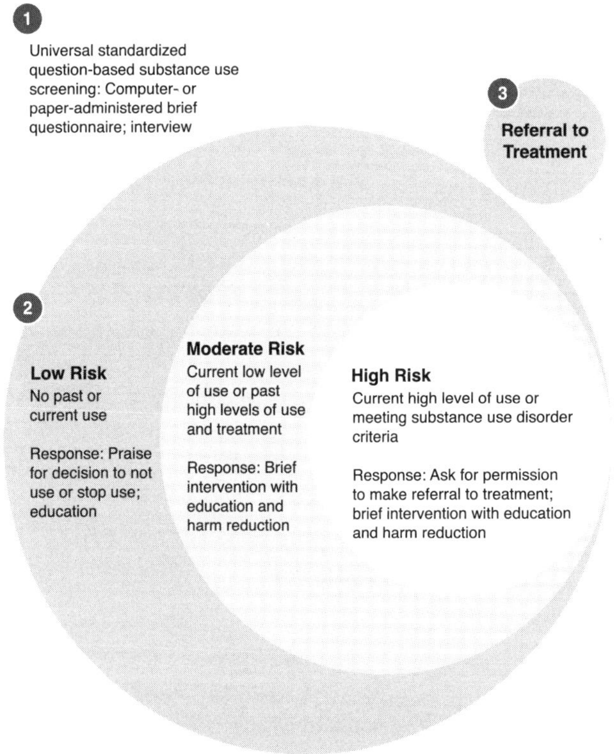

Figure 21–1. A conceptual model illustrating the stratification of adolescents based on their responses to Screening, Brief Intervention, and Referral to Treatment (SBIRT). The first step of SBIRT is universal screening, and the second step includes interpretation of patient's responses as the patient being at low, moderate, or high risk. The interpretation of patient's answers allows pediatricians to praise, provide a brief intervention, or transition to step 3, which is to provide a referral to treatment.

Preparing to Talk to Adolescents and Young Adults About Substance Use

Pediatricians should eliminate barriers to adolescents' honest conversations about their substance use to promote effective screening. This may include ensuring confidentiality, increasing knowledge of available resources to effectively screen for and respond to substance use, addressing biases about substance use in adolescence, and becoming more confident and competent discussing substance use.[24] Strategies to address some of these gaps are detailed in the following sections.

Confidentiality

Confidentiality in adolescent health care is evolving, and pediatricians need to be aware of current policies and practices for ensuring confidentiality, including guidance from the American Academy of Pediatrics (AAP).[25] For adolescents in foster care, maintaining confidentiality can be even more complex. Pediatricians should ask young people what information they want to be shared with their caregivers, caseworkers, or family of origin. When disclosure is necessary (for example, to facilitate access to follow-up treatment or intervention), clinicians should work with patients to create a supportive environment for the young person to disclose their use to the individual who needs to be informed. An important consideration for youth in foster care is that their caregivers are not their legal guardians unless court ordered, so caseworkers must typically provide consent for all treatments or interventions. Clinicians may also need to confirm that substance use documentation in the medical record follows confidentiality expectations and applicable local and federal laws. This is particularly important because medical record requests can include substance use documentation and are often entered into evidence as part of a child's case or shared with caregivers at the time of permanency.

Resource Availability

Before administering question-based substance use screening, it is important to know what resources are available to support the next steps. Clinicians should determine the answers to the following questions:

- What will you do if a patient screens positive for substance use?
- Are you trained in or competent in motivational interviewing to support abstinence or harm reduction?
- Is someone else in your practice trained in motivational interviewing?
- What resources are available for a referral to substance use treatment, if needed?

Bias

Substance use can be a challenging subject to discuss; self-awareness is important to identify potential biases that might decrease a patient's willingness to discuss their substance use. Biases are introduced by targeting screening to adolescents who "look like" they might be using substances, rather than screening all young people. Another way to introduce bias is to ask about substances in a way that makes youth not want to answer honestly. For example, leading questions such as "You are not using any substances, are you?" or "You don't drink more than a couple of drinks at a time, do you?" can contribute to adolescents recognizing the clinician's bias and therefore not engaging honestly. Additionally, adolescents in foster care might be aware of how parental substance use is negatively perceived by pediatricians and become reluctant to disclose their own use. Pediatricians can reduce bias by ensuring they and their staff are trained in using validated question-based substance use screening tools with all patients, asking open-ended questions without judgment to invite young people to answer honestly (for example, "How often do you use cannabis?"), eliminating the use of biasing language (such as making jokes about patients, caregivers, or others who use substances or are intoxicated), avoiding judgmental language (for example, "Don't you know using alcohol is bad for you?"), and ensuring resources are available to address substance use with respect and compassion for the young person receiving care.[26,27]

Discussing Substance Use

Intentional and specific use of language is important when talking to adolescents about substance use and documenting substance use in the medical record. Person-first language (such as "an adolescent who uses substances" rather than a "druggie" or a "smoker") should be used during direct patient care and documentation and is supported by the AAP[28] and the National Institute on Drug Abuse.[29] Consistent with AAP policy,[28] the use of person-first language increases patients' willingness to engage in conversations about substance use and decreases negative bias. Additionally, pediatricians should ensure that they are communicating in the language that the youth is most proficient in, even if they can speak and understand English, and should use terminology familiar to the young person, or ask young people what terms they use to describe a particular substance. In medical settings, physicians' nonverbal cues (body language, facial expressions, eye contact, and tone and volume of speech) have been found to affect patients' clinical outcomes,[30] which makes monitoring nonverbal body language and movement even more important during conversations about substance use. Strategies for initiating dialogues about substance use include[31,32]

- Open-ended questions (eg, "Tell me more about your use of alcohol.")
- Curiosity (eg, "What are some of the things you like or don't like about using nicotine?")
- Nonjudgmental statements (eg, "Some people who drink alcohol notice an impact on their ability to function the next day due to hangovers.")
- Seeking permission from the youth (eg, "Can I tell you some facts about cannabis use?")
- Reflecting the youth's own speech (eg, "What I hear you saying is that you dislike how you feel the day after drinking, and sometimes you don't like the actions you engage in when you drink too much alcohol.")

Screening: Asking Adolescents in Foster Care About Substance Use

Multiple professional organizations include question-based substance use screening (comprehensive and for specific types of substances [such as e-cigarettes]) in their guidelines for confidential adolescent health care service delivery. This includes the AAP[33,34] and the Society for Adolescent Health and Medicine.[35,36] Specifically, AAP guidelines[33] recommend that all adolescents receive question-based screening at least annually using standardized and validated instruments, such as the Screening to Brief Intervention[37]; the Brief Screener for Tobacco, Alcohol, and other Drugs[38]; the Car, Relax, Alone, Forget, Friends, Trouble (CRAFFT)[39]; the Alcohol Use Disorders Identification Test (AUDIT)[40]; or similar validated measures. Substance use screening is also an important component of the confidential adolescent interview.[41] These recommendations are no different for adolescents in foster care. Using standardized questions delivered via tablet and integrated into the electronic health record has been shown to be the most effective and acceptable screening method for adolescent patients.[42] However, only 60% of pediatricians reported routinely asking substance use questions of all adolescents, and only 42% reported using standardized questionnaires.[24]

Responding to Question-Based Screening Results Indicating No Substance Use

Praise Youth for Abstaining From Substances

It is important to reinforce healthy behaviors by praising young people when they indicate they are not using substances on question-based screens.

Ask Youth About Their Rationale for Abstaining

After offering praise, follow up with youth by asking about their rationale for not using substances. This provides additional reinforcement for positive behaviors and helps youth develop and practice expressing their justification for remaining abstinent. It also provides an opportunity for youth to clarify their responses and disclose substance use.

Responding to Question-Based Screening Results Indicating Substance Use

Ask for Permission to Share Information

Before educating young people about substance use, request permission from the patient to share information with them. This positions a young person as part of the decision-making process and creates a collaborative discussion between the patient and clinician. If the patient declines to engage in conversation, pediatricians should follow patient preferences and provide opportunities for the young person to discuss substance use during future appointments.

Provide Resources to Support Substance Use Education

Substance use education is important to correct misinformation and help youth make informed decisions. It is important to provide factual, developmentally appropriate education about how substance use can affect the patient, contextualized to make information meaningful for them (relevant to daily activities or future goals). For example, with a patient who is an athlete, the pediatrician could explain how substance use can affect athletic performance in the short term and long term; for a patient expressing interest in a career in health care, the pediatrician could explain the consequence of a substance use conviction to this career path. Often, if young people in foster care have had numerous placements, pediatricians can be a source of reliable health education that case workers or caregivers might not feel competent delivering.

Brief Intervention

A brief intervention is designed to be short in duration and aimed at reducing or stopping substance use. Brief interventions support substance use reduction outside the context of SUD treatment. Brief intervention uses motivational interviewing strategies; for that reason, pediatricians may want to complete training in motivational interviewing. Motivational interviewing was designed to help patients balance their ambivalence toward change and their reasons for change related to health behaviors in order to increase their willingness to engage in behavior change.[31] There are 4 key principles of motivational interviewing that inform the components of brief intervention (through the brief negotiated interview[43]).

1. Focus the patient's attention on the current and potential future negative impacts of health behaviors (eg, engaging with patients about their personal goals, discussing the pros and cons of substance use).
2. Decrease the emphasis on labeling, and helping the patient recognize the current impact of their health behavior (eg, feedback reflecting how young people connect their substance use to negative potential outcomes).
3. Give the patient responsibility for their current condition and desire for change (eg, readiness ruler reflecting behavior change).
4. Identify how the patient's behavior is inconsistent with their own beliefs or values (eg, creating an action plan to align behavior to values).

Through this process, the brief negotiated interview helps the adolescent explore their own substance use, identify a plan they are willing to implement, and address barriers to implementing their plan. In some practices, interdisciplinary teams have professionals with training in motivational interviewing (such as a psychologist or social worker) who are best suited to deliver brief interventions. It may also be necessary for a pediatrician to complete training, and resources are available.[44–46]

Encourage Youth to Reduce or Eliminate Substance Use

Adolescents should be encouraged to stop using substances because of the known health and legal consequences. If a young person is not ready to abstain from substances, pediatricians should discuss their willingness to reduce the frequency or quantity of substance use and explore other harm-reduction strategies (contexts of substance use). For example, a 2-week reduction challenge can engage the young person in conversations about what they need to accomplish that goal, including what type of support, and possible follow-up. Before engaging youth who are willing in a conversation about harm-reduction strategies, it is beneficial to have a few strategies to suggest if adolescents are unable to generate their own ideas (such as drinking no more than 3 drinks in one sitting). Targeting factors that decrease the risk of overdose (such as using fentanyl test strips) or identifying other negative consequences (such as intoxicated driving) can also be useful for harm reduction, even if youth are not willing to decrease the quantity or frequency of substance use. Harm-reduction strategies include not using substances alone, drinking water while using substances, buying substances from a single safe individual instead of strangers, monitoring one's drink when around other people, and keeping naloxone nearby.

Signs of an Overdose

For young people who engage in substance use, it is important to review with them and anyone who may accompany them to their appointment (including caregivers, group home workers, case workers, family of origin, friends, romantic partners) the symptoms of an overdose, contextualized to the substance they are using. For example, signs of an opioid overdose include blue or purple lips or fingernails, cold and clammy skin, slow or no breathing, and slow or no heart rate.[47] Signs of an alcohol overdose include difficulty remaining conscious, slow heart rate, vomiting, and seizures.[48] Pediatricians who feel confident discussing common symptoms of an overdose may also choose to incorporate those discussions into routine care with all adolescents.

Naloxone

Naloxone comes in a nasal spray and an injectable form, both of which can be administered to someone who is overdosing on opioids.[49] Naloxone is most effective when administered immediately during an overdose and can be repeatedly administered if needed. All young people known to use opioids should be prescribed naloxone. Pediatricians should teach youth and anyone who may accompany them to their appointment how to use naloxone properly. By discussing naloxone and ensuring it is available in clinic spaces and to young people and their caregivers, pediatricians are contributing to reducing the stigma attached to naloxone and eliminating barriers to patient access.

Diagnosing SUD

Pediatricians should use the *Diagnostic and Statistical Manual of Mental Disorders, 5th Edition,*[50] criteria when identifying and diagnosing youth with an SUD. Specific criteria include the following:

- Substances used in increasingly larger amounts
- Unsuccessful attempts to decrease substance use
- Spending significant amounts of time taking steps to obtain, use, or recover from using substances
- Cravings
- Repeated substance use that prevents fulfillment of academic, work, or familial obligations
- Continual substance use despite repeated social, interpersonal, physical, or psychological difficulties that are caused or intensified by substance use
- Decreased engagement in social, occupational, or recreational activities due to substance use

- Consistent substance use in physically dangerous situations
- Tolerance (a need for larger amounts of the substance to reach intoxication or the desired effect or decreased effects when using the same amount of the substance)
- Use of the substance to avoid withdrawal symptoms

Referrals

Clinicians Who Treat SUD

It is important to identify local clinicians in the community who treat SUD, as well as the age range served by the clinician and the types of treatment they provide. Research shows that it is beneficial to facilitate a warm hand-off to individuals interested in treatment.[51]

When to Refer

Youth who are experiencing negative effects of substance use (within social, familial, academic, or recreational domains) and are willing to engage in treatment should be referred to SUD treatment, which can include pharmacotherapy (ie, medication-assisted treatment) and behavioral therapy.[52] Individuals may choose to participate in either or both types of treatment, depending on the substance and the negative effects they are experiencing.

Medications can be used when treating withdrawal symptoms, helping patients remain in treatment and preventing their return to use.[52–54] The AAP recommends that pediatricians consider offering medications that can be used to treat opioid use disorder in pediatric settings, including methadone (typically reserved for those older than 18 years who are treated outside of pediatric settings), buprenorphine, and naltrexone.[55] Behavioral therapies that can be used to treat SUD include cognitive behavioral therapy, contingency management, family-based therapy, 12-step facilitation, and motivational enhancement therapy.[52]

Foster Care Considerations When Implementing SBIRT

There are unique challenges in implementing SBIRT with young people in foster care. Screening tools are validated in the general population and not specifically in youth in foster care, which can alter the interpretation of and response to specific screening items. For example, on the CRAFFT, a positive response to the question "Have you ever ridden in a car driven by someone (including yourself) who was 'high' or had been using alcohol or drugs?" for the general adolescent population often is due to youth driving or riding in the car with peers using substances. For youth in foster care, due to high levels of parental substance use, the response to this question can be positive due to youth being in the car with parents who are using substances, which requires a different response than for self- or peer-intoxicated driving. In addition, there are many unique barriers to accessing SUD treatment for youth in foster care. For example, substance use may need to be disclosed to a caseworker to obtain treatment, which may increase the court's awareness of the adolescent's substance use. Participating in any type of family therapy is also complex, because it is not always clear whom to include in treatment with the youth (such as foster family, family of origin, group home staff, or independent-living worker). Additionally, when young people move from one placement setting to another (for example, from a kinship caregiver to a group home), their access to ongoing treatment and available resources is often disrupted, and young people can be lost to follow-up or required to return to a waiting list to get access to a program in their new community. Notably, substance use and associated behavioral challenges can contribute to placement changes. Finally, SUD treatment, and pharmacotherapy for SUD in particular, requires a caregiver, caseworker, or trusted adult who is motivated and able to bring the youth to consistent and frequent follow-up appointments, which can be challenging. Despite these unique challenges, conducting screening and providing brief interventions to all young people in foster care are effective strategies to reduce harm from substance use in an especially vulnerable population.[56]

Key Takeaways

- Young people in foster care should be screened for substance use using validated screening tools during foster care–specific health supervision visits (see Chapter 2, Health Care Visits: Type and Periodicity).
- Using the SBIRT framework to screen and deliver brief interventions can assist in reducing substance use by young people in foster care.
- Thoughtful considerations must be made when engaging young people in foster care in substance use treatment due to unique and complex challenges such as confidentiality concerns, potential treatment disruptions with placement changes, and engaging appropriate supportive adults in care.

CHAPTER 22

Pregnant and Parenting Teens

Yael Smiley, MD, FAAP
Bryn King, MSW, PhD

Teens in foster care who are pregnant and/or parenting experience significant challenges in terms of their experiences while in foster care as well as their prospects after transitioning from care. Accounting for their unique needs and contexts may improve outcomes for this group of youth as well as their children. Pediatricians have a critical role in safeguarding these young families.

Background: Pregnancy and Parenting in Foster Care

Youth in foster care are at greater risk of adolescent pregnancy leading to childbirth compared with adolescents in the general population, those experiencing poverty, and those receiving child welfare services while still living at home with their families.[1–3] The risk of teen pregnancy and childbirth among youth in foster care may be attributable to their childhood experiences of maltreatment,[4] as well as their experiences in foster care.[5] Research on the context of early pregnancy and parenting among youth in foster care indicates that entry or reentry into foster care during adolescence, placement instability (including running from care), behavioral health concerns, and disconnection from positive social supports (such as family and school) are contributors to adolescent pregnancy and childbirth. Prior to pregnancy, many youth in foster care have reported difficulty accessing and effectively using sexual and reproductive education and health care due to changes in placement, lack of knowledge, and difficulty trusting clinicians.[6] In addition to these challenges, research indicates that the larger socioeconomic context drives both foster care entry and early childbirth, such that youth in foster care who are pregnant or parenting are more likely to be Black, Latino, or Indigenous[7] and come from low-income households and communities.[1]

There may be limitations to strategies to prevent and support youth in delaying pregnancy, as they may enter care while pregnant or become pregnant shortly thereafter.[2] There is limited research about youth in foster care during pregnancy, but it suggests that many teens who are pregnant may not receive adequate prenatal care and may even leave foster care while they are pregnant or shortly after giving birth.[2,8,9] There is also some research indicating that birth outcomes (birth weight, for example) for children born to youth who have had involvement with child protective services are worse than for those born to other teen parents.[10] The stress of parenting while still in foster care is high,[11,12] and adolescent girls who were pregnant and gave birth while still in foster care have described a range of emotional challenges and opportunities, including pride in their capacity; a sense of hope, permanence, and renewal as expectant and new parents; social isolation as a result of little family and community support; and stigma related to their status as both a youth in foster care and an expectant or parenting teen.[11,13–16] Expectant and parenting youth in foster care also face significant adversity with respect to completing their education and securing and sustaining stable employment.[17–22] Because many have experienced so much uncertainty in their living arrangements, they are rightly concerned about the stability of their current placements and their prospects for housing once they leave care. There are few placement options specifically designed for pregnant and parenting teens, and interventions designed to support the needs of expectant and parenting teens are rarely adapted for youth in foster care.

Effective supports are critical to the health and well-being of pregnant and parenting teens and their young children. Rates of rapid repeat pregnancy are high among the foster care population,[23,24] and additional children can increase risks to children and their parents.[25] Rates of two-generation child welfare involvement are also high for this population.[26] While surveillance bias is a contributor, it nevertheless elevates concerns about the risk of intergenerational maltreatment as well as pregnant and new parents' fears that their children may be removed from them.[11,27] In one study, nearly 20% of children born to young mothers in foster care were removed and placed in foster care before 4 years of age, and many of the factors contributing to the likelihood of early childbirth, including maternal mental health needs, also increased the risk of child removal.[28] Postpartum depression is more common among teen parents than their older counterparts,[29] and those in foster care may be at higher risk than youth not in foster care.[30] Given their potential experiences with trauma and placement instability, adolescents in foster care have high rates of diagnosed mental health concerns and prescriptions for psychotropic medication,[31–33] and the need for treatment may increase during pregnancy and after birth. Former youth in foster care who became parents have reported that they stopped taking psychotropic medication during pregnancy, which increased their symptoms and contributed to worsened mental health.[30] Relationships that could buffer the impact of these circumstances are not always available or responsive to the needs of youth in foster care,[15] and research indicates that pregnant and parenting youth in foster care may be especially vulnerable to intimate partner violence.[34] In sum, these youth experience significant adversity before, during, and after pregnancy and childbirth; yet, there are potential opportunities to meaningfully address their needs and improve their health and well-being.

Providing Medical Care for Pregnant and Parenting Youth in Foster Care

It is important that services to pregnant and parenting youth in foster care account for the history and contexts that led to their placement in foster care, their pregnancy, and their decision to become a parent. Providing medical care to these youth should also be guided by an understanding of the cumulative burden of these circumstances as well as the substantial stigma they experience related to their identities as youth in foster care and adolescent parents. It is essential that language and interventions do not convey to these young people that they are incapable parents or represent a threat to their children. Pediatricians should employ a nonjudgmental, trauma-informed, strengths-based approach to caring for these families.[28,35]

Rights

Pediatricians working in primary care, emergency departments, and subspecialty clinics will encounter pregnant and parenting youth in foster care. It is important for clinical staff to know adolescents' rights to consent to health care, which vary based on type of health care service and jurisdiction. The Guttmacher Institute tracks adolescents' rights to consent to medical care based on state law for contraceptive services, sexually transmitted infection services, prenatal care, adoption, medical care for minor's child, and abortion services.[36] Pregnant and parenting youth in foster care have all the same rights as their counterparts in the general population; including medical decision-making for their own child's medical care if they retain parental rights, as shown in **Box 22–1**. Youth in foster care who are pregnant or parenting are entitled to high-quality, nonjudgmental health care services including sexual and reproductive health care. Given the potential for these youth to be affected by traumatic experiences and stigma, it is especially important for pediatricians to adopt a reproductive justice approach in their practice. They should avoid coercion by recognizing "every person's right to decide whether to have children, to decide the number and spacing of children, and to have the information, education, and access to health services to make these decisions."[37]

Box 22-1

Case Study #1

Diamond was placed in foster care at 9 years of age because of abuse and neglect. She had her first child when she was 15 years old and 2 more children while she was still an adolescent. She lived in supportive housing for young adult mothers in foster care and participated in a peer support group for young mothers until her 3 children were removed from her care after witnessing intimate partner violence with the father of her youngest child. After her children were removed, the clinical staff worked with her to obtain her own medical care. Although she did not have custody of her children, she did still have medical decision-making rights, so the clinical staff ensured that she could continue to coordinate and attend appointments for her children along with child welfare workers and the foster family.

Pregnancy

After a pregnancy is identified, youth in foster care should receive the same counseling about pregnancy options as any other adolescent, allowing them to make their own informed medical decisions in their own context. Pediatricians may be more trusted, neutral, and knowledgeable than other support people in the teen's life, including friends and child welfare staff, and they are particularly equipped to provide this counseling. The American Academy of Pediatrics (AAP) recommends that pediatricians inform pregnant teens about their pregnancy options, which include continuing the pregnancy and raising the child; continuing the pregnancy and making an adoption, kinship care, or foster care plan; or terminating the pregnancy.[37] After the teen chooses an option, it is essential for pediatricians to coordinate with child welfare staff to help facilitate access to prenatal care, adoption services, or abortion care as allowable by law.

Parenting Teens

Prior to the end of pregnancy, the AAP *Bright Futures: Guidelines for Health Supervision of Infants, Children, and Adolescents*, Fourth Edition, recommends a prenatal visit with the baby's future pediatrician.[38] This allows the pregnant adolescent to reestablish care with their pediatrician and develop plans to access community resources and support parental well-being.[39] It is important for pediatricians to recognize that adolescent parents often experience judgment and stigma.[39] **Table 22–1** lists AAP recommendations for providing care to adolescent parents, with additional considerations to help provide nonjudgmental, asset-focused care to expectant and parenting youth in foster care and their children in the domains of coordinated care, adolescent and perinatal health, relationships, and advocacy.

Coordinated Care

Pregnant and parenting youth in foster care receive support from various professionals and social service agencies, which can be fragmented and burdensome for the young person to manage. Youth in foster care benefit when care can be coordinated and streamlined among these parties, as highlighted in **Box 22–2**. When possible, coordinated teen–tot clinics, integrated mental health programs, and colocated social service programs can minimize access barriers to medical care and social services. It is especially important for clinicians to partner with child welfare staff to ensure pregnant and parenting teens in foster care are connected to relevant community support programs, including housing, food, education, employment, and transportation programs.

Health

It is critical to address adolescent and perinatal health care needs for expectant and parenting youth in foster care. The AAP recommends strategies to promote breastfeeding by adolescent parents, which can be supported in adolescents in foster care as well.[39] These youth may need additional support from community-based lactation services, as well as support in securing private breastfeeding spaces, especially if they are placed in congregate settings. Because 17% of adolescent pregnancies are repeat pregnancies, pediatricians should offer regular nonjudgmental counseling about pregnancy spacing and offer all contraceptive options, including long-acting methods.[39] Addressing mental health needs in the perinatal period is critical, given the high burden of preexisting mental health conditions for youth in foster care, including offering evidence-based counseling about the safety of taking psychotropic medications during this time, including while breastfeeding.

Relationships

Pediatricians and other clinicians can also support healthy, safe relationships for pregnant and parenting teens in foster care and their children.[40] In promoting safe relationships, pediatricians should be aware of higher rates of intimate partner violence among this population and screen and provide resources accordingly.

Table 22–1. Guidance for Pediatricians When Caring for Pregnant and Parenting Youth in Foster Care

AAP Guidance[39] for the Pediatrician: Caring for Adolescent Parents	Additional Considerations for Pregnant and Parenting Youth in Care (PPYIC)
Coordinated Care	
• Create a patient-centered medical home for adolescent parents and their children. Teen–tot clinics, in which both the adolescent parent or parents and their child complete appointments at the same visit, model this approach. • Provide a multidisciplinary and comprehensive approach to caring for parenting adolescents by using community resources, such as doulas, social services, and nurse home visitation programs. • Recognize that social determinants of health (SDOH), such as poverty and childhood adversity, contribute to health outcomes for adolescent parents and their children. Provide referrals to community resources to address these needs. • Become aware of programs in your community that support pregnant adolescents and adolescent parents.	• Partner with child welfare staff to ensure PPYIC have access to medical care. • Consider that PPYIC and their children could have changes in housing and neighborhood but may still want to stay connected to trusted medical homes and clinicians. • Include child welfare staff in a multidisciplinary approach for PPYIC. • Learn eligibility criteria and referral pathways to connect PPYIC to appropriate social support programs. • Know if there are specific programs for PPYIC (eg, housing, home visiting). • Recognize that SDOH are associated with PPYIC being in foster care and rates of pregnancy. • Leverage resources of the child welfare system to overcome barriers related to SDOH.
Perinatal and Adolescent Health	
• Promote breastfeeding initiation and continuation among adolescent mothers by providing lactation resources and encouraging partners and maternal grandmothers to be supportive around breastfeeding. • Provide contraceptive counseling during the prenatal and postnatal periods in partnership with obstetricians and in subsequent health supervision visits. Offer access to the full range of contraceptive services, including long-acting reversible contraceptives. Provide adolescent fathers with contraceptive counseling. • Use a validated screening tool for assessing postpartum depression in all adolescent parents and refer to mental health resources when indicated. • Screen for intimate partner violence (IPV) and provide community resources to address positive responses from pregnant and parenting adolescents.	• Recognize that breastfeeding for PPYIC may be affected by privacy considerations and that PPYIC may need support accessing designated breastfeeding spaces. • Offer resources and support people for lactation from outside of the family, such as public health nurses or lactation consultants. • Adapt an especially noncoercive approach to the provision of contraceptive counseling and ensure that PPYIC have access to contraceptive services. • Provide evidence-based counseling about safety of using psychotropic and contraceptive medications during postpartum and lactation periods. • Be aware that PPYIC have higher rates of psychotropic medication use. Employ shared decision-making in choosing mental health management plans. • Offer colocated mental health supports when possible. • Recognize increased risk of IPV for PPYIC (see **Box 22–1**). • Know the policies in relevant jurisdictions for mandated reporting of IPV. Leverage relationships with child welfare staff to identify concerns about potentially abusive relationships for PPYIC.

Table 22–1 *(continued)*

AAP Guidance[39] for the Pediatrician: Caring for Adolescent Parents	Additional Considerations for Pregnant and Parenting Youth in Care (PPYIC)
Relationships	
• Involve partners and families in the newborn period and infancy, actively supporting their involvement in their children's care. • Recognize all forms of parenting, including coparenting, and support the role of the adolescent father or partner. • Promote low-cost activities with high yield in improving the social and cognitive development of young children, such as play and reading.	• Ask PPYIC to introduce their support people and ask if any should have a role in making health care decisions. • Acknowledge that support people can include partners, biological family, foster family, child welfare staff, non-biological chosen family, friends, and mentors. • Recognize increased stigma experienced by PPYIC. • Applaud PPYIC for their parenting approaches and successes. • Understand resources available to the young parent before making recommendations so they are contextually appropriate and can be successfully implemented. • Promote parenting groups specifically for teens, especially if teen–tot programs are not available.
Advocacy	
• Emphasize the importance of completing high school and pursuing higher education or vocational training. Advocate for on-site child care in schools or training programs that can facilitate this goal. • Advocate for longitudinal, comprehensive solutions that are focused on primary prevention strategies to continue to decrease teen pregnancy rates. Push for funding of programs that support adolescent parents to reduce repeat pregnancies and optimize the health of both parent and child (eg, health care, food assistance, housing, home visitation programs). • Advocate for a 2-generational approach to improving outcomes for the dyad in areas such as poverty, education, and social-emotional development. • Coverage of, access to, and coordination of services among clinicians needs to be a priority for payers to assist pregnant and parenting adolescents.	• Recognize there are additional barriers to attaining educational goals for PPYIC. • Learn about specific resources to support PPYIC in schools, such as scholarships, staff supports, tutoring, and child care. • Recognize that the burden on PPYIC is even higher than on other pregnant and parenting teens due to absence of parent and family resources. • Advocate for creation of new programs and funding of existing programs specifically designed for PPYIC. • Refer to existing teen–tot medical homes for both parents and children. Consider expanding these services in areas where they are not currently available.

It is important to acknowledge that there may be a range of support people, including partners, biological family, foster family, child welfare staff, non-biological chosen family, friends, and mentors. Patients should be invited to bring their chosen support people to medical appointments. Clinicians can support positive parent–infant relationship development by applauding these young people's parenting approaches and successes. Clinicians can also refer these teens to parenting programs, as some may have grown up in families with significant stressors. It is important to address the teen's trauma history to reduce intergenerational transmission of trauma.

Advocacy

Pediatricians can advocate for pregnant and parenting youth in foster care in various ways. On the individual and community levels, pediatricians should learn about specific resources to support these youth in the community such as education programs, housing programs, child care, and doulas, as illustrated in **Box 22–3**. Awareness of eligibility criteria and referral pathways will allow pediatricians to effectively advocate for access to necessary services for their patients. Pediatricians can also partner with child welfare and local policy organizations to advocate for the development of new programs and funding for existing programs specifically designed for pregnant and parenting teens in foster care, including parenting programs, trauma-informed care, and mental health care.

Box 22–2

Case Study #2

Nia was in foster care before getting pregnant. She gave birth to her daughter when she was 16 years old and was referred to a teen–tot primary care clinical program. The clinic-based social worker helped manage her transitions as she moved between her biological mother's home, foster homes, and independent living. She also had several health concerns, and the clinic-based social worker was her medical advocate and coordinated with her child welfare worker on scheduling and transportation for her many appointments. After her 21st birthday, Nia moved into independent housing with her daughter, started working as a community support worker, and was accepted into a scholarship program to support young parents in higher education. She is now enrolled in a 4-year bachelor's degree program and plans to pursue a career in social work to work with young mothers and children in foster care.

Box 22–3

Case Study #3

Ana entered care at age 16 years due to concerns about exploitation after her biological father was deported. She had her first child the following year. There were allegations of neglect, and Ana's child was removed from her, but she was referred to a teen–tot clinic by child welfare staff. She had a second child at 19 years old and received support from a teen-focused doula during pregnancy and postpartum. Her younger child remains in her care as she balances parenting with finishing her GED, full-time employment, and working to regain custody of her older child.

Key Takeaways

- » Youth in foster care are at higher risk of teen pregnancy and childbirth than youth in the general population due to their experiences of maltreatment and being in foster care.
- » Parenting youth in foster care experience greater vulnerability and stigma than do other teen parents.
- » Pregnant and parenting youth in foster care retain the same rights as other adolescents and other parents and are able to make their own sexual and reproductive health decisions as well as medical decisions for their children.
- » Individual pediatricians can support parenting youth in foster care by providing nonjudgmental, strengths-based, and trauma-informed care.
- » Pregnant and parenting teens in foster care benefit from health care systems that are accessible, streamlined, and connected to community-based programs and supports.

CHAPTER

23

Commercial Sexual Exploitation of Children

Molly McHenry, FNP, PMHNP
Anish Raj, MD, FAAP

Over the past 2 decades, a growing awareness has developed around the various patterns of maltreatment that adolescents in foster care can experience. A subset of the child welfare population that has increasingly gained prominence are individuals involved in or at risk for the commercial sexual exploitation of children (CSEC). This umbrella term is broadly defined as any exchange of a sexual act for anything of perceived value (eg, money, shelter, and substances) involving a minor (an individual younger than 18 years).[1] It encompasses both domestic and transnational sex trafficking, survival sex, and numerous other forms of sexual exploitation.[2] The most common manifestation of CSEC in the United States is domestic minor sex trafficking (DMST), which more specifically denotes CSEC that involves a US citizen or legal resident within the territorial borders of the United States.[3] While federal legislation has determined that force, fraud, and coercion do not need to be demonstrated in cases involving minors and that survivors be identified as victims of crime, clinicians should familiarize themselves with their individual state's laws.[1] Given the clandestine nature of the sex industry and the lack of common databases consolidating information following identification, accurate epidemiological data regarding the prevalence of CSEC in the United States are not currently available.[4] Cases of CSEC have been reported in all 50 states, but estimates are not generally considered reliable enough to cite.[1] Although the vast majority of CSEC survivors seek medical care during the period of exploitation,[5] many clinicians report not having been trained on appropriate identification and corresponding resources.[6,7]

In addition to an overview of risk factors and health needs commonly associated with CSEC, this chapter describes approaches to properly screen and identify potential victims in the clinical setting and efforts to address both prevention and the aftercare response.

Biopsychosocial Vulnerabilities

By virtue of their age and neurodevelopmental immaturity, all children and adolescents are considered vulnerable to manipulation and exploitation.[2] Socioecological model research demonstrates that involvement in the commercial sex trade is inherently difficult to separate from challenging familial circumstances, poverty, housing instability, and systematic oppression based on racial, gender, and sexual identity.[8] Based on their cumulative life experiences, youth in foster care are often at higher risk for the exposures that may lead to CSEC involvement.[9,10]

The literature has identified the following factors as being associated with CSEC victimization:

- *Maltreatment:* A history of childhood sexual abuse is the strongest correlate of CSEC.[9]
- *Behavior:* Running away from home is noted to be a prominent risk factor and a key mediating variable between a history of childhood maltreatment and CSEC victimization.[9] Research has increasingly found that youth with CSEC involvement commonly have a history of mental health morbidity (eg, posttraumatic stress disorder, anxiety, depression).[9]
- *Demographics:* Systematic oppression and social discrimination, often experienced by individuals of minority race or sexual orientation (lesbian, gay, bisexual, transgender, and queer or questioning [LGBTQ+]), have been associated with higher rates of CSEC victimization.[10] While the proportion of female to male victims remains unknown, it is believed that the number of male victims remains underestimated.[2]
- *Environment:* Household dysfunction, especially experiences with poverty, homelessness, the child welfare system, and caregiver substance use are associated with increased CSEC victimization.[10]

It is imperative that individuals not be labeled a "trafficking victim or survivor" simply based on the presence or absence of research-based risk factors. Clinical correlation is essential.

Screening and Identification in Clinical Settings

When CSEC is suspected, rapport-building with the patient is of utmost importance.[2,3,11,12] Youth experiencing CSEC face multiple and layered barriers in disclosing the realities of their lives and therefore receiving comprehensive and appropriate health care.[13] Barriers include fear, shame, depression, trauma, intoxication, and mistrust of adults in positions of authority.[12,13] Youth who are being trafficked often do not identify as victims.[14] Part of the grooming process by traffickers can include imparting a false sense of control and consent to the youth, often done through subtle manipulation and coercive control. It is not uncommon for traffickers to convince the trafficked youth that they are in a romantic relationship and frame the sex acts that are traded for money as a sign of loyalty and love to the trafficker.[15] Youth who are being trafficked may also feel a need to protect their traffickers as well as others being trafficked in the same network whom they might see as family.[16] Youth may have been coached on what to say by their traffickers, or their traffickers may be listening to the visit via a cell phone.[3] The reality of who is trafficking the youth may further complicate the interaction. Types of traffickers and typical corresponding characteristics are shown in **Table 23–1**.[17] If the patient is accompanied by someone who is thought to be their trafficker, that person should be excluded from the interview and their presence avoided during the entirety of the appointment, if possible. However, it may be difficult to separate a trafficker from the suspected victim. If an accompanying adult is suspected of trafficking and they are resistant to leaving the room, this should raise further suspicion. All of this should be kept in mind while navigating interactions with youth suspected of CSEC involvement.

If CSEC is suspected, a single comprehensive evaluation should be performed by the most highly trained clinician in child sexual abuse available. Multiple interviews and redundant questioning are to be avoided to protect the youth from retraumatization. Before asking sensitive questions, the clinician should have a transparent discussion about what mandated reporting is and what answers might warrant a call to child protective services.[3] Youth who are experiencing CSEC have little to no control over their lives. Thus, helping them to feel in control during the visit will build rapport while allowing them to discern what they feel comfortable sharing.[3,12] Youth who are experiencing sexual exploitation may want to disclose their abuse and can feel discouraged when they are not given the opportunity.

Screening tools can be used to identify youth who are at increased risk for CSEC, including a 6-question brief screen.[14] In one study, use of the screen differentiated youth involved in CSEC from those who had experienced isolated sexual assault with a sensitivity of 92% and a specificity of 73%.[14] If the screen indicates the youth is at high risk for CSEC, a further discussion is warranted. Aside from using screeners, there may be other potential indicators that a child is involved in CSEC, as seen in **Box 23–1**.[2] Of note, one study found that the presence of any tattoo, not just those including a man's name or sexually explicit images or words, was significantly more frequent among youth experiencing CSEC when compared with youth reporting sexual assault alone.[14] If there are concerns for CSEC, the clinician should use open-ended questions to elicit further information. Examples can be found in **Table 23–2**.[12] Using a normalizing statement before direct questioning about sexual exploitation can help youth feel more comfortable answering questions while also increasing the likelihood of accurate reporting. A study by Covenant House[18] found that the following language on a written intake form increased disclosures of sexual exploitation:

> Sometimes young people who are homeless or who are having difficulties with their families have very few options to survive or fulfill their basic needs, such as food and shelter. Sometimes they are exploited or feel the need to use their sexuality to help them survive. Have you or anyone else ever received anything of value, such as money, a place to stay, food, drugs, gifts, or favors, in exchange for your performing a sexual activity?

Sexual exploitation of any type involves a loss of control and autonomy. Thus, it is crucial to be transparent with the youth seeking care that they are not required to answer any questions or submit to any physical examination with which they feel uncomfortable.[3]

Table 23–1. Overview of Victim–Trafficker Relationship Types

Relationship Type	Characteristics
Friend	Trafficker and victim consider themselves friends before DMST victimization; marked by mutual recruitment: trafficker seeking "worker," victim seeking protection; agreement to mutually share profits, whether this actually occurs or not
Romantic partner	Trafficker is boyfriend, girlfriend, or romantic interest of victim; trafficker may not view the relationship as romantic but uses romance as manipulation tool; marked by dynamics similar to domestic violence relationships: physical, psychological, emotional, financial abuse tactics used to exert control
Family member	Victim more likely to be used for trafficker's financial gain than any mutually agreed-upon benefit; more often rural location of trafficking; younger age of onset; victims have more experience with child abuse than other victim-trafficker relationship types
Stranger	Most commonly referenced relationship type in popular media; no relationship between victim and trafficker preceding the DMST victimization; trafficker viewed as predatory, manipulative, skilled
No outside trafficker	Marked by "survival sex"; victim does not have a trafficker or pimp; victim exchanges sex for money or goods; may view sex work as consensual or empowering; exploiter is "john" who purchases sex from victim, but no outside facilitator involved

Abbreviation: DMST, domestic minor sex trafficking.

Reproduced from Twis MK. Predicting different types of victim-trafficker relationships: a multinomial logistic regression analysis. *Journal of Human Trafficking.* 2019;6(4):1–17.

Box 23-1

Potential Indicators of Commercial Sexual Exploitation of Children

Initial Presentation

Child accompanied by domineering adult who does not allow child to answer questions

Child accompanied by unrelated adult

Child accompanied by other children and only 1 adult

Child provides changing information regarding demographics

Chief complaint is acute sexual assault or acute physical assault

Chief complaint is suicide attempt

Child is poor historian or disoriented from sleep deprivation or drug intoxication

Historical Factors

Multiple sexually transmitted infections (STIs)

Previous pregnancy/abortion

Frequent visits for emergency contraception

Chronic runaway behavior

Chronic truancy or problems in school

History of sexual abuse/physical abuse/neglect

Involvement of child protective services (especially foster care/group home)

Involvement with department of juvenile justice

Significantly older boyfriend

Frequent substance use/misuse

Lack of medical home and/or frequent emergency department visits

Physical Findings

Evidence suggestive of inflicted injury

Tattoos (sexually explicit, of man's name, gang affiliation)

Child withdrawn, fearful

Signs of substance misuse

Expensive items, clothing, hotel keys

Large amounts of cash

Poor dentition or obvious chronic lack of care

Reproduced from Greenbaum J, Crawford-Jakubiak JE; Committee on Child Abuse and Neglect. Child sex trafficking and commercial sexual exploitation: health care needs of victims. *Pediatrics.* 2015 Mar;135(3):566–74

Table 23–2. Advice and Wording Suggestions From Trafficking Survivors on How to Discuss Trafficking With Patients in the Pediatric Emergency Department

Practical Advice	Wording Suggestions
Show genuine concern about their emotional and mental state.	"Are you emotionally okay? Are you mentally okay?"
	"You look a little down. What's going on? How's everything going? Is everything okay?"
Reassure the patient that you are with them in the situation.	"You're not alone. I am here with you."
	"I understand the situation you went through was difficult, and I'm here to listen."
Ask the patient for permission to hear more about what is going on.	"It sounds like you're feeling like no one understands you. Are you willing to tell me more about it? What makes you feel this way?"
	"I'm trying to understand. May I ask some personal questions?"
	"How has your day gone? Is there anything you feel as though you would like to share with us about how you're feeling today?"
Empower the patient by referring to them in encouraging terms.	"You're not alone. You've been through a lot and shown you are strong, brave, and courageous."
Reiterate that you will not break their confidentiality unnecessarily.	"As we talk, I want you to know that I'm here for you. I will do my best to keep what you share confidential. And you can ask me anything. However, there are certain things I may need to report to keep you safe. I will always try to let you know if I need to share something and explain why."
Use the patient's symptoms to begin the conversation.	"I was reading your chart and I noticed that some of these things have happened to you. Do you feel comfortable sharing more about the circumstances?"
	"Where is your abdominal pain coming from? Have you experienced [this or that], or have you been going through anything you'd like to share?"
Check with the patient to see if they feel safe to share at the moment before proceeding.	"Some teens who share things like this feel unsafe where they are living or have felt unsafe in the past. Do you have any concerns about your safety or your well-being here and now, in the recent past or possibly the near future?"
	"Do you feel safe right now?"
Explicitly assure the patient they are in a safe place at the moment.	"This is a safe space. You are safe if you choose to share anything with me."
Validate the patient's feelings.	"Thank you for sharing this with me. You are right, that is a lot to go through, especially at such a young age."
	"It's not your fault you are going through what you are."
Ask direct and concrete questions regarding trauma, stress, and abuse.	"Have you ever been hurt? Have you ever been abused? Have you ever been mistreated?"
	"Are you being exploited? Has he tried to exploit you?"
	"Have you experienced trauma or anything? Have you been stressing?"
	"Are you comfortable where you live? Are you safe at home?"
Ask if the patient is hoping for change in circumstanc-es or has future hopes.	"Sometimes, when I hear about things like this, I find the patient is looking for a change in their life. Are you?"

Adapted from Wallace C, Schein Y, Carabelli G, et al. A survivor-derived approach to addressing trafficking in the pediatric ED. *Pediatrics*. 2020;147(1):e20200772

Health Care Needs

Prominent national and international guidelines generally promote a trauma-informed, survivor-centered, and rights-based approach.[19] Comprehensive screening for sexually transmitted infections (STIs), including chlamydia, gonorrhea, trichomonas, syphilis, HIV, hepatitis B, and hepatitis C, should be offered, as well as pregnancy tests when indicated.[3] If a youth is deemed to be at risk of CSEC but is denying involvement, preventive health care should be provided, including contraceptive care, preexposure prophylaxis and postexposure prophylaxis, access to mental health care, updating any overdue immunizations, and addressing any other chronic health issues.[3] If possible, scheduling follow-up appointments will allow for continued rapport building as well as afford time to continue to address health needs. With ongoing rapport building, youth may feel more comfortable disclosing sexual exploitation to a clinician. Follow-up appointments will also allow for repeat STI screening when indicated as well as further application of preventive measures and chronic disease management. STI screening usually should be repeated 3 months after the initial screen.

At this time, no single, consensus clinic model has been established to meet the unique health care needs of survivors of CSEC. In recent years, innovative models of health care delivery have included

- Medical home with integration of primary care, sexual/reproductive health, and mental health[20]
- Adolescent health clinic with specialized services for youth who have experienced or are at risk for CSEC[21,22]
- Primary care clinic within a community health center designed for survivors of sexual violence (PurpLE [Purpose: Listen and Engage][23–25])

If a youth discloses a sexual assault within the preceding 72 hours, a forensic examination should be offered. This can be done by a designated child abuse team or with trained pediatricians at an emergency department. Sexual assault nurse examiners are present in most emergency departments and increasingly can be reached through telehealth for real-time assistance in forensic interviews, examinations, and sample collection.[26]

Community Resources

Current best practice recommendations for the community response include a coordinated, multidisciplinary collaboration between child protective services, law enforcement, local child advocacy center, legal aid, and clinicians. Key health care personnel can include child abuse pediatricians, primary care physicians, social workers, and case managers. Youth involved in CSEC are referred to an average of 3 distinct agencies for ongoing care.[8] As such, research supports having a designated navigator to coordinate services across organizations as the preferred practice.[8] Health care professionals should familiarize themselves with any existing CSEC coalitions or task forces in their community.

National resources include

- National Human Trafficking Hotline: https://humantraffickinghotline.org; 1-888-373-7888
- Polaris Project: https://polarisproject.org/
- International Association of Forensic Nurses: https://www.forensicnurses.org/page/TeleSAFE

Key Takeaways

- *Commercial sexual exploitation of children* is an umbrella term that encompasses numerous forms of maltreatment in which a sex act is exchanged for something of value. The most common manifestation of CSEC is DMST, which involves US citizens or legal residents within the territorial borders of the United States.
- Socioecological research suggests that based on their cumulative life experiences, youth in foster care are often at higher risk for the exposures that may lead to CSEC involvement.
- Building a rapport with youth suspected of CSEC involvement is of the utmost importance. This includes using transparent language about what mandated reporting means and what kind of information shared would warrant a report being filed.
- Let the youth know that they are not required to answer any questions or submit to any physical examinations if they do not feel comfortable doing so. This will foster a sense of autonomy and control on the part of the youth, which will aid in rapport building.
- There are complex and layered barriers preventing youth from disclosing CSEC. Barriers include fear, shame, depression, trauma, intoxication, and mistrust of adults in positions of authority. On the other hand, many CSEC victims want to disclose when given a safe opportunity.
- If CSEC is suspected but a youth denies involvement, preventive health care should still be provided, such as contraceptive care, access to mental health care, updating immunizations, offering STI screening, offering preexposure prophylaxis and postexposure prophylaxis when indicated, and managing any existing chronic illnesses. Scheduling follow-up appointments will allow for further rapport building and give victims more opportunities to disclose CSEC involvement.

CHAPTER

24

Youth Who Have Run From Their Living Situation or Are Missing From Care

Ariel Kiyomi Daoud, MD
Mary Emily C. Haas, MD, FAAP
Joseph Kiesler, MD

Defining the Problem

When considering the specific health needs of children in foster care, it is important to account for the increased health risks for those who are missing from care from their homes or foster care placements. There are varying terms used to describe situations in which youth are missing from foster care. Child welfare agencies do not always agree on terminology or when to identify a child as missing from care. For example, some report a child missing as soon as a child has left their placement, while others do so only after 24 hours.[1]

The following definitions have been adopted for this chapter:

- A child is considered *runaway* when they (1) leave home without permission and stay away overnight or (2) are away with permission, choose not to come home, and stay away for one or more nights.
- Previously, literature used the term *thrown away* to refer to youth in a situation where an adult household member tells the child to leave or prevents them from returning home, the adult does not arrange for adequate alternative care, and the child is gone overnight.
- This chapter uses *missing from care*[2] as a less stigmatizing and more general term to describe both situations above.

Missing from care is the most prevalent category of missing children, compared with children who are missing due to abductions, involuntarily lost, stranded, or injured.[3] From 2010 to 2019, about 1% of the approximately 400,000 youth in foster care ran away each year.[2,4] The rate of children who are missing from care is higher among youth in foster care than in the general population, and youth in foster care are about twice as likely to run away compared with children in the general population.[4]

The population of youth missing from foster care overlaps significantly with unaccompanied youth living on the street. To help understand the larger scope of the problem, on a single night in 2023, 34,700 unaccompanied youth were found to be experiencing homelessness in the US Department of Housing and Urban Development's annual Point-in-Time Count. Homelessness has major effects on the health of young people, including barriers to resources such as housing, health care, and community educational supports. Further, those who are unhoused are more likely to belong to another historically marginalized group, including identifying as Black/African American, cis-female, transgender, not singularly female or male, or gender questioning.[5]

For those children missing from care, the risks of *living on the street*—staying in a place not designated for regular sleeping accommodation for humans or in abandoned buildings—has both acute and chronic effects. Leaving a foster care placement without permission has negative consequences for the young person including, but not limited to, difficulty with finding future placements, human trafficking, poor health outcomes, educational interruption or cessation, and future homelessness. In some instances, leaving care without permission may be the child's only perceived way of escaping an unsafe situation. It is important to consider assumptions associated with this interruption in out-of-home placement when providing care for youth with a history of being missing from care.[1,6]

This chapter reviews characteristics associated with youth missing from care, understanding why youth become missing from care, specific health risks for this population, consequences for future housing insecurity and future placement challenges, and guidance for clinicians taking care of youth in foster care and those experiencing homelessness.

Characteristics Associated With Youth Missing From Care

Database analyses of children in out-of-home care have been performed with varying findings regarding characteristics associated with youth missing from care. This chapter considers two state-level analyses and one national database analysis. The findings regarding identifiers such as gender and race are nuanced and unsatisfactory, given the complexities of these identities and the ill fit of data collection methods to consider these characteristics adequately. The most robust, national analysis suggested that female gender had increased association with missing-from-care youth when compared with male gender, though the two state analyses found no significant differences in their binary gender analyses. Considering the results regarding other identity characteristics, such as race, they suggest that individuals from historically marginalized groups are likely at higher risk of unstable placements. Data are less complex regarding placement factors or elements of patient histories associated with youth missing from care (**Box 24–1**).[2,7,8]

Box 24–1

Characteristics of Youth Missing from Care

Out-of-Home Care Placement Factors

- ▲ Older age when removed from family of origin
- ▲ Older age at time of running away
- ▲ Increased number of out-of-home placements
- ▲ More recently placed in current placement (ie, 4 months' less time in their current placement compared to those who did not run)[6]
- ▲ Placement in a group/congregate setting rather than a family
- ▲ Separation from siblings in placement

Patient History

- ▲ History of abandonment or neglect
- ▲ History of sexual abuse
- ▲ History of psychological abuse
- ▲ History of substance use

The literature identifies 3 drivers of youth behavior when missing from care in a foster placement: searching for social support, normalcy, and activities. Another conceptualization of why youth leave is that they are trying to access or "running to" something, such as family of origin, friends, a romantic partner, autonomy, independence, or activities such as sporting events, parties, alcohol use, sexual activity, or sex work. Youth also have avoidance drivers, or things they are "running away" from, such as negative social interactions with staff and peers, restrictive placements and hostile living environments, and boredom. Connecting with families of origin in search of social support and normalcy might be a driver, even if the youth realize these are not healthy and safe environments. Youth may reach for autonomy because they have been independent and taken on responsibilities of adults in the past. They may also seek to maintain peer relationships and activities.[6]

Health Effects Specific to Youth in Foster Care

There are many health consequences (**Box 24–2**) for youth missing from foster care, and these overlap with those for children who run away from any living situation. Some effects on health may be positive if the child is running away from something harmful, such as abuse. However, the negative health consequences of youth being missing from care are better documented. Adolescents who initiate foster care disruptions have increased rates of school absences, exposure to crime (both as victim and perpetrator), substance use and sales, and juvenile justice involvement.[9,10] More generally, adolescents who experience homelessness, which includes this population, have higher rates of both acute and chronic medical problems—especially those related to sexual and mental health. Adolescent females who are experiencing homelessness or living in shelters have much higher rates of pregnancy and sexual abuse than the housed population.[11] In fact, 44% of one sample of female youth reported sexual exploitation while missing from foster care.[12] Children who run away from their living situations, whether in foster care or not, are more likely to have increased mental health problems (eg, suicidal thoughts) and increased drug use (particularly tobacco and marijuana).[10,13,14] All of this is made worse by this population's decreased access to health care.

Only half of youth experiencing homelessness have regular access to health care; youth who are missing from foster care, depending on the length of their absence, may have similarly decreased access.[15] These children also lack regular access to school and educational services. Poor academic achievement is more common in children who are experiencing homelessness or who are highly mobile, even when compared with other low-income children.[16] Adolescents who have run away from any living situation have poorer ratings of overall health as adults than their peers who have not run. For clinicians, being aware of the characteristics of youth associated with being missing from care, and the health consequences, will allow better support for adolescents in foster care when they present for medical care in clinics and hospitals.

Box 24-2

Health Risks Associated With Being Missing From Care

- Exposure to drugs and alcohol
  - Using and selling (which can place youth at risk for justice involvement as well)
- Sexual health
  - Victimization
  - Trafficking
  - Sexually transmitted infections
  - Pregnancy
- Criminal activity/incarceration
- School disruption
  - Decreased education
  - Disruption of community supports
- Decreased access to health care (documented for youth experiencing homelessness more generally than youth in foster care)
  - Missing medications for chronic health conditions
- Higher rates of acute and chronic health problems (asthma, lice, dental caries) (documented for youth experiencing homelessness more generally than youth in foster care)

Housing Insecurity and Placement Challenges

The goal of foster placement is permanency, with a consistency in placement and supportive, ongoing relationships. Of children in long-term foster placement, 20% to 50% experience a premature ending to their placement rather than staying in a single placement until placement permanency is realized. The various situations in which a child may be missing from care are examples of placement instability.[17]

As a child moves across the child welfare care continuum (**Figure 24–1**), they move further from the preferred placement with families of origin. Running away increases the likelihood that a young person will move farther from this preferred placement. It is more difficult to find family or therapeutic foster care placements for young people who have run away, and these youth are more likely to be placed in group care, including residential treatment. As they "age out" and lose touch with the system, they may be unaware that their history in the child welfare system entitles them to services to remedy early adulthood housing insecurity, and they may have more difficulty accessing them.[1]

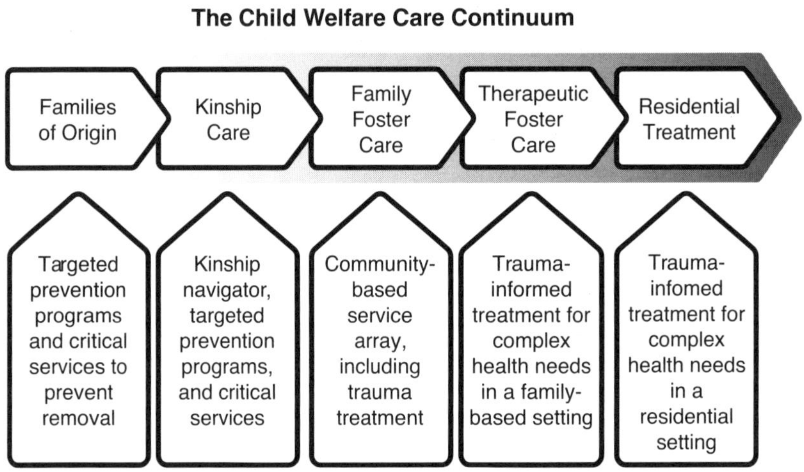

Figure 24–1. The child welfare continuum: a care support continuum with increasing complexity of care and services for children in foster care.

Reproduced from Capacity Building Center for States. Congregate care in the age of Family First: Overview. Children's Bureau, Administration for Children and Families, US Department of Health and Human Services. 2020. Accessed September 1, 2023. https://capacity.childwelfare.gov/states/resources/family-first-overview

While most of the roughly 600,000 children who spend time in the foster care system each year end up with a permanent placement, about 7% of children in foster care exit the system and are immediately emancipated. There is a racial disparity in those that enter the foster system and experience homelessness. Black youth are more likely to be placed in foster care (23% of youth in foster care versus 14% of the nation's youth) and more likely to experience homelessness (38% vs 13%, US population under 18).[18,19] Poverty significantly contributes to these disparities; Black children under 18 in the United States are overrepresented in poverty with a rate that is 1.8-times higher than their share of the general population.

Youth in foster care are more likely to experience homelessness after they leave or age out of the system compared with their peers who have not experienced foster care, with anywhere from 12% to 29% experiencing homelessness after foster care.[18]

Guidance for Clinicians

Pediatricians and other primary care clinicians are an important part of the team helping to keep children and adolescents in foster care safe and housed.

Box 24–3 presents clinical practice guidance for supporting youth in foster care who have been missing from care.[4,20]

Box 24–3

Guidance for Clinicians

Office Care: Prevention

- ▲ Ensure everyone in the office is providing trauma-informed care.
- ▲ Support strong family-caregiver connections at every visit.
- ▲ Be aware of characteristics associated with children missing from care as well as the health consequences that can follow. Conduct a thorough history to identify possible characteristics associated with youth missing from care and residing in unsafe environments (mental health concerns, substance use, history of sexual or physical abuse or exposure to trauma, behavior concerns, reproductive health).
- ▲ Provide appropriate care for any concerns noted (eg, discuss with patient the medical risks of leaving care, discuss how to access medication refills.
- ▲ Assess need for and, if needed, provide emergency contraception and sexually transmitted infection/HIV testing; offer/refer for placement of long-acting reversible contraception.
- ▲ Discuss safety plans with patients at risk for running away.
- ▲ Ask every patient about comfort with and safety in their current living situation.
- ▲ As children approach aging out of foster care, ensure there is a specific transition plan in place (ie, where they will live, with whom they will live, and how they will pay for housing).

Office Care After or During a Missing-From-Care Event

- ▲ Ensure everyone in the office is providing trauma-informed care.
- ▲ Consider using the term "missing from care" instead of "runaway" to reduce stigma.
- ▲ Rather than punishment, place an emphasis on what a child who has run away needs (providing medical and psychological care, such as emergency contraception and testing for sexually transmitted infections, family realignment, and possible change in placement if needed).
- ▲ Provide care for the whole family or caregiver unit after a missing-from-care event, caring for each family/caregiving member as well as the family or caregiver unit.
- ▲ Know the laws for your state regarding mandated reporting of sex trafficking to Child Protective Services and law enforcement.

In the Community

- ▲ Keep up-to-date on services and organizations that help children in unstable or transient living situations.
- ▲ Present information in your office on resources to support children who feel like they are not safe in their current living situation (eg, youth shelters, hotlines, basic need provision).
- ▲ Support organizations that provide services for children who have run away or are in unsafe living situations.

Key Takeaways

- There are multiple characteristics associated with youth missing from care, including foster history, substance use history, and social and abuse history. Pediatricians need to have a trauma-informed approach for screening and treating these patients.
- There are multiple driver's that contribute to children being missing from care (eg, social support, negative staff interaction, seeking independence). Understanding these will help the pediatrician counsel the child who has been missing from care and try to reduce health risks and negative outcomes of a child missing from care.
- Youth who exit foster care have an increased risk for homelessness in the years following their exit, and the racial disparities of homelessness are even more stark more for African Americans exiting foster care. Pediatricians have the opportunity and obligation to screen for the social drivers of health, especially housing needs, and advocate for these patients exiting the foster care system.

CHAPTER 25

Youth With Dual Involvement in the Justice and Child Welfare Systems

Jennifer Rodriguez, JD
Rachel Murphy, JD
Emmanuel L. Chandler, MD

Background and Systems Issues

Pediatricians must use intentional strategies to ensure the healthy development of adolescents navigating both the child welfare and juvenile justice systems—often termed *crossover* or *dual status youth*. Numerous studies have confirmed that youth in either the foster care or the juvenile justice system have higher rates of physical, developmental, and mental health conditions compared with the general population, and recent research shows that youth who move from one system to the other have even greater vulnerabilities. Pediatricians serving dual status youth should use a targeted approach that includes an understanding of both foster care and juvenile justice systems, increased efforts to address the unique health and developmental vulnerabilities these youth face, and a practice approach informed by equity and best practices for working with patients with complex trauma.

Most youth adjudicated in the juvenile justice system experience contact with the child welfare system at some point in their childhood. Studies have found that over 90% of dual status youth interacted with the child welfare system before the juvenile justice system,[1,2] and 7% to 30% of youth in foster care will exit to the juvenile justice system.[2] Involvement in multiple systems often results in exposure to multiple traumatic events and increases a youth's vulnerability and risks for poor adolescent and adult outcomes; however, these systems can work together to identify dual status youth and provide effective supports better tailored to their needs.[3,4] This chapter will discuss the effects dual status has on health outcomes during adolescence and adulthood, highlight a few systemic challenges and solutions, and provide tips for pediatricians to effectively work with dual status youth. Quotes from youth with dual status lived experience, shared in **Box 25–1**, powerfully encapsulate the core themes of this chapter, offering firsthand insights that illuminate the challenges, solutions, and complexities discussed throughout.

Box 25–1

Youth Quotes From Listening Session

On Health and Conditions/Access to Care in Facilities

"Addressing conditions issues in the facilities youth live in is so important for medical providers. Juvenile hall was dirty and caused us health problems. We were allowed two-and-a-half-minute showers, which was not enough time to wash your body; we suffered rashes and disease."

"I have migraines, and they get so bad I throw up. Because health care wasn't available, all they could give me in juvenile hall was Tylenol."

"To be healthy, I think it's important to have more time outside. Being locked indoors 23 hours of the day, every day, results in us feeling isolated and stuck and alone."

"If you have a physical injury, it's not taken seriously in facilities. We never received actual medical care in juvenile hall or our group homes and only got bad dental care. Later, group homes forced us to take psychotropic meds without any consideration of the impact on our physical health in the long term."

"For youth not in the system, usually parents make sure that doctor appointments are made, medications are taken, and care is given. We don't live with parents, so we don't get the proper attention and care, and no one does those things. For example, probation and group home staff said I needed a surgery, but I didn't, and no one listened. I just needed time to heal and rest, but I was forced into surgery."

On Doctor Best Practices

"One question I wish a medical provider would ask is, 'How is your life at home?' Often youth are in very bad situations, and if providers don't ask, we'll never share."

"Dual systems involved youth need a badge on our health file that signals to the provider that they will need more time and understanding in their care, and supports other patients don't need, such as help with life skills. They also need providers that know that the conditions in systems are going to cause behaviors that impact our health like running away and fighting, unless they are fixed."

"Doctors need to listen to us more, so they get individualized ideas of who we are and can give better treatment. Most youth distrust their doctors because they believe the doctors will listen to adults over them, causing long-term resentment towards all medical personnel throughout their lives. "

"In a perfect world, the physician would ask the youth what their history is, let the youth tell their story themselves, and determine what the problems are, and if they are in fact medical. If doctors saw a youth stressed out, they'd prescribe something without explaining the negative side effects. There's an automatic assumption that youth have mental health problems, but the diagnoses are incorrect; it's really PTSD and trauma. There's a reason these youth are in these systems, and no one gets down to the roots. They are thrown into a cage, foster home, or group home, and you as a doctor are adding to the trauma."

We would like to share our deep appreciation for the young people with lived experience who bravely and generously shared their stories and ideas for change with us for the purpose of writing this chapter and improving the health of their peers. Effectively serving adolescents requires professionals working with them to engage with, listen to, and act to solve the problems they identify.

Definitions of Terms

Dual status is a broad term that encompasses a range of circumstances. Jurisdictional terminology varies, but there are several terms that may be used to describe the varying levels of involvement a youth may have in each system.[5]

Dually identified is often used to describe youth who are currently involved in one system, either child welfare or juvenile justice, but were previously involved in the other system. *Dually involved* may refer to youth who are concurrently involved in both systems. Similarly, *dually adjudicated* youth may have formal, concurrent involvement in both systems, having been adjudicated both dependent and delinquent in the respective systems. The guidance in this chapter is meant to apply broadly to account for differences in terminology and different groups of youth.

Risk Factors for Dual Status

Systems involvement is inherently traumatic. Youth in the foster care system have, by definition, experienced trauma through abuse or neglect and removal from their family of origin. Youth detained in the juvenile justice system experience the trauma of incarceration or institutional placement.[6] Studies have found that up to 90% of children in the juvenile justice system have experienced at least 1 form of childhood trauma, and that justice-involved youth experience an average of 5 different forms of childhood trauma.[7] Systems-involved youth often have experienced more adverse childhood experiences than youth who are not involved in the child welfare or juvenile justice system and thus face increased risks of mental and physical health issues, substance use, and educational challenges.[8,9] Traumatic events can cause physiological changes in the brain and body, which may impact behavior.[10] In one study, childhood maltreatment was associated with a 59% increase in the likelihood of a juvenile arrest and a 28% increase in the likelihood of an adult arrest,[11] which mirrors the finding that child welfare-involved youth are 47% more likely to become involved in the juvenile justice system than their non-system-involved counterparts.[12]

Involvement in the child welfare and juvenile justice systems adds to these adverse experiences, including the trauma of being separated from one's family; loss of existing social bonds and support networks; reliance on institutional placements; and multiple moves. Both systems struggle to address grief, loss, and trauma but often do so poorly. Juvenile justice is more harmful because of the use of seclusion, restraint, and isolation and lack of focus on protective relationships. In addition, foster parents and group home staff may be more likely to call the police in response to adolescent behavior that may be handled differently within the family if the youth were not in the foster care or juvenile justice systems.[13,14] Once involved in the juvenile justice system, dual status youth are more likely to be detained or sent to a group home and less likely to receive probation or be diverted from juvenile court.[11,15] Dual status youth have longer histories in the child welfare system, more placements, and higher recidivism than do youth involved in only one of the two systems.[16]

Certain populations, including youth of color, girls, and lesbian, gay, bisexual, transgender, and questioning or queer youth, are more poorly served by these systems and, as a result, are at greater risk of dual status involvement. For example, systemic biases, including structural racism, lead to demographic disparities in both systems as well as in the dual status population. Youth of color in the child welfare system are less likely to receive mental health services than white youth and more likely to be referred to the juvenile justice system and enter secure facilities.[17] Similar to the child welfare system continuum, youth of color in the juvenile justice system are overrepresented at every stage of the delinquency process, with Black youth more likely than white youth to be formally charged, prosecuted for more serious crimes, and adjudicated delinquent, even when prior records are considered.[17,18] In particular, Black youth are 5 times more likely to be detained than their white peers and comprise nearly half of youth residing in juvenile facilities.[18,19]

Effects of Dual Status on Adolescent and Adult Outcomes

Studies have confirmed that dual-status youth experience the following disparities in outcomes compared with youth involved with a single system:

- ***Increased risk of mental health challenges.*** In the first few years after exiting care, dual-status youth are significantly more likely to receive outpatient mental health treatment, as well as treatment for a serious mental illness.[20] Dual-status youth are also more likely to experience complex trauma, which refers to exposure to multiple traumatic events and the long-term, extensive effects of that exposure on their physiological and emotional development.[18,21]
- ***Increased risk of substance use disorders (SUDs).*** Research shows that 4 out of 5 dual-status youth experience substance use problems, yet only a fraction receive treatment.[17] Dual-status youth are also more likely to need treatment for both a serious mental illness and an SUD.[20]
- ***Increased risk of further justice system involvement.*** Multiple studies have found that nearly two-thirds of dual-status youth experienced incarceration within 4 to 6 years of exiting care, compared to about half of justice-involved youth and a quarter or less of child welfare–involved youth.[20,22]

- ***Greater educational challenges.*** Due to trauma, disruption, and instability, most dual status youth struggle academically. One study found that more than 50% were more than 1 year behind in school, at least 44% required special education services, and 67% were identified as chronically truant.[18] Another study found that fewer than half had a high school diploma or equivalent.[18] Despite these increased educational risks, research has found that educational service referrals do not match this increased need.[23]
- ***Interference with typical developmental skill progress.*** The major developmental tasks of adolescents and young adults are to develop a more mature and integrated sense of self and sense of belonging in family, community, and the world; achieve increased independence and responsibility; develop increasing competency and self-efficacy across many life skills; and expand relationships to include healthy intimate relationships. Involvement in the juvenile justice system, in particular, removes a youth's voice and choice, interrupts the growth of competency and self-efficacy, and, through isolation, disrupts the development of healthy relational skills and relationships.
- ***Greater employment challenges.*** Dual-status youth experience lower rates of employment compared with their peers involved in only one system once they have exited care. Studies have found that only about one-third had either full-time or part-time employment, and that they are twice as likely to be unemployed.[10]
- ***Higher risk of poverty and need for public assistance.*** About half of dual-status youth experience periods of extreme poverty in the initial years after exiting care, compared with one-quarter of youth involved in the juvenile justice system and one-third of youth in the child welfare system.[20] Research also shows that youth with dual status are more reliant on public systems and assistance, such as cash aid, nutrition assistance, Medicaid, emergency departments, and housing shelters.[22]

Systemic Challenges and Solutions

In general, the child welfare system's stated mission is protecting youth, while the juvenile justice system's stated mission is balancing the safety of youth and the public. In addition to conflicting and sometimes reductive approaches, systems often do not communicate or share information that can help coordinate services and consider the youth's needs across intersecting domains. This may contribute to the adverse social, educational, and economic outcomes described in the previous section. Finally, access to adequate and necessary health care for youth while incarcerated and during the transition back into their communities is often impeded by long-standing Medicaid rules.

Information Sharing

To best serve the needs of a dual-status youth, it is vital to know about all of a youth's system involvement, which requires communication and cooperation between systems as well as clinicians and caregivers. For example, when a youth enters the juvenile justice system, their history of maltreatment, including past involvement in the child welfare system, is often lost. While it is critical to listen to young people about their experiences and goals, it also critical to remember that they are not adults and should not bear the burden alone of identifying their relevant needs and services. Youth with trauma may not always be able to explain what has happened to them or may not have access to all of the relevant clinical or administrative information. However, clinicians can be prepared with questions to elicit relevant history and can communicate with systems to obtain the necessary information to coordinate care and provide appropriate treatment.

The Effects of Incarceration on Medicaid Services

Many youth in foster care, and therefore many dual-status youth, receive Medicaid. Former youth in foster care can also receive Medicaid up to age 26 years. While incarcerated, these youth are subject to the Medicaid Inmate Exclusion Policy, which prohibits federal financial participation (FFP) under Medicaid to pay for health care provided to "inmates of public institutions."[24,25] Similarly, youth who are incarcerated in a public institution are not eligible for the Children's Health Insurance Program (CHIP), which provides low-cost health coverage to children in families that earn too much money to qualify for Medicaid. More information about CHIP is available from the Centers for Medicare and Medicaid Services.[26] An *inmate of a public institution* is defined as a person living in an institution that is the responsibility of a government unit or over which a governmental unit exercises administrative control,[27] with certain exceptions, including medical institutions and child care institutions for youth in foster care. This means that juvenile halls and other correctional facilities are responsible for covering the health care costs of incarcerated youth without any federal assistance. This provision has been included in the Medicaid statute since its inception, with the presumed rationale being that incarcerated people's needs were already being met and did not require additional assistance.[28]

An important distinction to note is that the inmate exclusion policy is a coverage exclusion and does not make incarcerated individuals ineligible for Medicaid outside of their confinement in a public institution, meaning that once they leave they should be able to resume receiving coverage of services immediately. Some states enacted policies to terminate Medicaid eligibility during incarceration, which required reapplication upon release and could lead to potential gaps in coverage. These policies were particularly detrimental to dual-status youth, who have higher recidivism rates and may enter and exit juvenile correctional facilities multiple times. Fortunately, in 2018, the federal Substance Use Disorder Prevention that Promotes Opioid Recovery and Treatment for Patients and Communities (SUPPORT) Act prohibited states from terminating Medicaid eligibility for "eligible juveniles," defined as youth younger than 21 years and former youth in foster care up to age 26 years who are enrolled in Medicaid at the time of incarceration or determined to be eligible for Medicaid while incarcerated.[29] To prevent interruption of care, states have the option to suspend eligibility for this population and are required to ensure timely determinations to enable full coverage upon release.[30]

There are also circumstances in which an incarcerated youth can receive Medicaid-funded services. Inpatient hospital stays are not subject to the inmate exclusion policy.[24] "Inpatient" means a patient who has been admitted to a medical institution as an inpatient on recommendation of a physician or dentist and who either stays or is expected to stay for at least 24 hours.[27] This allows youth who are currently incarcerated, but admitted to a hospital outside of their correctional facility, to receive services covered by Medicaid[31] during their inpatient admission. Similarly, youth who are in a juvenile correctional facility because they are awaiting an appropriate foster care placement are not subject to the payment exclusion policy. "An individual is not considered an inmate if … [h]e is in a public institution for a temporary period pending other arrangements appropriate to his needs."[27]

Next, under the Consolidated Appropriations Act (CAA) of 2023 and effective January 1, 2025, states have the option to provide Medicaid-covered services to eligible juveniles while they are incarcerated in a public institution but pending disposition of their charges.[32] States who choose to provide these preadjudication services to eligible juveniles must provide all mandatory and optional services to which they are otherwise entitled and will be able to receive FFP, essentially lifting the inmate exclusion during this period.[33]

Additionally, the CAA requires states to provide services to eligible juveniles before their release from a public institution.[34] Thirty days before release or not later than 1 week after release, or as soon as practicable, states must provide screening and diagnostic services, including for behavioral health, in accordance with Early and Periodic Screening, Diagnostic, and Treatment requirements.[33] Thirty days before release and for at least 30 days after release, states must also provide targeted case management services, including referrals to appropriate care and services available under the Medicaid state plan or waiver.[33] At least 24 states, as of May 2025, have sought innovative Reentry Demonstrations under Section 1115 of the Social Security Act (known as

Medicaid waivers), with many seeking to provide a broader scope of services up to 90 days before release.[35]

To maximize the provision of services for incarcerated youth, pediatricians should assume their patients are eligible and pursue Medicaid reimbursement as rigorously as possible. If youth are not receiving the care and services they need while in a juvenile facility, pediatricians can identify community-based alternatives and advocate for youth to be released from the facility in order to receive the services. Pediatricians can also advocate on a policy level if they believe that their states are not taking full advantage of flexibilities in Medicaid that would help improve access and care. See **Box 25–2** for a description of California's recent efforts to reduce barriers. Medicaid systems can also establish more nonclinical, billable provider classes that include family and youth peers, community health workers, and community violence prevention specialists to support youth and their families.

Box 25–2

California's Efforts to Remove Barriers and Increase Access to Care

California was the first state to receive approval to provide Medicaid services to incarcerated individuals before their release.[36] Through the Justice-Involved Initiative, youth and eligible adults who are incarcerated in correctional facilities will receive, up to 90 days before release, a targeted set of services to stabilize their health conditions and establish a community-based care plan. The Justice-Involved Initiative is part of California's recent efforts to reform their Medicaid program (known as California Advancing and Innovating Medi-Cal, or CalAIM), which includes several efforts to increase access to community-based services for youth in foster care and the juvenile justice system.[37]

Under CalAIM, youth with involvement in the foster care system or juvenile justice system or experiencing homelessness are categorically eligible for specialty mental health services. The access criteria have shifted from examining whether a young person has a mental health diagnosis to examining whether a young person has experienced trauma and recognizing that experience in these systems is inherently traumatic. When considering that most youth spend fewer than 30 days in juvenile hall, the practical effect of these 2 policy changes is that most youth in juvenile hall should be receiving specialty mental health services upon entry (because they are categorically eligible) and throughout their stay (because they will likely be released within 90 days).

In addition, CalAIM identified children and youth involved in the child welfare system and children and youth transitioning from a youth correctional facility as populations of focus for a new Enhanced Care Management (ECM) benefit provided by managed care plans. ECM is a community-based, interdisciplinary care approach that provides systemic coordination of clinical and nonclinical services and comprehensive case management for a person's needs across delivery systems. This policy change should increase care coordination for dual status youth and help prevent singularly involved youth from becoming dual status by identifying and providing the supports and services they need.

Common Challenges for Clinicians Serving Dual-Status Youth

While in foster care or the juvenile justice system, young people may experience disruptions to health care due to frequent placement changes or incarceration. Because of these gaps in care, these youth may have physical and mental health conditions that have not been addressed or adequately managed. For example, a youth diagnosed with asthma may have been without an inhaler for months because they have not seen their pediatrician to refill the prescription.

Transitions out of foster care or the juvenile justice system may also create challenges in accessing care. A lack of preventive care in the community, no primary care medical home, and disruption in insurance coverage may prevent continuity of care.[4] The health care system is complex and often opaque; youth may not have the health care literacy to navigate it on their own, and juvenile justice and child welfare systems staff may not provide any support before or after youth exit care. In addition, families may not have the resources, information, or training to manage their child's health care, such as reliable transportation, clinicians who speak their language, or the ability to prioritize mild health conditions over other necessities. For the many dual-status youth who exit detention to institutional care, the lack of a consistent, committed parent figure leaves them on their own to manage their health care.

Without parenting, these youth are often deprived of the knowledge, practical support, and advocacy experience required to maintain their health and access to health care. Additionally, youth may also be distrustful of clinicians based on negative past experiences. Dual status youth have reported feeling disregarded and inappropriately served by various professionals charged with helping them. They may have had their confidential health information shared without their permission, been ignored when they tried to explain their history, or been given medication without an explanation of side effects. Many youth have traumatic stress symptoms because of childhood experiences including multiple disruptions of relationships and transient living situations. Clinicians may misidentify traumatic stress symptoms that overlap with those of mental health conditions and provide medication for an incorrect diagnosis.

Administrative Best Practices for Clinicians

- Provide comprehensive medical services including but not limited to a comprehensive history and physical examination, preventive screenings (including screening for traumatic stress symptoms and suicidality), and management of chronic health conditions for all youth. If youth do not have a primary care physician, connect them with a primary care physician and medical home.[4,38]

- Assess each youth's individualized needs across domains. Make efforts to address needs related to social drivers of health (eg, housing, food) through a health care agency or other community agencies. Collaborate with other professionals treating or serving the youth to ensure that care is coordinated and all options are considered.
- Specific policies and procedures are needed to ensure that uninsured dual-status youth have access to insurance coverage as they reenter the community.[4,39]
- If youth have managed care insurance, use care management to connect them with community providers and necessary clinical services and handle case management.
- Clinicians can be a resource to help educate child welfare and juvenile justice professionals about care that promotes healthy development and coordinate health care upon a youth's transition. Physicians, nurse practitioners, nurses, therapists, and others can collaborate with probation officers, social workers, public defenders, dependency attorneys, judges, and others to explain what clinical services they currently provide to youth and what they can do once youth leave systems.

Tips for Providing Care to Dual-Status Youth

- Introductions matter! Say who you are, with whom you are affiliated, and what your goal is. Establish rapport, and reassure youth that their life and health are what matter to you, not why they are in the system.
- Use a trauma-informed approach. Be aware that you will need to diligently work to gain youths' trust due to past experiences where adults have failed them. Let them tell their story.
- Ensure that youth understand confidentiality and its limitations. Practice confidential care according to state and local laws.[4,40] Be sure to uphold confidentiality even when youth move between systems.
- Spend time gathering information to understand the youth's health history and current situation. Call every family member and agency case manager to get more details and context.
- Learn and understand how the child welfare and juvenile justice systems operate, and learn how to advocate within those systems for your patient.

Tips for Pediatricians Working With Families of Dual-Status Youth

- Remember that family involvement still matters, even though the youth is in the system. This includes birth families, kinship or foster families, and chosen families.

- Use a trauma-informed approach with families, similar to what you use with the youth. Many family members have similar experiences and histories as youth and may have hesitancy about engaging with a clinician.
- If family members identify needs related to social drivers of health, such as food or housing insecurity, provide them with referrals and work with them to engage social work resources. Aim to meet these needs of both youth and their families

Key Takeaways

- » The term *dual-status youth* includes youth who have had some level of contact with both the child welfare and juvenile justice systems.
- » Compared with youth involved in only one of these systems, dual-status youth experience more adverse outcomes in adolescence and adulthood across a range of domains, including mental health, education, employment, and involvement in the justice system.
- » Lack of communication and coordination between systems, as well as limitations on Medicaid services provided to incarcerated youth, may result in inadequate and disrupted care for the most vulnerable youth.
- » Dual-status youth often experience both adultification and restrictions on their autonomy over their health and well-being and may have to navigate societal systems, including health care, on their own. Youth may distrust clinicians due to past negative experiences and trauma.
- » Pediatricians should inquire about how a youth's living situation and experiences may be affecting their health, make extra effort to build rapport with youth, and provide space for them to tell their full story.
- » Pediatricians should collaborate with the other professionals working with the youth to optimize care and services, and be willing to engage in additional advocacy around individual and systems issues affecting the health of dual-status youth.

Part 4. Additional Considerations for Specific Populations

CHAPTER 26

American Indian and Alaska Native Youth

John (Jack) Hessburg (Anishinaabe), MD, PhD, FAAP
Raquel Vargas-Whale (Choctaw Nation of Oklahoma), MD, MSc, FAAP
Jason Deen (Blackfeet), MD, FAAP, FACC

To understand the current needs of American Indian and Alaska Native (AIAN)[a] youth in the foster care system, it is necessary to acknowledge the historical context that has created the disparities in care for AIAN children and adolescents and their disproportionate representation in the foster care system, as well as the framework of the current systems of protections in place for Native youth. This chapter provides that much-needed context for pediatricians and other clinicians who may encounter Indigenous children and adolescents in the foster care system and outlines considerations for improving care for this population.

Historical Context

Although estimates vary widely, between 1 and 12 million people were living in North America and speaking over 300 languages prior to European contact.[1,2] Due to the effects of wars, disease, genocidal policies, and structural racism, the AIAN population in what is now the United States decreased to a nadir of approximately 250,000 people in 1900.[1,3] Currently, there are around 950 tribal groups in what is now the United States, of which 574 sovereign Native nations are recognized by the US federal government.[4,5] As of the 2020 Census, approximately 1.1% of the US population identified as AIAN alone, with 2.9% (approximately 9.7 million people) identifying as AIAN either alone or in combination with another racial group.[6]

[a] Throughout this chapter, *Native* and *Indigenous* will be used as umbrella terms to refer to the current and historic descendants of the Americas, Hawaii, and the Pacific Islands. *American Indian* (AI) and *Alaska Native* (AN), or together AIAN, will be used more specifically to refer to groups and people from the contiguous United States and Alaska, respectively. Specific tribal names and affiliations will be used when applicable.

Considering the diversity of Native people in the precolonial era, any description of historic AIAN family structures and child-rearing practices is merely surface level. Some common themes from ethnographic and indigenist studies include guiding children by allowing some level of independence and learning from mistakes, conveying lessons through storytelling, and passing traditional knowledge and responsibilities on through ceremonies, traditions, and the teaching of skills.[7–9] It was common for children to stay with extended family or other community members, with a broad view of entire clans, communities, and tribes being responsible for the upbringing of children.[10]

European contact brought settler colonialism—the extractive relationship of colonial powers over the people they displace and the land into which they expand. Settler-colonial forces in the Americas relied on Native land for resources from food to mineral wealth, kidnapped people to work in slavery, waged wars that destroyed food sources and environments through scorched-earth policies, and drove AIAN people off of their land and away from known sources of food, resources, and significant spiritual and ceremonial landmarks.[1,3,11]

Treaties with Native nations were often established under false pretenses, with underlying problems related to differing cultural perceptions of land ownership and reciprocity of goods, and many were later violated by the US government.[3,12,13] During this period, AIAN Nations were treated as sovereign entities, and many were promised goods, protections, and land rights.[3,12] A series of Supreme Court decisions in the early 1800s established that the federal government was responsible for interactions between tribal governments and the United States.[14] This was the framework for the enshrinement of AIAN governments as sovereign entities physically located within the bounds of the United States but subject to federal control and not on equal footing with the US government.[13,14] Also included in these rulings was the trust doctrine between the US and AIAN groups, establishing a fiduciary responsibility of the federal government toward AIAN Nations.[15] However, these rulings did not specify what this responsibility entailed, and these broad uncertainties left much room for interpretation.[15]

Consistent with the standing view of the US government and its citizens that AIAN people were an outside force to be exterminated, or at least removed from their valuable lands, the Department of War was the initial governmental entity responsible for all matters pertaining to Native people under the purview of the United States.[12,13,16] The 1800s saw the forced removal of AIAN people in a number of regions under President Andrew Jackson during the Indian Removal period (including the Trail of Tears), the Indian Wars of the Great Plains, and the extermination of entire tribes through the effects of wars and disease brought by Spanish and later US colonial forces in California and the Pacific Northwest.[1,3]

Policies designed for cultural assimilation were intertwined with territorial dispossession in an attempt to subjugate AIAN people to the dominant US culture.[3,16,17] One of the earliest efforts was the Civilization Fund Act, steadily providing money to "civilize" Natives by funding education and missionary groups.[16] The General Allotment Act of 1887 ended historical practices of communally owned and tribally managed land, forcing reservations to allot regions of land to individual tribal members, disrupting Native lifestyles in the new environments into which they were forced.[1,3,18] These governmental policies were designed to remove AIAN people from their land, force the planting of western crops, and prioritize the learning of industrial trades in efforts to force assimilation.[3,11,16,19]

Assimilation Policies Targeting AIAN Youth

As Hand (Anishinaabe)[9] writes, "First Nations and Indigenous children were a special focus for colonial powers: children were viewed as more malleable, and hence, more susceptible to 'civilizing and christianizing' efforts than adults if they were removed from the corrupting influence of their parents and communities." Beginning in 1878 and based on the structure of the military prison at Fort Marion in Florida, boarding schools were created as a tool of assimilation, specifically targeting Native children, to remove them from their communities, sever traditional ties, and force them into the dominant US culture.[3,16] In the words of Richard Pratt, US military officer and founder of the Carlisle Indian Industrial School, the goal was to "[k]ill the Indian in him, and save the man."[20] This was attempted by placing schools prohibitively far away from communities; severely limiting contact with family members; enacting a strict military-inspired schedule of austerity, exercise, manual labor, and vocational training, and enforcing a curriculum emphasizing Euro-centric "American" culture and the importance of assimilation.[3,19,21] Children were pressured into attending boarding schools by the federal government through withholding rations (made necessary for survival once groups were forced from their homelands and away from traditional food sources) unless children were sent to boarding schools and outright kidnapping by the Indian Police.[16] Native youth were renamed with English names; their hair was cut, which was a great spiritual violation; and they were physically punished for speaking Native languages, practicing their religions, or attempting to uphold traditional practices.[16,21] In total, there were 417 boarding schools, including those in Alaska and Hawaii.[22] Over 950 children are known to have died in these schools, with 74 burial sites identified on school grounds as of 2024, though these numbers continue to rise through ongoing investigative efforts.[22] In addition to causing trauma to and disruption of families and communities, the schools negatively affected multiple generations of Native families.[23] Boarding schools remained active in the United States through the 1960s.[3,16]

Two major assimilationist policies were enacted in the 1950s: the Termination Act, which ended the federal recognition of many individual tribes, and the Indian Relocation Act, which created an influx of poor, largely young Natives into already underresourced urban minority working-class communities.[3,12,13] Concurrent with these assimilationist efforts, the Indian Adoption Project was started in 1958 by the Child Welfare League of America under the auspices of the Bureau of Indian Affairs (BIA).[19] The stated goals of this project were to remove AIAN children from their families and adopt them into non-Native families physically far away.[19,24] Thousands of children were removed and placed in largely white, well-off families, perpetuating "white savior" mentalities and Native stereotypes of children needing to be "saved" from their environments.[19] The legacy of these unjust assimilation practices remains today.

The Indian Child Welfare Act

Between 1969 and 1974, 25% to 35% of all AIAN children were in the child welfare system. More than 85% of those in foster care and adopted during this time were placed into non-Native families.[24,25] In response to the ongoing disruption of families and communities, through the efforts of AIAN activists, leaders, and lawmakers, the Indian Child Welfare Act (ICWA) was passed in 1978.[26] Stating in its text that "[t]here is no resource that is more vital to the continued existence and integrity of Indian tribes than their children," ICWA prioritizes placing AIAN children in AIAN families and communities and attempts to recognize the nation-to-nation relationship between the United States and tribal governments and the federal trust responsibilities to AIAN Nations.[25–27] The bill offers protections to enrolled members of federally recognized AIAN communities and their biological children who become involved in the child welfare system. If a child is not residing in a Tribal Nation, the tribe must be notified of child welfare proceedings in state courts. ICWA mandates that there must be "active efforts" made to support families in a culturally appropriate way before removing children from homes.[26] If a child is to be removed, then ICWA designates a priority list of foster care placements:

> 1) an extended family member; 2) a foster home licensed, approved, or specified by the child's Tribe; 3) an Indian

> foster home licensed or approved by an authorized non-Indian licensing authority; or 4) a children's institution approved by the Tribe or operated by a Tribal organization that can meet the child's needs.[25]

There is a similar hierarchy of prioritized placement preferences for adoptive families as well:

> 1) an extended family member; 2) another member of the child's Tribe; or 3) another Indian family.[25]

While this is arguably one of the strongest protections for Native children in the foster care system, ICWA has several limitations. Its protections are extended only to federally recognized tribes, and as such it excludes tribes that have been affected by termination policies and those that are recognized only on state levels, individuals with Native status outside of the United States, and children of mixed Native descent or heritage who are not enrolled members of a specific tribe.[25] Notably, there has been "systemic failure to use tribal citizenship to evaluate ICWA eligibility,"[28] including relying on stereotyped physical features (or the lack thereof) and failing to collect data on tribal enrollment or descendancy in order to bypass ICWA proceedings.[28] There is a shortage of AIAN foster parents as well, limiting available appropriate placements.[29] While there are few recent studies on foster care placement of AIAN children, the limited studies available indicate there are persistently high non–culturally congruent placements.[29]

Some states have expanded ICWA protections, including recognizing members of non-federally recognized tribes and further supporting kinship placement.[25] The BIA strengthened regulations in 2016, reaffirming that protections extend not only to enrolled tribal members but to those eligible for enrollment and the biological children of tribal members and prohibiting the use of certain pieces of information when deciding placement, such as blood quantum, participation in cultural events, or the prioritization of non-ICWA placement for perceived improvement in socioeconomic status.[25] There have been a number of legal challenges to ICWA, the latest being *Haaland v Brackeen* (2023) in which 3 non-Native families argued that it was racial discrimination to not allow them to adopt Native children when appropriate Native placements existed. However, ICWA was affirmed by the Supreme Court, upholding that determination of Native status is a political and not a racial classification due to the relationship between the US and tribal governments.[25,30]

While there are differences in colonial history throughout the Americas, there are similarities in the repercussions for other Indigenous youth in the United States. Native Hawaiians were similarly forced from their land, were subjected to boarding schools, and had their language and traditional ways of life banned.[16,31] Native Hawaiians are similarly disproportionally represented in the foster care system, both in Hawaii and, to a lesser extent, in some states in the mainland United States.[31,32] Additionally, a significant number of migrants and refugees from central America are of Indigenous descent, and unaccompanied or separated children do not have the same protections or provisions for culturally specific care as individuals from federally recognized US tribes.[33,34] In both circumstances, these youth are racially Indigenous but not represented by political entities recognized under ICWA.

Disparities and Disproportionality

Native youth experience disparities in health, including greater mean exposures to adverse childhood experiences (ACEs) and higher rates of infant mortality, dental problems, type 2 diabetes, and suicide,[35,36] although biases in identification and reporting may play a role in these high numbers. AIAN people in the United States experience higher rates of physical and sexual abuse as well, with the Indian Health Service estimating that 20% of AIAN children experience physical or sexual abuse before 18 years of age, with the highest rates among women and two-spirit and other gender-diverse youth.[37] AIAN people face the highest rates of violence of any ethnic group in the United States; as illustrated by the Missing and Murdered Indigenous Women, Girls, and Two-Spirit movement, the true rates are likely underreported.[38,39]

There is also disproportionality with respect to Native youth in foster care, as AIAN youth enter at higher rates and remain longer than do white youth.[40,41] This disproportionality is more pronounced in certain states: those with the greatest disproportionality have AIAN youth representing more than 50% of the foster care population, a rate 3 to 4 times greater than the Native populations of those states.[40] As outlined by Cross (Seneca), there is disproportionality at every stage of the child welfare process for Native youth.[39] From reporting to investigating, to substantiating, to removal, Native youth are overrepresented compared with white youth in the United States.[39] Native children are 4 times more likely than white children to be removed from their birth families after controlling for reasons for removal, have a greater number of placements on average, are less likely to meet the goal of family reunification, and are more likely to "age out" of the foster care system without attaining permanency.[24,25,41] AIAN families are less likely to receive preventive health services or substance use treatment prior to a child's removal.[24] Native youth in the foster care system are more likely to report substance use, self-harm, suicidality, and physical and sexual abuse (outside of the reason for placement) than those not in care.[25,42] Additionally, there is disproportionality with respect to dual system-involved Native youth (that is, those with exposure to both the foster care and juvenile justice systems), though widespread research on this population is lacking.[43] There is a lack of outcomes studies for Native youth with a history of foster care involvement; however, given the disparities in health and exposures to adverse events, there are likely lifelong disparities as well.

Compounding the traumatic experience of removal from their family of origin, removal from their community can lead to a "profound sense of loss throughout their lives, as well as estrangement in their adoptive homes and communities and stress related to parenting the next generation."[25] As Linjean (Cherokee Nation) and Weaver (Lakota) wrote, "[w]hen Native adoptees are disconnected from the kinships and stories that contextualize their trauma repercussions, which simultaneously convey the shared history of resilience, they lack a frame of reference to understand themselves, which is detrimental to their identity and wellness."[25] While these authors discussed the experience of adoptees, similarities can be drawn with youth in foster care in non-Native homes.

Best Practices for Health Care

Accurate identification of Native youth is crucial to ensure ICWA protections are upheld and to connect them with available resources. AIAN children can be identified as such at any point in child welfare proceedings, but doing so early provides a greater opportunity for family support prior to removal, with fewer placements.[24] For those families who identify by a tribal collective name, notices should be sent to all relevant tribes and, as Grinnell et al[24] have asserted, to culturally and historically linked tribes as well. Major barriers to identifying AIAN children are the lack of a nationwide data collection system and consistent underfunding of welfare organizations.[24,26] Mechanisms intended to detail ICWA compliance in the Adoption and Foster Care Analysis and Reporting System proposed in 2016 were abandoned in 2020 after states argued this would be too resource intensive for too small of a population affected, which, as Grinnell et al[24] state, represents "ongoing, tacit complicity in the erasure of Indian children and their families." In 2024, the US Department of Health and Human Services again proposed a similar rule to enhance data collection on this population, which was ultimately folded into a broader child welfare bill that became law on January 4, 2025.[44,45]

Avoiding removal from the home and supporting reunification efforts are important goals. Some communities have improved outcomes by integrating

Indigenous community-based programs with Child Protective Services to create more culturally specific and strengths-based programs that are informed both by historical trauma as well as the individual and personal traumas unique to Native youth in foster care.[46] By creating these culturally specific ties and additional sources of support, some of these programs have demonstrated decreased rates of removals and re-referrals within families and increased kinship placements after removal.[46] These programs work to address what Bussey and Lucero[46] (Choctaw) described as the "three challenges [American Indian families face] when involved with the child welfare system: (a) overcoming the fear they will lose their children like countless Native people before them; (b) prevailing over their caseworker's lack of cultural knowledge; and (c) being judged as an adequate parent using dominant culture." Fostering this strengths-based approach, acknowledging the historical and individual challenges Native parents face when navigating US governmental institutions (such as child protection agencies), and empowering families to connect with resources are potential roles for the pediatrician. As Haight et al[47] described, "Indigenous ways draw our attention to the potential of less coercive, and more extended family-, community-, and strengths-based approaches broadly relevant to reforming poorly functioning child welfare systems." An additional promising alternative structure is Family Group Conferencing, a restorative model originating in New Zealand to better serve the Māori population and adopted by some Alaska Native and Native Hawaiian communities. It uses a structured model centering families and community members to identify root causes leading to concerns for child welfare and support families in addressing those concerns.[31,32,48] In a meta-analysis of the effectiveness of ICWA, Francis (Haliwa-Saponi) et al[29] emphasized the particular importance of including ongoing feedback from tribes and including them as important stakeholders in the development and implementation of any program regarding foster youth.

On a systemic and individual level, Bell (Cherokee) et al[35] provided recommendations for pediatric health professionals caring for Native patients. Given the disparities outlined earlier in this chapter, recommendations with particular relevance to Native youth in foster care are detailed in **Box 26-1**. Another important protective factor is to prioritize and support connecting youth in foster care to their communities. As Linjean and Weaver[25] noted, "participation in Tribal traditions and day-to-day cultural practices in community with others imparts a sense of belonging and permanence, an essential grounding in one's personal identity as a Native person, which is inseparably linked with being part of a collective with a shared identity." Learning Native languages, participating in ceremonies, and attending powwows are independent protective factors, and maintaining cultural traditions and community ties is associated with lower rates of substance use, depression, and suicide, as well as improved school attendance.[39]

Box 26–1

Opportunities for Pediatricians in Practice

- ▲ Partner with local tribes and communities to set health priorities, understand historical experiences, and combine efforts already underway, such as cultural enrichment and preservation programs.
- ▲ Provide opportunities for adequate training of clinical and office staff in culturally sensitive and trauma-informed care practices. Advocate for local and regional models that incorporate culturally and linguistically appropriate services tailored for local tribes.
- ▲ Provide evidence-based supports for parents and young children by promoting the use of home visiting models, high-quality child care, and early childhood programs, such as Early Head Start, Head Start, and Nurse-Family Partnership; Start a Reach Out and Read program in AIAN clinics and any clinic serving these families. Include books representing AIAN and Indigenous children and families.
- ▲ Use a trauma-informed approach to identify and respond to traumatic stress symptoms and address social drivers of health (eg, poverty, food insecurity, homelessness, lack of neighborhood safety, incarceration of parents or other family members, mental health conditions of parents or other household family members, housing inequity, access to schools, academic achievement, intimate partner violence, child abuse and neglect, and involvement with the juvenile legal system) to help families identify and implement practical solutions.
- ▲ Identify strengths and screen youth and families for protective factors to promote positive youth development.
- ▲ Create efforts to promote and strengthen protective factors for youth, focusing on cultural preservation-based efforts.
- ▲ Create a medical home that acknowledges and is sensitive to discrimination in clinical settings and generations of unresolved traumas and racism that AIAN children and families experience.
- ▲ Assess patients for mental health conditions, including signs of posttraumatic stress, anxiety, grief, depressive symptoms, and suicidality, as well as their mothers for perinatal depression using validated screening tools and a trauma-informed approach.
- ▲ Participate in strengths-based, community-driven, and culturally centered suicide prevention programs.
- ▲ Offer gender-affirming care in accordance with published American Academy of Pediatrics policy.[49]
- ▲ Screen AIAN youth for substance use; if identified, conduct a brief intervention and then refer for ongoing treatment.
- ▲ Work to prevent, identify, and address sex trafficking in AIAN youth.

Adapted from Bell S, Deen JF, Fuentes M, Moore K; American Academy of Pediatrics Committee on Native American Child Health. Caring for American Indian and Alaska Native children and adolescents. *Pediatrics.* 2021;147(4):e2021050498.

Conclusion

The Wiindigo is a cannibal creature from Anishinaabe folklore that is doomed to grow larger and more gaunt with every meal, perpetually driven to consume.[50,51] LaDuke (Anishinaabe)[52] writes of "Wiindigo infrastructure," furthering the traditional metaphor to describe the "economic system predicated on accumulation and dispossession, that denigrates the sacred in all of us." The Wiindigo of settler colonialism has consumed ecosystems and communities and targeted Native youth through boarding schools, adoption policies, and disproportionate involvement with the foster care system. To move forward in a good way, to work to end the disruption of AIAN families and away from perpetuating these extractive and destructive policies, it is important for non-Native organizations and pediatric health professionals to support and partner with Native communities and organizations to provide culturally specific care, work to reduce out-of-home placements for Native youth and support reunification, and prioritize placement (when it is necessary) with kin and in community. Native voices must be prioritized and Native people involved at every stage of the analysis, development, and implementation processes. Rather than perpetuating and continuing settler-colonial policies leading to the further destruction of Native families, communities, and ways of being, there must be a shift to investing in and building systems that will help Native youth in the foster care system, embracing the Haudenosaunee Seven Generations philosophy of not just looking for a temporary fix, but working to create a world to benefit the seven generations to come.[47,53]

Key Takeaways

» Native youth were particularly vulnerable and targeted throughout the settler-colonial history of the United States. Current protections for AIAN youth in the foster care system are in response to this historical and ongoing trauma and are rooted in their political status as members of sovereign tribal entities.

» Fostering the connections between Native youth and their communities is an important protective factor and leads to improved physical and mental health outcomes.

» Pediatricians can partner with local tribes and communities to improve identification of AIAN youth in foster care, provide culturally specific support to families and patients, and implement trauma-informed care.

CHAPTER
27

Children and Youth Who Identify as LGBTQ+

Kirsten Simonton, MD
Amanda Scully, MD, MEd, FAAP

Children and youth who identify as sexual or gender minorities are overrepresented in the child welfare system. This chapter uses the term *LGBTQ+* to represent individuals who identify as lesbian, gay, bisexual, transgender, queer or questioning, and/or any of the innumerable identities other than exclusively heterosexual *and* cisgender. Approximately one-third of youth in foster care identify as LGBTQ+.[1,2] Despite their high prevalence in child welfare, these vulnerable children are likely to go through the foster care system and medical settings unrecognized, likely related to bias, discrimination, barriers to disclosure, and poor data collection. The vulnerabilities experienced by unsupported LGBTQ+ children compound with the vulnerabilities experienced by all children in the child welfare system, placing them at an even greater risk of adverse health outcomes.[3] It is therefore essential for social service and medical professionals to understand the issues unique to this population to assist them in successfully navigating their health and identity. This chapter discusses important considerations for all LGBTQ+ children in foster care, with special attention to issues related to sexual orientation. Considerations unique to transgender and gender diverse youth, including gender-affirming care, are discussed in Chapter 28, Additional Considerations for Transgender and Gender Diverse Children and Youth.

Overrepresentation in the Foster Care System

According to the Centers for Disease Control and Prevention Youth Risk Behavior Surveillance Survey data, an estimated 9.5% of youth age 13 to 17 years in the United States identify as lesbian, gay, or bisexual, and 0.73% are transgender.[4,5] Although gender and sexuality data are not uniformly assessed within child welfare systems, existing data demonstrate an overrepresentation of LGBTQ+ youth in foster care. Since the early 2010s, regional prevalence studies have estimated that LGBTQ+ youth represent 1 in 3 to 1 in 5 youth in the child welfare system (**Table 27–1**). For example, 19% of youth in Los Angeles County foster care identify as LGBTQ+,[6] 34% of youth in New York City foster care identify as LGBTQ+,[2] and 32% of youth in the Cuyahoga County, Ohio, foster care system identify as LGBTQ+.[8] A statewide study in California found that 30.4% of youth in foster care and 25% of youth in unstable housing were LGBTQ+, compared with only 12% of youth in stable housing.[1] In all regional studies, most youth in foster care, including those who identify as LGBTQ+, were youth of color. In New York City, LGBTQ+ youth were less likely to be white and more likely to be Latinx compared with cisgender, heterosexual youth in foster care.[2] Family rejection and violence is an often-cited reason that LGBTQ+ youth experience homelessness or child welfare involvement.[6] The marginalization and disrupted social supports that accompany discrimination, violence, out-of-home placement, and homelessness leave LGBTQ+ adolescents particularly vulnerable to exploitation, including forced labor and sex trafficking.[9]

Table 27–1. Studies Assessing Prevalence of LGBTQ+ Youth in Foster Care

Reference	Population	Methodology	Prevalence
Wilson et al, 2014[6]	Los Angeles County foster care	Telephone interview of 786 youth 12–21 years old	19%
Sandfort et al, 2020[2]	New York City foster care	Telephone survey of 659 youth 13–21 years old	34%
Matarese et al, 2024[7]	Cuyahoga County, OH foster care	Telephone and text message surveys of 251 youth 12–21 years old	32%
Baams et al, 2019[1]	Data from ~500,000 students age 10–18 years in the California Healthy Kids Survey (2013–2015)	Data from 2 multiple-choice items that assessed (1) gender identity and sexual orientation and (2) living situation, including foster care	30.4%

Risks for Health and Psychosocial Disparities

Clinicians may feel discomfort when interacting with LGBTQ+ populations or, conversely, may dismiss LGBTQ+ identity as unimportant to health care.[10] Neither of these is a constructive approach. Being a member of the LGBTQ+ community is neither a pathology nor a risk behavior for adverse health outcomes. Furthermore, LGBTQ+ children may enter foster care for reasons unrelated to their sexual or gender identity.

However, the effects of homophobia, transphobia, and heteronormative/cis-normative bias contribute to a vast array of health disparities in this population, including disparities in mental health, sexual health, and interpersonal health.[11] Even clinicians who approach LGBTQ+ populations with acceptance and without trepidation will have patients who choose not to disclose their sexual or gender identity. This may be due to previous discriminatory encounters in the health care system, concerns about clinician competency in LGBTQ+ topics, or concerns about confidentiality, which may be compounded for patients in the child welfare system.[12] Physicians should recognize that LGBTQ+ youth, regardless of whether they disclose their sexual or gender identity in the health care setting, are at higher risk of experiencing certain adverse events and health outcomes including interpersonal violence, mental health disorders, and substance use disorders (SUDs) as the result of homophobia and heterosexism.[13]

The Experience of LGBTQ+ Youth in Foster Care

As observed in the general population, LGBTQ+ youth within the foster care system face a heightened risk of health disparities, such as interpersonal violence including school violence and mental health concerns including SUDs.[1] These risks are further compounded by the existing disparities experienced broadly by youth within the child welfare system, including higher rates of chronic medical, developmental, and mental health conditions and inadequate access to health care services. Therefore, perceived, fear of, or actual rejection and maltreatment faced by LGBTQ+ youth can precipitate engagement in the foster care system as well as subsequent placement disruptions, transitions to congregate care settings, homelessness, survival crimes, and juvenile justice involvement.[14,15]

During nationwide listening forums conducted by the Child Welfare League of America, LGBTQ+ youth in foster care reported negative stereotypes; unsafe and unsupportive placements, including verbal and physical harassment; and lack of access to affirming support and health care.[16] Regional studies have demonstrated similar disparities. LGBTQ+ youth report gender- or sexual identity–related discrimination within the child welfare system and experience a greater number of placement changes, increased rates of group home placement versus family placement, a higher likelihood of mental health hospitalization, and an increased risk of becoming homeless while in foster care.[6] Other studies found that LGBTQ+ youth were more likely to be placed in group homes or residential care, reported lower satisfaction with their current placements, were more likely to be homeless and to have negative confrontations with police, and exhibited a higher rate of depressive symptoms.[2] Lesbian, gay, and bisexual youth in the child welfare system were significantly more likely to meet clinical thresholds for depression, trauma, and SUDs and to report more overall mental health and behavioral difficulties compared with heterosexual youth.[17] These adverse educational, safety, and health outcomes influence all aspects of LGBTQ+ youth well-being, including their likelihood of family permanency.

LGBTQ+ youth are more than twice as likely to be moved from their first placement at the request of the family and are more likely to experience periods of homelessness either during their time in foster care or when exiting foster care.[16] A national survey found that the primary reasons for homelessness among LGBTQ+ youth include being forced out or running away due to sexual orientation or gender identity, family issues including violence, and aging out of the foster care system.[18]

The intersectionality of race and sexual minority status is robust in foster care, likely perpetuated by structural racism and LGBTQ+ stigma. LGBTQ+ girls of color are particularly overrepresented in foster care. Compared with other groups in the child welfare system, LGBTQ+ youth of color experience increased discrimination, violence, and longer stays in foster care.[19,20] This reflects the interplay between the stress and discrimination faced by LGBTQ+ youth of color, which increases their risk for out-of-home placement, and the racial inequities that exist along all points of the child welfare continuum, including disparities in maltreatment reporting, child protective services investigations, and placement decisions.[21]

Legal Barriers and Supports

There is currently no federal law guaranteeing nondiscrimination protections for LGBTQ+ people across most categories. The Civil Rights Act of 1964 includes protections on the basis of sex, which has been interpreted to include sexual and gender identity in select instances, although this is not explicitly enumerated. Therefore, specific protections are left to state legislatures. At the time of this writing, fewer than half of US states offer broad LGBTQ+ nondiscrimination protections; in many states, there are no laws protecting individuals on the bases of sexual orientation and gender identity. Since the mid-2010s there has been a national surge in anti-LGBTQ+ legislative attacks, with hundreds of bills being introduced to restrict LGBTQ+ youth access to athletics, school instruction, gender-affirming care, and public facilities such as restrooms.

Even without explicitly addressing a marginalized population, laws can exacerbate existing disparities. One illustration is the 2022 Supreme Court case *Dobbs v Jackson Women's Health Organization*, which reversed *Roe v Wade*. This ruling broadly restricted reproductive rights in many states, disproportionately affecting LGBTQ+ individuals, who seek abortion services at increased rates compared with their cisgender, heterosexual peers and who are more likely to report physical or sexual abuse when accessing these services.[22,23] Along with abortion services, other types of health care are affected by these restrictions. States have relied on the Supreme Court reasoning in the *Dobbs* case to issue restrictions or bans on gender-affirming health care, which have passed in over half of US states as of 2024.[24]

Over a dozen states permit state-licensed child welfare agencies to refuse to place and provide services to children and families, including LGBTQ+ people, if doing so conflicts with their religious beliefs. Conversely, as of 2023, more than half of US states have policies that prohibit discrimination based on both sexual orientation and gender identity.[25] Many states have enacted a bill of rights for children in foster care, including specific protections such as educational consistency, access to extracurricular activities, and information-sharing and placement considerations.[26] Some state systems and agencies have developed youth bills of rights, which explicitly prohibit discrimination and outline specific protections for LGBTQ+ youth in foster care, including access to activities and assistance available to their cisgender, heterosexual counterparts. While rights granted by individual state policies vary, federal law dictates that all children receiving state child welfare services have a right to be safe in their placement; receive protection from physical, emotional, and sexual abuse; and have their physical, mental health, and educational needs met.

Providing Affirmative Care in Pediatric Practice

All youth need nurturing environments in which they can express their full selves, including their gender and sexual identities, without discrimination, harassment, or fear of rejection. LGBTQ+ youth in foster care face housing instability and permanency challenges that create barriers to a stable, nurturing home and healthy relationships. Health care professionals can help caregivers embrace and support youth as well as create welcoming and inclusive environments in their own practices. Open and affirming spaces can start with visible indicators of safety, respect, and support, which may include

- Employee badges or stickers that include symbols of LGBTQ+ allyship
- Employee badges that identify personal pronouns

- Posted nondiscrimination policies that specifically include gender and sexual identities
- Medical forms that ask for pronouns and preferred names along with separate fields for sex assigned at birth and gender identity
- Brochures or educational materials addressing LGBTQ+ health topics

It is important to normalize conversations around sexual and gender identities in the health care system and to avoid assumptions regarding any youth's identity. Available guidance on documenting sexual and gender identities in the pediatric medical record recommends that screening is standardized among all demographic and socioeconomic populations, inclusive language is used, and patient-affirmed names and pronouns are visible across encounters.[27] Clinicians should limit information gathering to what is necessary for the context. For instance, it may be useful to understand a youth's sexual behaviors to determine relevant counseling and testing; however, attempting to define or label their sexual orientation may not be crucial to provide appropriate health care. Sexual orientation and gender identity may be fluid or evolving for some youth, and the extent to which they are comfortable sharing this information may evolve. It is therefore critical for clinicians to ask about these topics at subsequent visits rather than assume there have been no changes in the interim.

The American Academy of Pediatrics has issued guidance on the comprehensive office-based health care of LGBTQ+ youth.[28] This report outlines elements of comprehensive sexual health and psychosocial histories and emphasizes the mental health, reproductive health, victimization, and substance use disparities among LGBTQ+ youth that necessitate intentional screening and monitoring.

Appropriate environmental and process changes, information gathering, and documentation start with clinician education. All adults who interact with youth in a health care setting should receive training on culturally effective language, supportive communication, and issues related to confidentiality when working with LGBTQ+ patients, in addition to training on trauma-informed care.[12] Web-based and in-person training opportunities on LGBTQ+ patient-centered care are available for health care practices (**Table 27–2**) to address knowledge gaps, identify biases, and alleviate the discomfort that can prevent affirming care. Because racial disparities in child welfare persist among LGBTQ+ youth in foster care, clinician education must address the marginalization that occurs at the intersection of race (culture, ethnicity) and sexual identity. Clinicians should be aware of confidentiality considerations for patients based on state and federal laws. Practices can support patients' privacy rights by standardizing a process to assess youth's information-sharing preferences and identify areas of the medical record to document information in a way that respects those preferences.

Working With Caregivers in Pediatric Practice

Protective factors at the family level should be carefully considered for LGBTQ+ children in foster care. Family and caregiver reaction to the disclosure of sexual or gender identity is closely correlated with children's levels of depression and self-esteem.[29] For children in foster care, clinicians should model LGBTQ+-affirming attitudes and language when interacting with biological and foster families alike, regardless of whether a child has disclosed their sexual or gender identity to the clinician or their caregivers. When a patient has disclosed such information to their foster parents or caregivers, clinicians should ask caregivers about their feelings regarding the youth's identity or expression. All indicators of acceptance and warmth toward youth in their care should be praised. Clinicians can provide information and support for caregivers who may be experiencing difficult emotions, confusion, or discomfort with the youth's identity.

Pediatricians can also assess and advocate for affirming placements for their LGBTQ+ patients in foster care. At the same time, pediatricians must recognize that affirming placements are not always possible and that a child may ultimately be reunified with non-affirming family members. Therefore, clinicians should assess youth preferences regarding when and how sexual and gender identity information can be safely shared. Patient safety should remain the priority when deciding whether to share or document this information, and clinicians should understand the limits of confidentiality within their electronic health records and within their state legislation.

Resilience and Advocacy

The disparate outcomes experienced by LGBTQ+ youth, especially LGBTQ+ youth in foster care, are not related to some intrinsic quality of sexual or gender identity, but rather are related to the disproportionate number of adverse experiences that this population faces. Perhaps more striking than the number of LGBTQ+ youth who experience negative health and social outcomes is the number of LGBTQ+ youth who overcome their adverse experiences and live healthy lives. Clearly, this group of children has a high level of resilience.[30]

Table 27–2. Select Resources for LGBTQ+ Youth and Clinicians

Topic	Organization	Website
Health care	American Academy of Pediatrics	https://www.aap.org/en/patient-care/lgbtq-health-and-wellness/
	Centers for Disease Control and Prevention	https://www.cdc.gov/healthy-youth/lgbtq-youth/
	American Psychological Association	https://www.apa.org/topics/lgbtq
Staff training	Human Rights Campaign: staff training	https://www.thehrcfoundation.org/professional-resources/staff-training
	National LGBTQIA+ Health Education Center	https://www.lgbtqiahealtheducation.org/
Legal/advocacy	Lambda Legal	https://lambdalegal.org/
	American Civil Liberties Union	https://www.aclu.org/
	GLAAD	https://glaad.org/
	Human Rights Campaign	https://www.hrc.org/
	Advocates for Youth	https://www.advocatesforyouth.org/issue/lgbtq-health-and-rights/
	Movement Advancement Project: national and state policy maps	https://www.lgbtmap.org/

Like any child, an LGBTQ+ child's level of resilience depends on numerous individual, family, community, and societal factors.[31] At the individual level, internalized homophobia is an independent risk factor for adverse outcomes, and resolution of internalized homophobia is associated with positive health outcomes.[32] Thus, clinicians should seek opportunities to encourage their patients' self-acceptance and positive self-image. This may include affirmative office-based practices and language during patient encounters as discussed in the previous section. When used at every encounter for every patient, these practices demonstrate to children and families that their sexual and gender identities are normal and accepted, even if they have not disclosed this information yet. When a patient does identify as LGBTQ+, clinicians should reaffirm their support of this identity and carefully screen for evidence of depression or anxiety, which may be related to internalized homophobia or gender dysphoria. Referral to LGBTQ+-affirming mental health services may improve self-acceptance and lead to improved outcomes for these children.[33]

At the community level, affirming attitudes and policies within schools and access to LGBTQ+ alliances or other communities can greatly affect the resilience of LGBTQ+ youth. School programs that emphasize acceptance and anti-bullying policies inclusive of LGBTQ+ students decrease victimization of LGBTQ+ students; peer support further decreases victimization as well as depressive symptoms among LGBTQ+ youth.[34,35]

Unfortunately, recent attitude and legislative changes against LGBTQ+ individuals at the societal level have resulted in numerous statewide policies that preempt discussion or affirmation of LGBTQ+ identities in schools and decrease children's access to LGBTQ+ peers and role models both within and outside of schools. Other policies have codified familial rejection of LGBTQ+ children, requiring child protective services to investigate families that affirm their LGBTQ+ children. There are limited data on how these policies will affect the resilience of LGBTQ+ youth. Clinicians who wish to advocate for policies that support resilience among their LGBTQ+ patients can do so at the school, district, state, and national levels. Pediatricians should be knowledgeable about these opportunities as well as resources to assist LGBTQ+ youth in foster care and their caregivers. Select organizations and their associated websites are listed in **Table 27–2**.

Conclusion

Awareness of the unique issues affecting LGBTQ+ youth and the way these issues compound those that affect all children in foster care enables clinicians to provide the most informed and affirmative care to all of their patients in foster care, regardless of whether any particular patient has disclosed their sexual or gender identity. Clinicians can cultivate awareness of the unique adverse experiences and outcomes that their LGBTQ+ patients face and can advocate for these children within their practices and communities. In this way, progress toward improving the health of this especially vulnerable population can be made.

Key Takeaways

- LGBTQ+ children, especially those who belong to racial and ethnic minorities, are overrepresented in foster care.
- The adversities experienced by LGBTQ+ children compound the adversities experienced broadly by children in foster care, placing LGBTQ+ children in foster care at greater risk of interpersonal violence, unstable placements and housing, and risk-taking behaviors than either group alone.
- Affirming office-based practices may encourage youth to address their sexual and gender identity–related health concerns with their physicians.
- Advocacy at the individual, family, community, and state levels, as well as advocacy for affirming placements, can increase the resilience of LGBTQ+ youth and improve the health of this vulnerable population.

Chapter 28

Additional Considerations for Transgender and Gender Diverse Children and Youth

Joseph R. Rojas, MD, MSHPM, FAAP
Jason Rafferty, MD, MPH, EdM, FAAP

Transgender or gender diverse (TGD or "trans") youth have gender identities that do not entirely align with the sex they were assigned at birth[1–4] (see **Table 28–1** for discussion of relevant terms). While an exact accounting is difficult, most sources suggest that similar to lesbian, gay, bisexual, and questioning or queer (LGBTQ+) youth, TGD youth are overrepresented in the foster care population. The Williams Institute estimates 1.43% of youth age 13 to 17 years in the general population are TGD,[5] whereas Baams et al[6] found that 5.04% of youth age 10 to 18 years in foster care are TGD. While some youth enter foster care due to parental rejection and/or maltreatment related to their gender identity, it is critical to also realize that not all TGD youth enter foster care for reasons related to their gender identity.

Among the many youth in foster care, TGD youth face additional barriers to safe, supportive placements and medically appropriate care. Pediatricians who care for youth in foster care should therefore be familiar with the needs and challenges faced by this group to best promote positive development.

Gender-Affirming Care Model

Given the limited education and training many pediatricians have received in caring for TGD youth, some may feel ill-equipped to address the needs of TGD youth in foster care. However, as outlined in Chapter 27, Children and Youth Who Identify as LGBTQ+, every pediatrician is capable of creating a safe and open space for youth to address their health needs; in fact, this is our professional mandate for all patients. The gender-affirming care (GAC) model offers pediatricians general guidance on promoting the health and positive

Table 28–1. Relevant Terms and Definitions Related to the Care of Transgender and Gender Diverse Individuals[2–4]

Term	Definition
Sex	An assignment made at birth (usually male or female), typically on the basis of external genital anatomy but sometimes informed by internal gonads, chromosomes, or hormone levels
Gender identity	A person's deep internal sense of being female, male, a combination of both, somewhere in-between, or neither, resulting from a multifaceted interaction of biological traits, environmental factors, self-understanding, and cultural expectations
Gender expression	The external way a person expresses their gender, such as with clothing, hair, mannerisms, activities, or social roles
Gender perception	The way others interpret a person's gender expression
Gender diverse	A term used to describe people with gender behaviors, appearances, or identities that are incongruent with those culturally assigned to their birth sex; gender-diverse individuals may refer to themselves with many different terms, such as *transgender, nonbinary, genderqueer, gender fluid, gender creative, gender independent*, or *noncisgender. Gender diverse* is used to acknowledge and include the vast diversity of gender identities that exist. It replaces the former term *gender nonconforming*, which has a negative and exclusionary connotation.
Transgender	A subset of gender-diverse individuals whose gender identity does not match their assigned sex and generally remains persistent and consistent over time; the term *transgender* also encompasses many other labels individuals may use to refer to themselves.
Cisgender	A term that is used to describe a person who identifies or expresses a gender that is consistent with the sex they were assigned at birth
Nonbinary	The gender of a person who does not identify as exclusively male or female. They may identify as both male and female, somewhere in between, or completely outside of those categories.
Agender	A term that is used to describe a person who does not identify as having a particular gender
Affirmed gender	A person's true gender identity, particularly when validated as authentic
Affirmed female; trans female	Terms that are used to describe individuals who were assigned male sex at birth but who have a gender identity that is asserted to be more feminine. It replaces the former and potentially stigmatizing term *MTF (male to female).*
Affirmed male; trans male	Terms that are used to describe individuals who were assigned female sex at birth but who have a gender identity that is asserted to be more masculine. It replaces the former and potentially stigmatizing term *FTM (female to male).*
Gender dysphoria	A clinical symptom characterized by a sense of alienation to some or all of the physical characteristics or social roles of one's assigned gender; also, gender dysphoria is a psychiatric diagnosis in the *DSM-5*, focusing on the distress that stems from the incongruence between one's expressed or experienced (affirmed) gender and the sex assigned at birth.

Abbreviation: DSM-5, Diagnostic and Statistical Manual of Mental Disorders, 5th Edition.

For a more comprehensive glossary of terms, please see https://www.hrc.org/resources/glossary-of-terms or https://pflag.org/glossary/.

development of LGBTQ+ youth. For TGD youth, the GAC model encourages pediatricians to partner with youth and families to offer nonjudgmental dialogue and education on gender diversity, facilitate access to care, and advocate for safer community spaces where children can develop and explore their gender identities.[2]

Asking all adolescent patients direct and nonjudgmental questions about gender identity and expression allows youth the opportunity to define their own experiences. Rather than focusing on labels and terms (which are ever-evolving), pediatricians should seek to understand and appreciate the youth's own gender experience while understanding that identity and expression can evolve throughout development. From this starting point, pediatricians can then explore with the youth any related stressors, sources of support, and additional considerations for GAC while weighing the risks and benefits in a family-centered shared decision-making approach.[7]

As health professionals, pediatricians can help to destigmatize gender diversity through education of caregivers, families, and child welfare personnel. Key messages pediatricians can share include the following:

1. Gender development is a normal process for all children, and diversity in gender identity and expression is normal.
2. Gender identity evolves as an interplay of biology, development, socialization, and culture.
3. Trans identities and diverse gender expressions do not constitute a mental disorder.
4. If mental health concerns exist, they often stem from stigma and negative experiences and are not intrinsic to TGD identity.[8]

Role of the Pediatrician

Pediatricians and other clinicians can serve a vital role in facilitating communication and understanding between youth and their caregivers. Some parents and caregivers may struggle to understand and accept their child's TGD identity, and some may not know their child's gender identity. Questions parents and caregivers may have include "Is my/this child too young to understand gender identity?" or "What if their identity changes in the future?" Pediatricians can provide education and dispel myths about normal development, identity exploration, and any applicable interventions. They can also provide empathy and alliance as caregivers cope with uncertainty. Youth, on the other hand, may feel unsafe disclosing their gender identity to a caregiver, including if they are concerned that their placement would be in jeopardy, or they may be frustrated when a caregiver does not immediately support their gender identity. In this setting, pediatricians can help youth assess their safety in the home, identify sources of support, and develop a safety plan if they are feeling unsafe. Pediatricians can also facilitate open family discussions exploring differing perspectives, emotions, and goals to build understanding and inform relevant decision-making. When medical interventions are involved, these discussions must be accompanied by information on realistic expectations, risks, and current research.

Some youth in foster care may not have caregivers who are engaged, particularly if they have had multiple placements or parental rights have been restricted or terminated. In these cases, pediatricians may find themselves needing to engage with the youth's social worker, Court Appointed Special Advocate, court-appointed attorney, or judge to facilitate mutual understanding of the youth's wishes and needs related to gender identity and expression. The same process of education and dialogue can help when collaborating with these important individuals in the youth's life.

Social and Legal Affirmation

It is important that pediatricians keep in mind that the process of gender affirmation looks different for every youth. There is no prescribed path or sequence that every individual must follow or a predetermined end point that they must reach. With this in mind, pediatricians should be broadly familiar with the forms of GAC available, as outlined in **Table 28–2**.[2,9] While an in-depth discussion of medical management is beyond the scope of this chapter, it is essential to recognize the particular importance of supporting social affirmation for youth in foster care. Pediatricians can help families advocate for the use of one's asserted name, pronouns, and identity at school or in the community; identify sources of support; and address any stressors that may arise, such as bullying or discrimination based on gender. Resources like Gender Spectrum's gender support plan (www.genderspectrum.org) can provide a framework for these discussions. Pediatricians should also be aware of resources in their area for TGD youth, including referral options if the youth is considering options for medical affirmation.

One area in which youth in foster care may have some advantages compared with the general population is legal affirmation. The adoption process and family court involvement may offer opportunities to legally change a child's given name and, depending on the state, the sex or gender identifier listed on their birth certificate. In some areas or institutions, youth cannot be affirmed with their identifiers unless this process is completed. Therefore, it is important that pediatricians are knowledgeable about local legal processes in which these youth may be involved. Additional resources on legal affirmation can be found through the National Center for Transgender Equality's ID Documents Center (www.transequality.org/documents).

Pediatricians should be aware of the evolving legal landscape for TGD-affirming care, including that in their own state. State laws and regulations limiting access to TGD care and full participation in society for TGD youth may take several forms. Resources such as LGBTmap.org can help pediatricians stay up-to-date on the latest legal barriers and protections for youth in their state. In addition, state chapters of the American Academy of Pediatrics (AAP), the AAP Division of State Government Affairs, and GLBTQ Legal Advocates and Defenders, also known as GLAD (www.glad.org) can be helpful resources on local laws and referral networks.

Barriers for Youth in Foster Care

TGD youth and their families face barriers to care, regardless of their child welfare status. A 2022 study by Weixel and Wildman[10] demonstrated significant geographic barriers to care, with fewer TGD clinical care programs and mental health clinicians located in the South and Midwest regions of the United States compared with the Northeast and West. In fact, as many as one-third of states may have no TGD youth clinic. Medicaid recipients, including youth in foster care, residing in states without TGD clinical programs may be limited in their ability to access out-of-state care because Medicaid coverage does not cross state lines. Youth in foster care may be further limited by restrictions on out-of-state travel or limited transportation options. Even in states with TGD care clinicians, Medicaid coverage of services may be restricted based on state policy. In some cases, pediatricians may be able to help youth and families overcome financial barriers by requesting child welfare agencies directly cover the cost of appropriate and necessary TGD care, but this is not always an option.

Youth in foster care may face additional challenges around consent for appropriate GAC. For youth under 18 years of age seeking medical or surgical treatment, a parent or legal guardian must provide consent; if the parents' legal rights have been restricted or terminated, the court must provide consent. Adolescents in some states may be able to consent to outpatient behavioral health counseling and treatment, including gender-affirming mental health

Table 28–2. Forms of Gender Affirmation[2,9]

Component		Definition	General Age Range[a]	Reversibility[a]
Social affirmation		Adopting gender-affirming hairstyles, clothing, name, gender pronouns, and restrooms and other facilities	Any	Reversible
Medical affirmation	Puberty blockers	Gonadotropin-releasing hormone analogues, such as leuprolide and histrelin	During puberty (Tanner stage 2–5)	Reversible[b]
	Cross-sex hormone therapy	Testosterone (for those who were assigned female at birth and desire masculinization; estrogen plus androgen inhibitor (for those who were assigned male at birth and desire feminization)	Early adolescence onward	Partially reversible (skin texture, muscle mass, and fat deposition); irreversible once developed (testosterone: Adam's apple protrusion, voice changes, clitoral enlargement, and male pattern baldness; estrogen: breast development); unknown reversibility (effect on fertility)
Gender-affirming surgeries or surgical affirmation		"Top" surgery (to create a male-typical chest shape or enhance breasts); "bottom" surgery (surgery on genitals or reproductive organs); facial feminization and other procedures	Typically adults (adolescents on case-by-case basis[c])	Not reversible
Legal affirmation		Changing gender and name recorded on birth certificate, school records, and other documents	Any	Reversible

[a] The provided age range and reversibility are based on the little data currently available.

[b] The effect of sustained puberty suppression on fertility is unknown. Pubertal suppression can be, and often is indicated to be, followed by cross-sex hormone treatment. However, when cross-sex hormones are indicated without endogenous hormones, fertility may be decreased.[9]

[c] Eligibility criteria for gender-affirming surgical interventions among adolescents are not clearly defined between established protocols and practice. When applicable, eligibility is usually determined on a case-by-case basis with the adolescent and the family along with input from medical, mental health, and surgical pediatricians.[9]

care, though the age of consent varies by state. Preadolescent minorsrequire parent or legal guardian consent, or court order, to access outpatient mental health services. This system can be confusing, especially for youth, so pediatricians should confirm who is responsible for medical decision-making early on or refer youth and caregivers to resources such as GLAD to help them navigate this process. These additional barriers for youth in foster care may delay GAC when consent is needed, especially if a court order is required.

Conclusion

Transgender and gender diverse children and youth in foster care require the support and understanding of pediatricians to help them reach their developmental potential. Within the framework of the GAC model, pediatricians can assess gender concerns and provide evidence-based information to youth and families, while supporting them in navigating complex medical and legal systems.

Key Takeaways

» GAC is essential for TGD youth, particularly those involved in the foster care system where gender diversity is overrepresented compared with the general population.

» TGD youth in the foster care system face significant barriers to GAC, including consent, insurance, availability of services, and complex legal and medical systems.

» Pediatricians can help youth and caregivers explore identity and emotions, advocate, provide education, dispel myths, and connect them to relevant local resources.

CHAPTER

29

Children Exposed to Substances in Pregnancy

Barbara H. Chaiyachati, MD, PhD, FAAP
Yuan He, MD, MPH, FAAP

Introduction

Caregiver substance use was a risk factor for more than 1 in 4 substantiated cases of child maltreatment in 2021,[1] with national trends indicating significant increases in maltreatment associated with caregiver use of substances other than alcohol.[2] Childhood exposure to substances can be associated with significant ramifications for child development, physical and mental health, and overall well-being, with most studies examining prenatal exposure. These children may also experience familial disruptions and discontinuity in caregiving situations during their lifetime, placing them at increased risk of adverse childhood experiences and trauma. Given the increasing prevalence of prenatal substance exposure,[3] it is important that primary care physicians and other pediatricians feel comfortable with the identification, diagnosis, and management of clinical manifestations of prenatal substance exposure.

This chapter describes the epidemiology of substance use during pregnancy, recognition of clinical manifestations and early management of substance-exposed infants, and outpatient management within the pediatric primary care setting. In all care interactions and settings, pediatricians should use person-first language regarding substance use, with attention to modeling nonstigmatizing language that is consistent with American Academy of Pediatricians (AAP) recommendations.[4] Stigmatizing language in medicine can be particularly harmful by creating barriers to care and exacerbating cycles of disengagement, hesitancy to access treatment, and poor health. Using medically accurate language in all circumstances, including related to substance use, is an important component in respecting the dignity of children and families. Respect of the patient and family's dignity, regardless of custody status or family structure, is an intrinsic component in modeling emotional safety and establishing trusting care relationships.

Epidemiology of Substance Use During Pregnancy

Prenatal substance exposure is not uncommon, with estimates of self-reported substance use during pregnancy varying from up to 20% reporting alcohol use to 7% of reporting the use of prescription opioids for pain at any time during gestation in the United States.[5,6] Recent trends indicate increasing prenatal cannabis exposure,[7] likely due to growing acceptability, increasing legalization, and decreased perception of harms.[8] Prenatal exposure to opioids is also increasing—particularly to fentanyl, which has surged in the drug supply since 2013 and further increased during the COVID-19 pandemic,[9] and to buprenorphine, which is used to treat opioid use disorder in pregnant patients. When prenatal substance exposure is present, polysubstance exposure is common. For example, among people who disclosed current alcohol use during pregnancy, almost 40% also reported the use of 1 or more additional substances, most commonly tobacco and cannabis.[5] Overall, substantial decreases in tobacco use in pregnancy have been documented, from greater than 20% in the early 2000s to approximately 5% 20 years later.[10,11]

Racism has contributed to disparity and disproportionality in the identification of and response to prenatal substance exposure. Critical comparisons can be made between the societal and media responses to crack cocaine use being framed as a problem within Black communities versus opioid emergence within suburban white communities.[12] Among Black families, multiple studies have identified an increased likelihood of both substance use screening during pregnancy and urine toxicology testing at or after delivery, regardless of history of substance use (eg, prenatal disclosures and testing).[13–15]

Reducing prenatal substance exposure requires accessible reproductive, pregnancy, and substance use care to facilitate agency in pregnancy; identification of prenatal substance use; and connection to treatment resources.[16] Punitive societal approaches to substance use in pregnancy have been shown to be a barrier to substance use disclosure and receipt of care.[17–19] In addition, drug overdose is an increasing cause of morbidity and mortality among pregnant and postpartum people, with disparate impacts on American Indian and Alaska Native populations.[18–21]

Diagnoses of neonatal abstinence syndrome (NAS) and neonatal opioid withdrawal syndrome (NOWS) increased almost fivefold between 2004 and 2014[22] and continued to increase through 2017, albeit at a slower pace.[23] The effects of prenatal substance exposure on neonatal and child health outcomes differ depending on multiple factors, including substance type and the frequency, magnitude, and timing of exposures.

Caregiver substance use, including prenatal substance exposure, is associated with an increased likelihood of child protective services reports and out-of-home placement.[24,25] In a 2006 birth cohort, almost one-third of infants medically diagnosed with prenatal substance exposure were placed in foster care within their first year after birth.[25] Nationally, out-of-home placements related to parental substance use increased substantially from 2000 to 2017.[26] Regarding the intersection with race and racism, studies have demonstrated mixed results regarding the association between race and ethnicity and child protective services involvement for prenatal substance exposure; however, disentangling and fully elucidating the complex layers of this association is difficult in these studies.[27–29]

The study of associations between parental substance use and child maltreatment is complicated by the multiplicity of potential connections, including statutory definitions.[24] Pediatricians should be aware of relevant regulations at this intersection. Federally, the augmentations of the Child Abuse Prevention and Treatment Act in the 2016 Comprehensive Addiction and Recovery Act set out Plans of Safe Care to facilitate identification of need and coordination of resources to support families affected by prenatal substance exposure.[30] As of 2024, approximately half of states in the United States reference prenatal substance use as instances or evidence of child abuse and/or neglect in statute,[31] risking a punitive approach that limits help-seeking behaviors[17,32] and engagement in medical care. Furthermore, birthing parents on methadone or buprenorphine for treatment of opioid use disorder may face stigma and increased child protective surveillance, which can jeopardize the birthing parent's recovery.[33] Physicians play an important role in developing Plans of Safe Care and should be aware of local processes.

Neonatal Manifestations of Prenatal Substance Exposure

Presentations of prenatal substance exposure can vary, depending on the substance, dose, and timing of exposure, as well as parental physical and mental health, access and engagement in health care, and socioeconomic supports. Clinicians should be knowledgeable about potential experiences that children in foster care may have related to prenatal substance exposure.

Clinicians caring for children affected by prenatal substance exposure may discover a history of birth complications, which are more common in pregnancies affected by substance use, including preterm birth and low birth weight.[34,35] Prenatal exposure to specific substances, if known, should alert the clinician to assess for associated manifestations. For instance, prenatal tobacco exposure increases the risks of low birth weight, prematurity, and other poor birth outcomes, as well as sudden infant death syndrome (SIDS).[36] Opioid exposure (alone or with other substances) is associated with NAS and NOWS, which can manifest in myriad ways.[37,38]

Management of NAS and NOWS includes both nonpharmacological and, in some cases, pharmacological interventions to address infant symptoms.[38,39] Nonpharmacological care is a mainstay of treatment and includes modifications of the infant care environment and supportive interventions such as rooming with the parent, swaddling, gentle transitions, and pacifier use. Pharmacological care, when required, utilizes medications such as morphine or buprenorphine in settings where nonpharmacological management is inadequate to address infant needs. Medications are titrated to effect, allowing the infant to achieve basic early functions, and are subsequently titrated downward. Depending on the institutional practice, infants may complete medication weaning on either an inpatient or an outpatient basis. Clinicians should familiarize themselves with local practices to be able to best support families in the early days after discharge, including the potential to continue to support medication weaning plans, continued support and implementation of Plans of Safe Care, and fostering connections to desired and needed services, including developmental surveillance, social services to address concrete needs, and parental supports as necessary.

Children Exposed to Alcohol in Pregnancy

Fetal alcohol spectrum disorders (FASD) is an umbrella term that encapsulates the wide range of clinical manifestations associated with prenatal alcohol exposure.[40–42] It does not in itself represent a clinical diagnosis, but rather encompasses several diagnoses: fetal alcohol syndrome (FAS), partial fetal alcohol syndrome, alcohol-related neurodevelopmental disorder (ARND), alcohol-related birth defects (ARBD), and neurobehavioral disorder associated with prenatal alcohol exposure (ND-PAE).

The AAP has clinical guidelines to support assessment for FASD,[42] which is best done through a structured, multidisciplinary approach that ideally includes expertise in general pediatrics, genetic dysmorphology, and psychological/neuropsychological assessment. Diagnosis of an FASD is best accomplished by multidimensional assessment, to address the significant variability and wide range of symptom severity[43]:

1. Documented prenatal alcohol exposure
   a. Absence of prenatal alcohol exposure history by absent disclosure or

inaccessible birth records does not preclude a diagnosis of all FASD, but it does limit application of some diagnoses, such as ARND and ARBD.

2. Neurodevelopmental assessment and neuropsychology evaluation to evaluate for deficits in neurocognition, self-regulation, and adaptive function
   a. To meet FAS diagnostic criteria, structural (microcephaly and/or neuroimaging abnormality), neurological (seizure or abnormal neurological examination), or functional (global developmental delay less than the third percentile or deficits below the 16th percentile in 3 or more specific domains) central nervous system abnormalities must be documented.
3. Dysmorphology evaluation to assess for 3 cardinal facial characteristics of FAS
   a. The 3 features are smooth philtrum, thin upper lip, and reduced palpebral fissure length. Standardized images for grading are available for use in the diagnostic process.[44]
4. Evaluation for growth deficits and/or structural anomalies
   a. Adjusted prenatal and/or postnatal growth failure (height, weight, and/or head circumference) less than the 10th percentile.
   b. Microcephaly can also be characterized as a structural central nervous system abnormality.
5. Physical health differences associated with prenatal alcohol exposure include congenital renal, cardiac, skeletal, and ocular anomalies. Conductive and sensorineural hearing loss can also be seen.[42,45,46]

Outpatient Presentations and Management

Prenatal substance exposure has been associated with reduced attendance to health supervision visits, setting the stage for tenuous continuity of care, which may further delay recognition of medical and developmental issues, if present, once a child enters foster care.[47,48] At the first pediatric visit, pediatricians should ask caregivers and child welfare case workers about any known history of prenatal substance exposure to understand factors that may affect a child's health. Pediatricians should also be familiar with regulations and practices to address confidentiality of maternal medical history, particularly at the convergence of pregnancy, substance use, and infant medical documentation.

Ideally, accurate documentation of medically actionable exposure history will be available to inform future evaluations and diagnoses. This can be challenging for children in foster care, because records may not be complete or the birthing parent may not be available to provide a history. With the exception of FASD, which is diagnosed contingent upon documented alcohol exposure, diagnosis and management related to other prenatal substance exposure rarely requires specific knowledge of substance type. In all cases, medical management should address physical and developmental manifestations at the time of presentation, which are likely multifactorial in etiology.

For infants, anticipatory guidance in the first days and weeks after birth includes continued attention to supporting infant self-regulation and organized response to environmental stimuli, because infants may have persistent dysregulation during the first weeks and months after birth. Nonpharmacological approaches (swaddling, for example) and environmental modifications (such as soft ambient or white noise) should be reviewed. Referrals to early intervention and other developmental surveillance and support programs should also be made, if not already completed at the time of birth.

Support of breastfeeding should be informed by prenatal substance use per guidelines available, including potential for toxicity to infants if substances are transmitted via human milk.[49,50] Of note, while the use of cannabis products may be legal for medical and/or recreational purposes, current data are inadequate to determine the effects of exposure via breastfeeding or human milk for infants.[51]

History of prenatal infectious exposures, or associated negative test results, should also be routinely documented. This includes recognition of increased risk of infectious exposures related to illicit substance use, such as HIV, syphilis, hepatitis C, hepatitis B, and tuberculosis.[52–54] If negative prenatal or perinatal maternal infectious test results are not available or cannot be confirmed, counseling should be conducted to describe possible health and developmental risks posed by perinatal infectious exposures and engage in shared decision-making to develop a postnatal testing plan for the child. For example, infants born to parents with hepatitis C can be tested for hepatitis C as early as 2 months after birth.[55] Moreover, negative test results only at the time of birth, in the presence of risk factors such as the absence of prenatal care and reported high-risk exposures (eg, injection drug use), may warrant further postnatal testing if additional health information about the birthing parent is not available. Specific testing plans should be informed by local prevalence, test characteristics, and prenatal substance exposures to balance risk and benefit with resource utilization and predictive value.

Other behavioral and physical health challenges related to prenatal substance exposure are varied and may not manifest until later in childhood. Most studies on long-term outcomes after prenatal substance exposure are limited by confounders. Outcomes are likely to represent multiple contributing factors, including parental substance use history, co-occurring parental mental health conditions (such as depression and anxiety), exposure to intimate partner violence or other forms of trauma, and other environmental factors (such as poverty, social and structural drivers of health, and systemic racism). Care should be taken in all discussions and documentation to use nonstigmatizing language.

Examples of behavioral considerations include the following:

- Tobacco exposure throughout pregnancy is linked with increased irritability, inattention, and hyperactivity,[56] with an increased likelihood of attention-deficit/hyperactivity disorder and anxiety symptoms in adolescence and young adulthood.[57]
- Prenatal cannabis exposure is associated with externalizing behavior problems, such as impulsivity and inattention,[58] as well as earlier initiation of cannabis use in adolescence,[59] which can be associated with lower academic achievement, lower educational attainment, and psychotic symptoms.[60,61] When providing age-appropriate counseling regarding the risks of substance use at routine physical examinations, pediatricians should consider the risks of dual cannabis and other substance exposure (exposure during pregnancy and use during adolescence).
- FASD includes differences such as impaired neurocognitive function (eg, global developmental delay or domain-specific impairments in learning, memory, or reasoning), impaired self-regulation (eg, poor attention or impulse control), and impaired adaptive functioning, which requires at least one challenge in communication-related tasks as well as another skill deficit.[42,43] Absent prenatal history should not exclude consideration of FASD, with the exception of ND-PAE.[62] Children with FASD can be best supported through integrated care in a medical home,[63] as well as with an individualized education program or 504 plan at school, depending on needs.

Best Practices

- To address pervasive distrust, fear, and marginalization and promote engagement in care, clinicians caring for children should use nonstigmatizing language and a compassionate approach, which facilitate the best outcomes for children and families.
- Coordination of care should take into account physical, mental, and socioemotional health needs, including awareness of psychosocial factors

(including both social and structural drivers of health) that influence and shape outcomes and are difficult to disentangle from teratogenic effects of prenatal substance use.

- Comprehensive attention within an established medical home that includes collaboration with all who care for the child (including biological parents, kinship and foster caregivers, and child welfare caseworkers) can optimize a child's health and developmental trajectories, regardless of the custody situation.

Key Takeaways

- Prenatal substance exposure is unfortunately common and associated with an increased risk of adverse health outcomes, developmental challenges, and child maltreatment.
- Supportive, nonstigmatizing approaches that respect the dignity of children and caregivers are critical for continued engagement in health care and other services.
- Optimal care for children with a history of prenatal substance exposure includes established care in a medical home that incorporates developmental surveillance, behavioral health support, and close collaboration with community-based services that may be needed to support family well-being.

CHAPTER 30

Neurodevelopmental Disorders: Identification and Intervention

Douglas Waite, MD, FAAP

The neurodevelopmental disorders are a group of often-overlapping developmental challenges in early childhood that often become apparent before a child enters school. These developmental challenges present as delays in one or more areas of the child's development, including social interaction, adaptive function, speech and language development, gross and fine motor development, and cognitive disabilities. The broad category of neurodevelopmental disorders spans challenges in communication such as isolated speech delay, autism, global developmental delay, intellectual disability, fetal alcohol spectrum disorders (FASD), gross and fine motor disabilities, learning disabilities, and attention-deficit/hyperactivity disorder.[1]

Multiple causes during both the prenatal and postnatal periods place children in foster care at especially high risk for having a neurodevelopmental disorder. For example, the rates of autism and intellectual disability among youth in foster care are 2 to 5 times greater than the rates found in the general US population, with likelihood of foster care involvement increasing with age.[2] Similarly, the prevalence of FASD in foster care is estimated to be 18.8%, with nearly one-third of children who are diagnosed with FASD being placed into foster care.[3] In addition, children with disabilities such as autism and FASD are at a greater risk of maltreatment than children without disabilities.[4,5] For these reasons, routine screening to improve the identification of infants and children with developmental delays and neurodevelopmental disorders is the first step toward interventions to maximize child development and the stability of permanency planning. The following sections review each of the risk factors that contribute to developmental challenges as well as essential components of the prenatal and postnatal developmental history that facilitate identification of children who require interventions.

Risk Factors for Developmental Challenges Among Children in Foster Care

Child Abuse and Neglect

Neglect, a risk factor for developmental challenges, is the primary reason for child welfare referral and placement. Early childhood neglect, though often the most clinically difficult form of maltreatment to recognize, has a profound effect on child development. Children experiencing neglect over the first 4 years after birth show a progressive decline in cognitive functioning and a significantly reduced head circumference at 2 and 4 years of age.[6] Child maltreatment, particularly emotional abuse and neglect, is associated with a wide range of long-term adverse health and developmental outcomes. The effects of early childhood abuse and neglect can last far beyond childhood. Child maltreatment poses substantial risk for undermining the broad spectrum of developmental domains, including emotional and behavioral regulation, development of attachment relationships, self-organization and self-esteem, peer relations, and adaptation to school.[7] The impact of child abuse and neglect on child development has led to the concept of developmental trauma disorder.[8,9] While currently not recognized as a neurodevelopmental disorder, this concept emphasizes the effects of severe postnatal adverse experiences on child development.

Chapter 17, Childhood Trauma and Resilience, details mechanisms through which neglect affects brain development. Child abuse and neglect disrupt brain development not only through the persistent absence of responsive care that reinforces neurodevelopment but also through activation of the body's stress response.[10,11] Research over the past 50 years has led to the evolving concept of toxic stress, which directly affects brain architecture and function.[12] Early exposure to abuse and neglect shape neuronal networks through synaptic pruning, putting maltreated children at risk for emotional dysregulation in early life.[13,14]

Early exposure to child abuse or neglect, family turmoil, neighborhood violence, extreme poverty, racial discrimination, or other hardships can prime biological systems to become hyperresponsive to adversity. Deprivation, neglect, or emotional abuse, though less visible and easier to ignore than overt physical abuse, can cause more harm to a young child's development, with effects including subsequent cognitive delays, impairments in executive functioning, and increased risk of a wide range of health problems over a lifetime. Severe neglect has been associated with decreased development of the prefrontal cortex as well as abnormal activities in areas of the brain associated with emotion, stress regulation, attention, and self-control.[15]

Research examining the impact of toxic stress and adversity on children's developing neuroendocrine and immune systems is a rapidly growing field of study. Prolonged exposure to toxic stress can contribute to dysregulation of the hypothalamic-pituitary-adrenal axis and cortisol levels over time, contributing to decreased cerebral volumes in the prefrontal cortex and hippocampus with increased neurogenesis in the amygdala. These neuroendocrine changes increase the risk of developmental delays and later difficulties in learning, attention, and self-regulation.[12] Studies examining immune system biomarkers as related to toxic stress and adversity in children found higher levels of biomarkers for chronic disease compared with nonaffected peers.[16] In contrast, secure positive attachments result in increases in oxytocin, which improves ongoing attachment and brain development.[17] Early identification and referral of children at risk of developmental delays can markedly change the trajectory of development.[18]

Alcohol and Substance Use

While parental alcohol or substance use is often a major cause of neglect, in many cases it is not captured on intake to child welfare services.[19] An elevated risk for both prenatal substance and alcohol exposure, in addition to child abuse and neglect, synergistically places children in foster care at exceptional risk for developmental challenges.[5] States are mandated to establish a plan of safe care for these children under the Comprehensive Addiction and Recovery Act.[20] The sum of these risk factors makes the identification and treatment of the developmental challenges of children in foster care an urgent task pertinent to all who work in the field of child welfare.

Assessment of Factors That Could Challenge Development

A brief review of prenatal and postnatal influences on child development provides a framework for obtaining a complete medical history to identify specific risk factors that can threaten the development of children in foster care. A complete medical history encompasses the prenatal, birth, and postnatal periods, beginning with conception, a mother's discovery of her pregnancy, prenatal factors that affect brain development, birth-associated risks, and postnatal developmental milestones. In addition, a review of the family history should include the birth families' medical history as well as the biological parents' personal histories of developmental and learning challenges, school achievement and employment histories, and past and current mental health issues and substance use disorders. The family history should also include the histories of siblings, half-siblings, and grandparents, because mental health and substance disorders are often present across generations.

Most children entering foster care have experienced adversity. For this reason, the Adverse Childhood Experiences (ACE) questionnaire is less useful in identifying children with histories of severe traumatic experiences. The International Society for Traumatic Stress Studies website has information for specific screens for traumatic experiences, such as the Child Trauma Screen, which are more appropriate for use with children in foster care. These can be found at https://istss.org/clinical-resources/child-trauma-assessments. Further information can be found at the American Academy of Pediatrics (AAP) site "Supporting Children who have Experienced Trauma": https://www.aap.org/en/patient-care/foster-care/supporting-children-who-have-experienced-trauma/. While such screens are helpful, integrating trauma-informed practices into developmental assessments should be done with the recognition that each child may experience and show developmental and behavioral challenges resulting from trauma differently. Chapter 10, Assessing Risk and Protective Factors, provides further discussion.

Figure 30–1 highlights common challenges that can influence child development across the prenatal, birth, and postnatal periods.

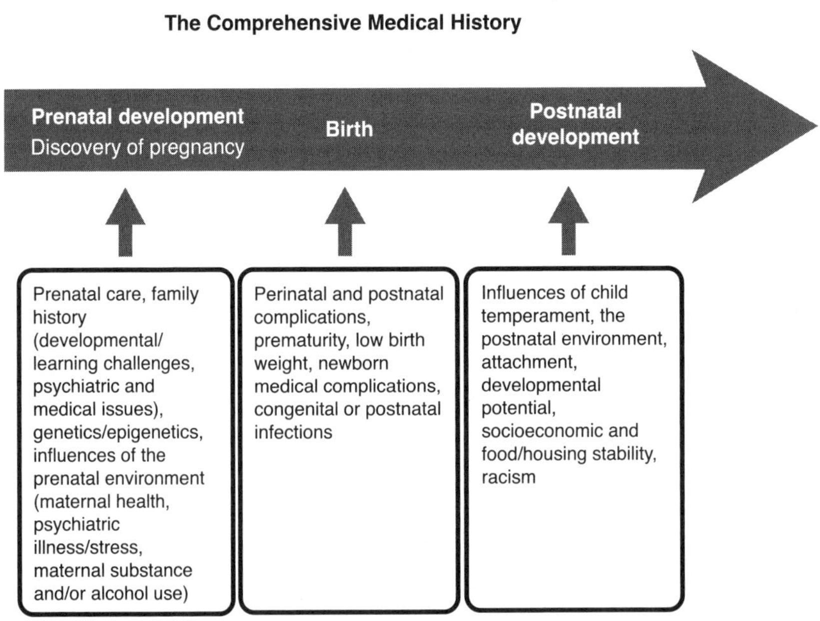

Figure 30–1. Timeline illustrating essential elements in each period of the comprehensive medical history.

Influences on Prenatal Development

Research over the past 50 years has highlighted the important influence of prenatal brain development on later developmental milestones. This history is often difficult to obtain for children in foster care because of gaps in information that foster care agencies, foster parents, and biological parents have provided to pediatricians. In addition, because of the stigma associated with involvement in the child welfare system and concerns that the information biological parents disclose may prevent the return of the child to their care, many parents are not forthcoming in providing this important information. Awareness of this dynamic can help pediatricians gain trust over time to develop an alliance and a working relationship with biological and foster parents toward the common goal of helping the child attain their developmental potential while maximizing chances for reunification of families.

Pediatricians are adept at obtaining a birth history at the time new patients enter their practice yet may feel uncomfortable inquiring about alcohol and substance use during pregnancy. **Box 30–1** includes pertinent parts of the prenatal history that can be included in the initial developmental assessment of all children in foster care. These should be documented in the medical chart for ongoing reference. In addition, many of these open-ended questions can serve as an opening for ongoing dialogue that can be revisited by either the pediatrician or the biological parent as a relationship of trust develops between the pediatrician and parents over the course of health supervision. In addition, these data can often be obtained from the foster care agency, as it may have access to information lacking to the foster parent and not disclosed by the biological parent.

Birth History

Box 30–2 highlights pertinent historical facts that can influence child development, which should be obtained when a child enters foster care. Obtaining this information is often complicated by Health Insurance Portability and Accountability Act (commonly known as HIPAA) regulations that prohibit review of maternal obstetric history. In addition, biological parents may not be available to provide a birth history otherwise unknown to the foster parent or foster care agency. Nonetheless, foster care placement can be seen as an opportunity to gather and synthesize information that might otherwise become lost with the passage of time. Every effort should be made to obtain and document the birth history in the medical record.

Box 30-1

The Prenatal History (Ideally Obtained From the Birth Parent)

- How far into your pregnancy did you discover you were pregnant?
- What medical problems did you have during your pregnancy?
- What medications were you prescribed during your pregnancy?
- Did you experience any stressful events during your pregnancy?
- How much alcohol did you drink prior to discovering you were pregnant?
- How much alcohol did you drink after you discovered you were pregnant?
- What other substances (cannabis, opioids, tobacco, or others) did you use prior to and after discovering you were pregnant?
- What medical, developmental, and behavioral challenges do the siblings of your child have?
- Do any persons in either the maternal or paternal family have developmental difficulties such as autism, speech delay, problems learning, or behavioral/psychiatric issues?

Box 30-2

Birth History

- Gestational age
- Birth weight
- Type of birth (vaginal, cesarean section)
- Obstetric history or documentation of prenatal exposure to infections such as HIV and other sexually transmitted infections
- Any known prenatal maternal substance use
- Perinatal or postnatal complications (past laboratory test results or radiographic evaluations, subspecialty evaluations following birth)

Influences on Postnatal Child Development

Multiple factors shape child development after birth. **Figure 30–2** describes a pyramid of typical child development milestones that begins with adaptation of the infant to the environment. This includes the temperament of the child, the ability of the child to be soothed, and the development of emotional self-regulation that comes with attachment.

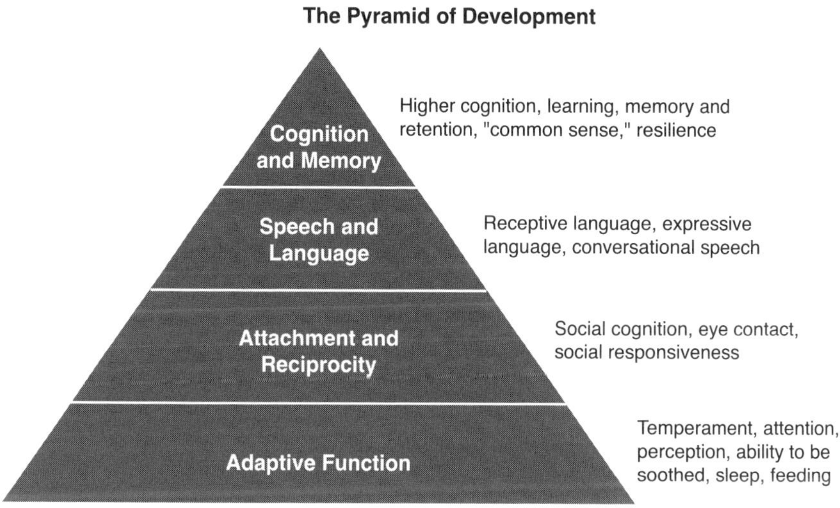

Figure 30–2. The pyramid of child development. Milestones at the base of the pyramid form the basis upon which subsequent milestones are developed.

While the basic structural and functional frameworks of the human brain are established by the second year after birth, subsequent brain development continues through reorganization and remodeling of already established neural networks shaped by the environment.[21] Adaptive function, including the development of attention, social cognition, and social responsiveness, is the foundation of attachment, which encourages reciprocal vocalizations and the development of speech and language.[22] A child's temperament, ability to be soothed, and sleep patterns also affect parent–child attachment. Social interaction occurring in the first months after birth, such as eye contact and social smile, reinforce attachment, which is the basis of acquisition of social learning, speech, and language. Speech and language support subsequent social development, emotional and behavioral regulation, memory, cognitive development, and learning.[10]

Figure 30–3 describes the typical developmental trajectory of a child.

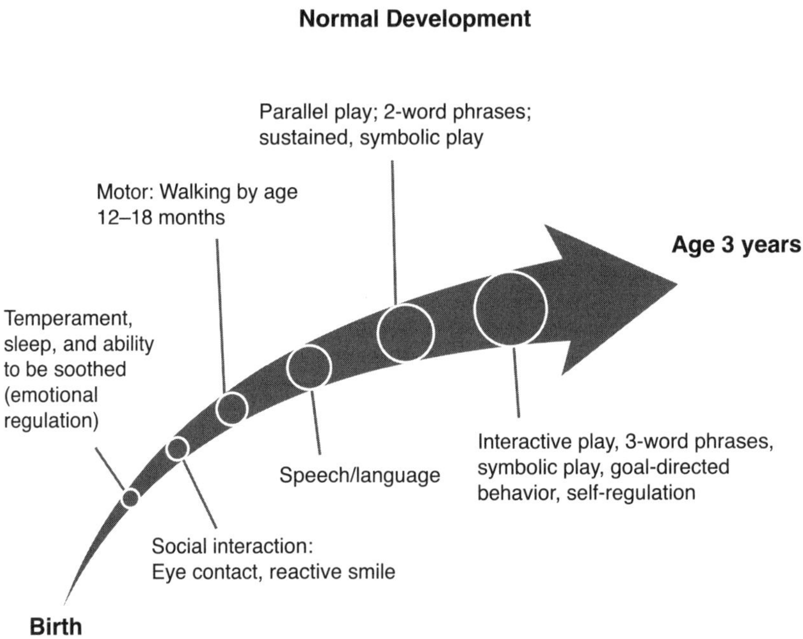

Figure 30–3. Typical developmental trajectory in the context of a safe, nurturing relationship with a caregiver who is stable over time in a child's life.

The relatively new field of epigenetics studies the influence of the social and physical environment on genetic expression and the subsequent shaping of brain development and function through experience-dependent adaptation or maladaptation.[23] The potentially deleterious sequelae that accompany child maltreatment not only result in adverse consequences during infancy and childhood but often initiate a negative developmental cascade that can reach across the lifespan. At the same time, children's development is shaped by experience, and positive changes in their environment remain possible throughout their lifetime.[13] Thus, interventions such as foster care placement, early intervention and educational interventions, and child and family support interventions can positively affect a child's developmental trajectory.

Starting from the base of the developmental pyramid described in **Figure 30-2**, the potential challenges to typical development faced by children in the child welfare system become multifactorial, with each new step of development influenced by previous developmental accomplishments or challenges (**Figure 30–4**).

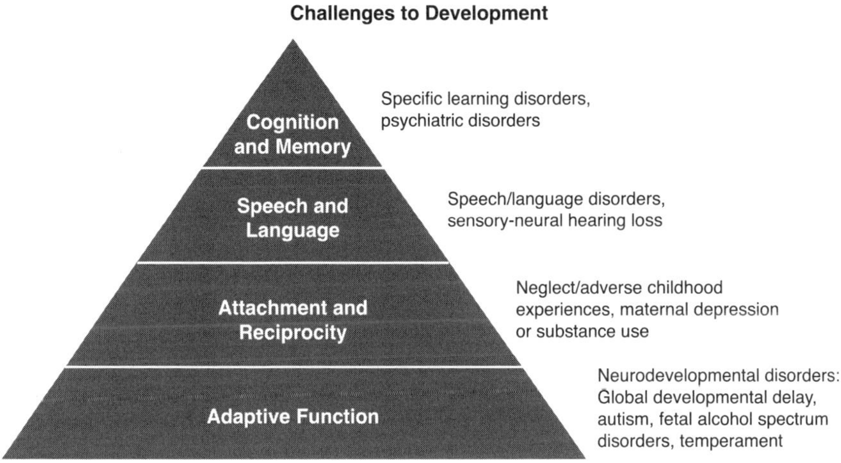

Figure 30–4. Challenges to typical development. Multiple risk factors that are common among children in foster care have the synergistic potential to adversely affect child development.

Challenges to development can become apparent soon after birth among children with a neurodevelopmental disorder and become more apparent over time as a child's developmental trajectory lags from expected developmental milestones. Subsequent parent–child interactions and environmental supports or adversities further shape development. Each of these factors will be considered separately in the rest of this chapter.

Common Developmental Trajectories Among the Neurodevelopmental Disorders

Overview

Children with a neurodevelopmental disorder such as autism, global developmental delay, or FASD have developmental delays that shape further developmental stages. These challenges may manifest as difficulty being consoled, intense temperament, difficulties sleeping and feeding, and failure to engage in reciprocal social interactions that reinforce parent–child attachment.[24] The complex dynamic of difficult-to-soothe crying can lead to a sense of parental helplessness and inefficacy, affect parental attachment, and increase the risk of child abuse or neglect. For example, the peak period of infant crying in the first 3 months after birth correlates with the highest rates of abusive head trauma,[25] and children with a neurodevelopmental disorder are at greater risk of child abuse and neglect.[26]

Children with neurodevelopmental disorders typically present with developmental delays in the preschool years, ranging from excessive crying with difficulty being consoled to lack of social interaction, failure to gain speech and language, and subsequent emotional, behavioral, and cognitive challenges. This trajectory is highlighted in **Figure 30–5**.

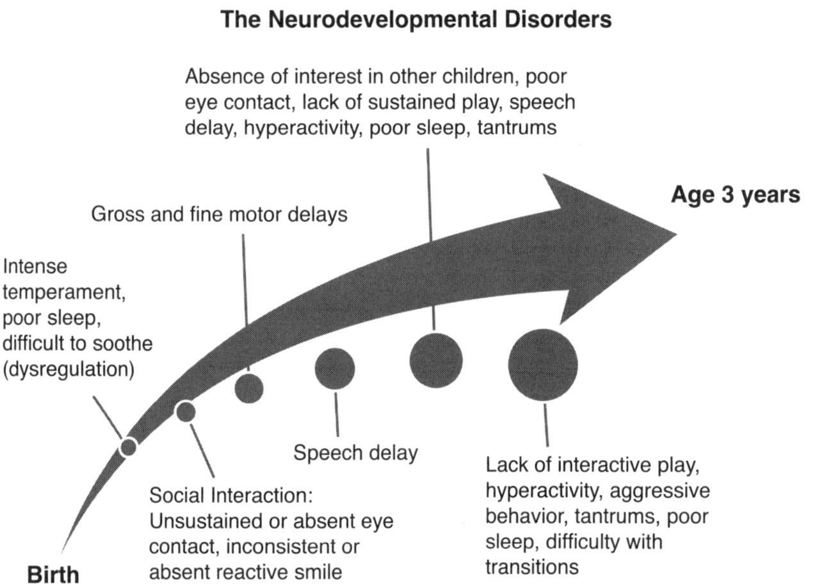

Figure 30–5. Developmental challenges common among children with neurodevelopmental disorders.

While children in foster care may present with symptoms of psychiatric disorders in early childhood, a comprehensive developmental history that includes screening for underlying neurodevelopmental disorders should precede psychiatric diagnoses such as attention-deficit disorder and oppositional defiant disorder. Historically, children in foster care receive prescriptions for psychiatric medications at a rate far greater than that of children who are not in foster care.[27] In many cases, multiple psychiatric diagnoses and prescriptions for multiple psychiatric medications are used to treat behavioral manifestations that often eclipse greater undiagnosed neurodevelopmental challenges (see Chapter 38, Psychotropic Medication Oversight, for a detailed discussion).

The AAP recommends developmental surveillance at every health visit as well as the administration of standardized screening tests at all health supervision visits up to age 60 months for children in foster care, given their high prevalence of trauma and high mobility among placements. Special attention to surveillance is recommended at the 4- to 5-year health supervision visit, prior to entry into elementary education, with referral if there are developmental or behavioral concerns.[28] Given the elevated risk for developmental challenges of children in foster care, a lower threshold for referral for further evaluation recognizes the complex relationship between child–parent attachment and child development that is disrupted by foster care placement. In addition to screening for delays across developmental domains, assessment of a child's attachment to their caregiver guides environmental interventions to support child development while in foster care. This includes training on parenting skills and the effects of trauma on brain development, as well as education about developmental milestones to ensure parents understand their child's current developmental ability and have realistic expectations for their behaviors. The diagnosis of a developmental disability can provide a basis to educate parents about specific developmental challenges common to children with a neurodevelopmental disorder, such as autism. This reframing of behavior to "can't" instead of "won't" is one of the cornerstones of discussions that allow parents to better understand that their child's behavior is not willful but secondary to their developmental disability.

FASD

Since a specific pattern of facial features, growth deficiency, and developmental delays was first described as fetal alcohol syndrome (FAS), neurodevelopmental impairments associated with prenatal alcohol exposure, even in the absence of physical findings of FAS, have come to be recognized as FASD.[29] While the prevalence of FASD in the general population is estimated to be 1.1% to 5%, the estimated prevalence of FASD among children in foster care is 18.8%. [3,30,31] Thus, about 1 in 5 children in foster care have FASD, most of whom are never identified or diagnosed with this disorder. For example, 80% of children in foster care who were referred and subsequently diagnosed with FASD had never been previously diagnosed.[32] Children with FASD are frequently overprescribed psychiatric medications while their underlying neurodevelopmental disabilities go unrecognized. In this case, diagnosis helps inform parent education, interventions, treatment, and medication management.[33,34] Prenatal alcohol and substance exposure place children at higher risk of involvement in the child welfare system, multiple foster home placements, and poorer long-term outcomes. For this reason, pediatricians caring for children in foster care should consider this diagnosis when evaluating children in foster care with developmental and/or behavioral challenges.

The developmental challenges of children with prenatal alcohol exposure and FASD have been well reviewed elsewhere.[35,36] Further information can be found in the AAP FASD Toolkit (https://www.aap.org/en/patient-care/fetal-alcohol-spectrum-disorders/). The new diagnostic classification of neurodevelopmental disorder associated with prenatal alcohol exposure provides a path for general pediatricians to diagnose FASD.[37,38] The diagnosis of all FASD other than FAS is dependent on obtaining a history of prenatal alcohol exposure.[39] Because of the prevalence of FASD among children in foster care, it is especially important that all children in foster care be screened for prenatal alcohol exposure. This history should be revisited if children present with developmental delays, behavioral challenges, or psychiatric diagnoses.

Ongoing Care From Childhood to Adolescence

Pediatric care of children in foster care with developmental disabilities is especially challenging. Challenges with attachment, loss, and transitioning to adulthood place a greater burden on pediatricians to coordinate care in the medical home across multiple disciplines.[40] Specific supports include advocacy for early intervention, special education services (often advocating against the educational mandates for placement in the least restrictive environment when schools may not recognize the exceptional needs of a child), and state disability services provided under the Individuals with Disabilities Education Act. State-based disability services provide day programs after adolescents "age out" of school, job training and job linkage, and care coordinators to help facilitate home-based services and supportive housing. Finally, because many children in foster care who are subsequently adopted may have disabilities that inhibit their ability to make life choices, adoptive parents may need to seek guardianship to safeguard their young adult's well-being.

Identification of a child's developmental needs must be integrated into a plan of care that ensures the safety and well-being of the child into adulthood, independent of whether the permanency plan is reunification with their parent or adoption. This plan of care should include transition planning that recognizes an adolescent and young adult's disability and builds environmental supports toward maximizing independence while recognizing that many young adults may require support across their lifespan.

Key Takeaways

- The developmental history for children in foster care should include prenatal, birth, and postnatal risks for challenges in child development. Elements of the family history include developmental and learning challenges, psychiatric illness, and substance and alcohol use disorders in parents, grandparents, and siblings.
- All children in foster care should have developmental screening as recommended by the AAP at entry to care and at every health supervision visit until age 60 months.
- All children in foster care should be screened for prenatal alcohol exposure.
- All children in foster care should be screened for the effects of traumatic experiences on their development.
- Foster care placement provides an opportunity to gather and integrate information, diagnose developmental disabilities, and recommend interventions for children in foster care. The pediatric medical home can serve as the point of coordination of services and advocacy across disciplines to support child development through adolescence.

CHAPTER 31

Children With Medical Complexity

Rebecca R. Seltzer, MD, MHS, FAAP

Introduction

Children with medical complexity are a diverse population with chronic medical conditions that are associated with high rates of health care use, high health service needs, and functional limitations.[1,2] With advances in pediatric medical care and medical technology, a growing number of children are surviving once fatal diagnoses (eg, congenital anomalies, extreme prematurity, neuromuscular disorders, genetic syndromes) and may require intensive daily care regimens, such as medications, treatments, and often dependence on medical technology and equipment (eg, ventilator, feeding tube, wheelchair).[1,3] While children with medical complexity represent less than 1% of US children, they account for up to one-third of pediatric health care spending and over half of pediatric inpatient charges.[2–5] They typically receive care from multiple pediatric specialists (eg, neurology, gastroenterology, pulmonology, physical therapy, speech therapy) and across various sites of care (eg, inpatient, outpatient, emergency department, rehabilitation, and school). Many have prolonged and recurrent hospitalizations due to exacerbations or declines in their conditions.

The care needs of children with medical complexity pose significant demands on the health care system and family caregivers. Navigating this complex network of care amidst a fragmented health care system places children at risk of significant unmet needs.[5,6] Additionally, the daily care needs of this population impose significant and often unrealistic demands on family caregivers. Families report spending a median of 2 hours per week on care coordination and 11 to 20 hours per week on direct medical home care.[5] Due to home nursing shortages and a lack of respite care options, caregivers are rarely given a break in their responsibilities.[7,8] Parents often report having to quit a job or cut back on hours to care for their child.[5] Subsequently, many caregivers experience financial stress, burnout, and adverse physical and mental health effects,[5,9,10] which may affect their ability to provide the intensive daily care that their children require. Such family stressors can also be risk factors for maltreatment.[11] When families of origin are unable to safely meet a child's needs, concerns for neglect or abuse may arise and result in child welfare system involvement.[12,13]

This chapter covers health care and child welfare system considerations for children with medical complexity in foster care, including placements, care coordination, medical decision-making, consents, and practical considerations for pediatricians.

Child Welfare System Involvement for Children With Medical Complexity

Prior research shows that, compared with their healthy peers, children with complex medical needs and disabilities experience higher rates of maltreatment and are disproportionately represented in the child welfare system.[12,14–17] As previously mentioned, children with medical complexity represent less than 1% of children in the United States,[2,4] yet they account for an estimated 10% of children in foster care.[18] A Canadian study found that children with medical complexity had disproportionately higher rates of child welfare system involvement and placement in out-of-home care compared with the general pediatric population.[19] In that study, nearly one-quarter of children with medical complexity had involvement with the child welfare system and over one-third of those children were placed in out-of-home placement after the investigation. A meta-analysis found that rates of maltreatment for children with disabilities were over 3.5 times higher than for children without disabilities.[15] While neglect is the most common form of maltreatment experienced by children with disabilities, other types of maltreatment (such as sexual abuse and physical abuse) are also experienced at higher rates in this population.[15–17] Victims of maltreatment who are nonverbal or have intellectual or developmental disabilities that limit their ability to recognize or disclose maltreatment may go unidentified, leading to underreporting.[11]

In a recent survey of US child welfare agencies, medical neglect was reported as the most common reason that children with medical complexity come to the agency's attention for both family support services and out-of-home placement (unpublished data). Most children reported to child protective services for medical neglect have serious chronic medical conditions.[20] Several factors place children with medical complexity at increased risk of being reported for neglect: complex medical care plans are difficult to follow, medical fragility increases the risks of morbidity and mortality if the care plan is not followed, and frequent appointments with clinicians are difficult to maintain. The financial and psychosocial stressors experienced by these families further complicate their ability to follow a complex care plan.

The relationship between medical complexity and maltreatment is bidirectional. Not only are children with complex medical needs at higher risk of maltreatment, but abuse and neglect can result in permanent disability and medical complexity.[11] For example, studies have shown that children with abusive head trauma are at significant risk of long-term disability, including neurodevelopmental disability, visual impairment, epilepsy, feeding difficulties, communication deficits, and motor impairment.[21,22]

Placement Considerations

Children with medical complexity whose daily care needs cannot be met by their parents or who have been maltreated may be placed in the foster care system.[13] While most enter foster care involuntarily due to concerns for abuse or neglect, some families may enter through a voluntary placement agreement to support their child's care needs. Voluntary placements are not available in all states. Once it is determined that a child will be placed in foster care, the agency must determine an appropriate placement that is equipped to provide the child's specific level of care.

Many children with medical complexity are placed in a specialized medical or therapeutic foster care home with foster parents who have received additional training based on the child's identified medical needs (for example, how to manage a feeding tube or tracheostomy).[13,23,24] Not only does the availability of such specialized placements vary by state, but the criteria used to determine what children qualify for a specialized medical placement also vary.[25] Additionally, state variation exists regarding regulations for training requirements, foster parent payment, and number of children with medical complexity permitted in one foster home.

Due to challenges with recruitment and retention of medical foster parents, children with medical complexity may be placed in congregate care settings (group homes or residential nursing facilities). They are more likely to be placed in a congregate care setting than children in foster care without medical complexity.[26] In fact, 1 in 5 surveyed agencies reported that more than 20% of children with medical complexity in their care are placed in congregate care settings (unpublished data). For hospitalized children in need of a new placement or change in placement, limited availability of appropriate placements can result in delays in discharge from days to months.[27] If no other options exist, some children may be sent to placements out of state, creating additional barriers to the child engaging with their family of origin.

Outcomes for Children With Medical Complexity in Foster Care

Medical complexity is considered a primary determinant of unmet health care needs, regardless of family income, primary language, or Medicaid enrollment.[6] Because children in foster care are also known to experience unmet health care needs, those with medical complexity in foster care may be particularly vulnerable to poor health outcomes. Yet, the ability to track outcomes for children with medical complexity in foster care is limited by the lack of linked child welfare and health data. Additionally, agencies do not have a uniform definition for children with medical complexity or required field for medical complexity in mandatory state and federal foster care and adoption reporting systems.[28] The available data demonstrate that children with medical complexity are more likely to experience poor child welfare–related outcomes, such as placement instability, prolonged time in care, and lack of permanency (reunification, adoption, or guardianship).[26]

Special Considerations for the Pediatrician Caring for Children With Medical Complexity in Foster Care

Care Coordination

Children with medical complexity are at risk of fragmented care due to the many clinicians they see and systems involved in their care.[29] When in foster care, they are at even greater risk due to the additional systems and services involved (**Figure 31–1**). Research has shown that once children with medical complexity enter foster care, many remain in the foster care system for prolonged periods of time and have frequent changes in foster parents and other care providers.[23,24,26,30] Changes in foster home placements threaten access to established clinicians, home nursing services, school-based services, and medical equipment deliveries. While disrupted health care continuity is problematic for all children in foster care, it is particularly concerning for children with medical complexity, whose medical stability depends on coordinated care with varied clinicians. If medical care plans are not followed, these children may face serious negative outcomes, such as acute decompensation of chronic conditions, hospitalization, or death.

Recognizing the critical importance of care coordination for children with medical complexity in foster care, pediatricians should openly communicate with child welfare agencies, caregivers (foster parent or group home staff), and families of origin (as appropriate) to ensure that all involved parties understand the child's care plan and are addressing any unmet needs. Because caregiver transition (ie, new removal, reunification, change in placement) places children at risk of fragmented care, these may be key time points to maintain more frequent follow-up with the medical team. In some states, special care coordinators through Medicaid or Title V programs may be able to assist with care coordination. Chapter 7, Care Coordination and Case Management, covers these topics in detail.

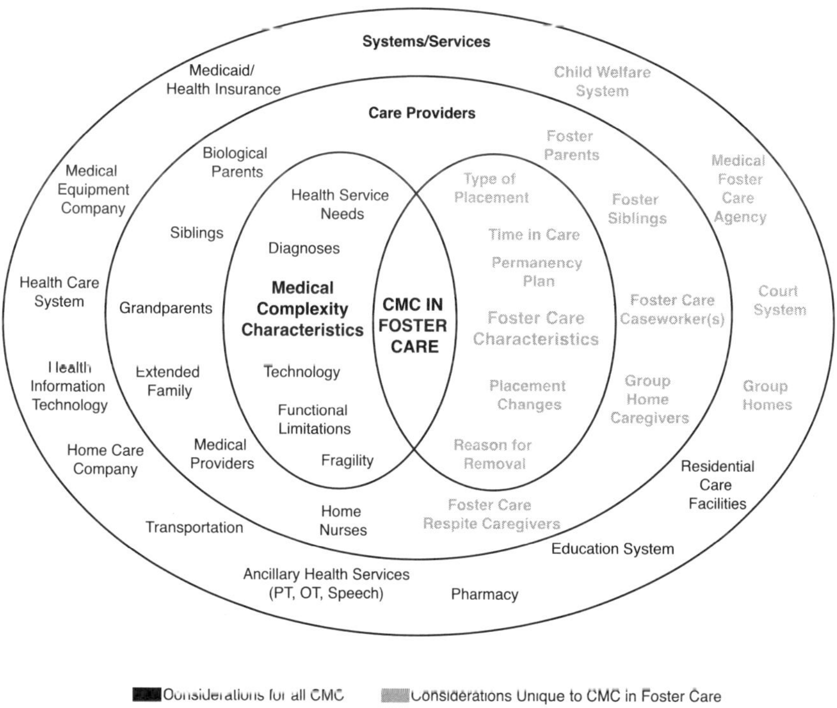

Figure 31–1. Delivery-of-care considerations for children with medical complexity in foster care. Abbreviations: CMC, children with medical complexity; OT, occupational therapy; PT, physical therapy.

Medical Decision-Making and Consent

Children with medical complexity interact frequently with the health care system, both for planned and unplanned visits. Because children younger than 18 years are not allowed to consent to their own medical care, with some minor exceptions, it is important to clarify who is legally authorized to consent on behalf of a patient in foster care. The court order that outlines such decision-making authority should be included in the patient's medical record. While policies related to consent vary by state or local child welfare agency, the foster parent is often permitted to consent to routine care, including health supervision visits, standard vaccines, and routine screening laboratory tests. Much of the care received by children with medical complexity is considered nonroutine, such as medical procedures, surgery, and anesthesia. Nonroutine care may require the consent of the biological parent (if termination of parental rights [TPR] has not occurred) or the child welfare agency. For some children, value-sensitive decisions about end-of-life care and do-not-resuscitate orders may become relevant; the authority to make these serious decisions is often limited to the biological parents (if no TPR) or a judge.[31] Guardians ad litem can be additional resources when navigating complex medical decisions. **Box 31–1** highlights some key considerations for medical decision-making for children in foster care.[31]

Hospital Discharge Planning

Hospital discharge is often delayed for children entering a new foster care placement, especially children with complex medical or behavioral needs. Common barriers to discharge cited by hospital clinicians include waiting for the court and child welfare agency to determine the child's discharge disposition and finding an appropriate foster care placement.[27] Additionally, ensuring a safe discharge requires more time-intensive coordination among child welfare workers, medical team members, and caregivers. Research has shown that foster caregivers often receive inadequate training about the child's medical care needs.[32] This can have significant implications for children with medical complexity, whose daily care is particularly complex.[33] As such, it is important for inpatient teams to tailor discharge practices to ensure that new foster caregivers are aware of the child's specific needs, routines, and postdischarge care plan and that they feel well trained and prepared to deliver this care.[27] Other strategies for safe discharge planning include confirming that the child's insurance is active, medications are ordered and picked up before discharge, and any recommended medical equipment, supplies, home nursing services, therapies, and follow-up care with clinicians and specialists are arranged before discharge. Additional recommendations for discharge planning have been previously published.[27]

Box 31–1

Key Considerations When Faced With Nonroutine Decisions for a Child in Foster Care

1. What is the seriousness/uncertainty of decision under consideration?

- For example, anesthesia for MRI versus surgery for tracheostomy versus withdrawal of care

2. Confirm with hospital/clinic social worker or child welfare worker the following:

- Have parental rights been terminated for the biological parents?
  - If no, then biological parents typically retain medical decision-making rights and should be involved in discussions.
- What is stated in the court order regarding decision-making authority for this child?
  - A copy of court order should be reviewed and placed in medical record

3. Once legal decision-maker(s) is confirmed, document information in the medical record:

- The name and contact information for all legally authorized decision-makers should be documented, in addition to the order they should be contacted.
  - For example, "Contact biological mom first at [phone number]. If biological mom unable to be reached in [set amount of time], then contact child welfare worker at [phone number]. If child welfare worker cannot be reached in [set amount of time], then contact the child welfare agency supervisor/director at [phone number], etc."

Avoid the "game of telephone" between care team members

- Ensure that the person(s) authorized to make medical decisions/provide informed consent on behalf of the child is *directly counseled by medical team* about the risks, benefits, long-term impacts, and alternatives of the medical decision at hand.
- Identify and seek input from other team members (ie, foster parent and medical foster care nurse) that are actively involved in the child's care and can speak to the child's best interests. If there is any uncertainty about the decision at hand, invite these individuals, the legal decision-maker(s), and any relevant medical team members to take part in a physician-facilitated care team conference.

If team members cannot reach consensus on a decision, despite a care team conference where all information can be collectively discussed, then consider involvement of a hospital ethics or legal consult.

Abbreviations: MRI, magnetic resonance imaging.

Reproduced from Seltzer RR, Raisanen JC, da Silva T, et al. Medical decision-making in foster care: considerations for the care of children with medical complexity. *Acad Pediatr.* 2020;20(3):333–340.

Aging Out of Foster Care

Because many children with medical complexity now live into adulthood, there are unique challenges to consider for those who age out of foster care without achieving permanency. It is necessary to develop a transition plan of care from child to adult clinicians and systems of care well before the child's 18th birthday. This should be done not by physicians alone, but in partnership with child welfare, the education system, and other involved state agencies (ie, disabilities administration). The American Academy of Pediatrics has published guidelines on health care transitions for adolescents and young adults.[34] An additional consideration for those in foster care is whether they can remain in their current placement as they transition from the custody of child welfare to adult protective services. Additionally, upon turning 18 years old, there is a need to determine what level of support, if any, the youth needs in making medical, financial, and other life decisions. While full guardianship is needed for some, many youths with medical complexity can do well with less restrictive decision-making supports (power of attorney or supported decision-making).[35] Consultation with a lawyer through a medicolegal partnership or other legal aid resource can be helpful during this time of transition.

Practical Considerations for Pediatricians

- Recognize that children with medical complexity and disabilities experience higher rates of maltreatment and are disproportionately represented in the child welfare system. Some risk factors for abuse and neglect include the child's complex daily care needs and the financial, emotional, physical, and social challenges that these families experience.
- Pediatricians can work to prevent maltreatment and promote stable placements (whether with the biological or foster family) by proactively supporting families in addressing any unmet needs.
  - If a child is not showing up to appointments or following their care plan as prescribed, work with the family to identify and address modifiable factors (eg, lack of transportation, lack of training, concern about medication side effects) rather than waiting until concerns rise to the threshold for neglect.
  - Attempt to simplify care plans and prioritize follow-up needs (eg, medical appointments, imaging) as much as possible to avoid overwhelming a family. When creating care plans, actively engage the family and consider what is feasible for the child and family's situation, along with what is culturally appropriate and sensitive to their health care beliefs.

- Collaborate with clinical and child welfare social workers, along with community organizations, to create a routinely vetted and updated list of local resources for children with medical complexity and their families.
- Refer families to clinic or hospital social workers and appropriate state- and community-based resources to identify supports (eg, supplemental security income, energy assistance, housing modifications, education advocates, respite). Parent advocacy organizations for children with medical complexity, such as Family Voices and Family-to-Family Health Information Centers, are another helpful resource (www.familyvoices.org).

► Children with medical complexity in foster care are at risk of fragmented care, which has serious implications for their health and well-being.

- When children with medical complexity newly enter foster care, attempt to track down and synthesize as much medical history as possible to share with the caregiver and child welfare team. Be a resource to educate them about the child's medical conditions and care plan.
- Regular communication among clinicians, child welfare staff, caregivers, and other key team members is critical to ensure continuous, coordinated care.
- Maintain close follow-up, especially during caregiver and placement transitions. When appropriate, allow the caregiver to choose whether they prefer in-person or telemedicine visits.

► Become familiar with what placement options are available for children with medical complexity in your state and advocate for the child being placed in the least restrictive setting that is equipped to safely meet their care needs.

► Clearly document the following information in the child's medical record:

- Contact information (name, phone number, backup phone number) for key team members in the child's care, such as the child's caregivers (resource parent or group home), biological parent (if involved), and child welfare caseworker.
- The name and contact information for all legally authorized medical decision-makers. If there is a hierarchy in the order they should be contacted (for example, biological parent and then child welfare worker), that should also be documented.
- A copy of the most recent court order related to the child being in foster care.

Key Takeaways

- Children with medical complexity and disabilities experience higher rates of maltreatment and are disproportionately represented in the child welfare system.
- Pediatricians can work to prevent maltreatment and promote stable placements (whether with the family of origin or foster family) by proactively supporting families in addressing any unmet needs.

CHAPTER 32

Children and Youth Living With or Affected by HIV

Susana Williams Keeshin, MD

Introduction

Globally, there were 1.3 million new HIV infections in 2022, 130,000 of which were among children.[1] Young people age 15 to 24 years account for over a quarter of new infections. In the United States, there were 36,740 new diagnoses in 2021, nearly 21% of which were in young people age 0 to 24.[2] Between 2010 and 2017, approximately 15% of adults and children living with HIV in the United States were foreign born.[3]

Recent decades have seen great strides in the treatment and prevention of HIV in children and youth, both in the United States and globally. Despite these successes, children are still affected by the HIV epidemic due to either their own infection, the loss of a parent or guardian due to HIV, or the heightened risks of racism, poverty, homelessness, dropping out of school, stigma, and discrimination that many people with HIV experience. Children and youth in foster care living with or affected by HIV have significant health needs and are at increased risk for chronic physical problems, developmental delays, and mental health issues. Pediatricians and foster parents face specific challenges related to HIV infection, which can include an initial adjustment period after a new diagnosis, decisions about disclosure of infection status, accessing past medical history, management of medication regimens, and identifying appropriate health care services.

With the advancements in antiretroviral therapy (ART), people living with HIV who have an early diagnosis and access to health care, are able to follow a healthy lifestyle, and achieve an undetectable HIV viral load, can have a lifespan comparable to those without HIV. However, because children and adolescents in foster care experience medical care interruptions, this population is at increased risk of having a detectable HIV viral load. It is important to discuss this prognosis and the importance of care continuity with youth in foster care living with HIV, along with caregivers, any trusted support people, and child welfare professionals.

This chapter discusses a few of the most common scenarios in which a pediatrician may encounter a child in foster care who is living with HIV, as well as considerations for prevention and disclosure.

Perinatal Transmission

Perinatal HIV transmission can occur during gestation, during delivery, and while breastfeeding. In 1992, new infant infections peaked at 2,000 in the United States.[2,4] This coincided with the overall peak of HIV infection among all ages in the United States. From the late 1970s through 1994 (most of this era was prior to ART), an estimated 14,920 infants were born with perinatally acquired HIV in the United States.[2,4] Due to prenatal testing, treatment, and pre-exposure prophylaxis (PrEP), the number of new HIV infections in infants is fewer than 150 annually since 2015, and the most recent data show fewer than 100 per year, which is less than 1% of all new HIV diagnoses.[2,4] Between 2015 and 2019, perinatal infections decreased by 41%.[2] Notably, approximately 12,000 children born in the United States between 2017 and 2020 were exposed to but did not perinatally acquire HIV.[5] Despite this decrease in HIV acquisition, perinatal transmission of HIV in the United States does occur and is still the most common route that children younger than 13 years acquire HIV. Thus, some children in foster care will have perinatally transmitted HIV.

Refugee and Immigrant Children

In 2022, approximately 43.3 million children worldwide were displaced as a consequence of conflict and violence.[6] Children comprise less than one-third of the global population but more than 41% of the world's refugees.[6] The US Office of Refugee Resettlement has 2 programs for unaccompanied children: the Unaccompanied Refugee Minors Program and the Unaccompanied Children Program. Both can result in refugee and immigrant children entering the foster care system. In the United States, as many as 35% of unaccompanied children are placed in long-term foster care while in the custody of the federal Office of Refugee Resettlement.[7] The number of child refugees or immigrants entering foster care each year is unfortunately unknown due to limitations in data collection.[8]

The link between HIV and refugee or immigrant status is complex. Some children may have been living in countries with a high HIV prevalence, which is a risk factor for HIV infection. Some children are known to have HIV before arriving in the United States, and some are diagnosed years after settlement because HIV screening was not conducted before or on their arrival in the United States. As of 2010, refugees are no longer tested for HIV infection before their arrival to the United States. Thus, refugee and immigrant youth should be screened on entry into foster care. Fourth-generation HIV-1/2 antigen/antibody testing should be conducted for children age 18 months or older and an HIV quantitative polymerase chain reaction test (measuring the amount of HIV RNA, also known as viral load) should be used for screening in children younger than 18 months.[9] Repeat screening 3 to 6 months after resettlement is advisable for those with a recent exposure or risk behavior. HIV risk factors specific to refugee and immigrant children include HIV prevalence greater than 1% in the child's region or country of origin, birth mother deceased due to known or suspected AIDS-related illness, exposure to sexual or gender-based violence, substance use, limited access to health care and education, and food insecurity. Although HIV-1 is the most common type of HIV worldwide, HIV-2 should be assessed in children from Angola, Benin, Burkina Faso, Cabo Verde, Côte d'Ivoire (Ivory Coast), Gambia, Ghana, Guinea, Guinea-Bissau, Liberia, Mali, Mauritania, Mozambique, Niger, São Tomé and Príncipe, Senegal, Sierra Leone, and Togo.[4]

There are instances in which refugee children in foster care are diagnosed with HIV years after entry into the United States. These situations are often traumatic for the child, foster family or caregiver, and physician. Some of these children are rehomed because of stigma or because the foster family does not feel equipped to deal with the diagnosis. Children who are diagnosed late with HIV may have slowed growth, developmental delay, unexplained malnutrition, anemia, pancytopenia, prolonged fever of unknown origin, hepatosplenomegaly, lymphadenopathy, intermittent or persistent skin rash, intermittent or persistent diarrhea, recurrent bacterial infections, and thrush. The time it takes to present with HIV symptoms is variable for those with untreated perinatal HIV. Some children may become symptomatic within the first 2 years after birth, but some do not become symptomatic until the second decade after birth.

Adolescents

Most adolescents, like adults, acquire HIV due to condomless sex and less often through sharing syringes and other injection equipment with someone with HIV. Adolescents in foster care are at higher risk for acquiring sexually transmitted infections (STIs) and HIV compared with their peers who are not in foster care.[10–12] Thus, reviewing sexual risk factors at each visit is important. Furthermore, the American Academy of Pediatrics (AAP) recommends that all adolescents age 15 to 21 years should be screened for HIV at least once in a health care setting.[13] After the initial screening, adolescents at increased risk of HIV infection should be retested annually or more frequently. Those who are at increased risk include men who have sex with men; youth of all genders having condomless sex with multiple partners or who have an STI or a partner with an STI; youth who inject drugs either currently or in the past; youth who engage in transactional sex or trade sex for money, drugs, or other commodities; youth with past or present sex partners who are living with HIV, are bisexual, or inject drugs; and youth who engage in receptive anal sex, regardless of sexual orientation. These recommendations remain the same for adolescents in foster care.[14]

Given the increased risk of HIV among adolescents in foster care, pediatricians must adeptly identify acute HIV infection, which is a nonspecific viral syndrome similar to mononucleosis, influenza, and hepatitis. Common symptoms include fever, fatigue, myalgia, arthralgia, lymphadenopathy, pharyngitis, oral ulcers, and rash. However, the range of possible presentations is wide and encompasses neurological syndromes (meningitis and encephalitis), hepatitis, and gastrointestinal symptoms.[15–17] Acute HIV infection is often not recognized by primary care and emergency physicians because the symptoms mimic those of other common, typically self-limited viral illnesses. Occasionally, youth may be asymptomatic with acute HIV infection or have very mild nonspecific symptoms that are very short-lived, thus increasing the risk of remaining undetected. This may be especially true for youth in foster care if their medical care is fragmented.

Pre-Exposure Prophylaxis

Pre-exposure prophylaxis is the use of ART to prevent the acquisition of HIV by those who are at increased risk for infection. Despite the availability of PrEP since 2012, there is an enormous gap in PrEP utilization: from 2019 to 2022, only 26% of individuals with an indication for PrEP were using it.[18] Many barriers to utilization, adherence, and maintenance exist along the continuum, from awareness to an individual's willingness to take PrEP to prescription by a clinician. However, PrEP prescriptions for adolescents have increased almost annually since 2018,[19] when PrEP was authorized for all individuals weighing at least 35 kg. However, there are racial and ethnic disparities in PrEP utilization, as youth of color are less likely to discuss PrEP with their physician or use PrEP.[20,21]

PrEP consists of 1 or 2 ART agents but not a complete regimen that would be used to treat HIV. The combination of emtricitabine/tenofovir disoproxil fumarate (F/TDF) was the first FDA-approved medication for PrEP in 2012, followed by combined emtricitabine/tenofovir alafenamide (F/TAF) in 2019 and the first long-acting (LA) injectable medication, cabotegravir-LA (CAB-LA), in 2021. F/TDF and CAB-LA are approved for everyone weighing at least 35 kg, while F/TAF is approved for those weighing at least 35 kg, excluding individuals at risk for HIV acquisition through receptive vaginal sex. When taken as directed, all forms of PrEP are approximately 99% effective in reducing sexual transmission of HIV, and oral PrEP is 74% to 84% effective in reducing HIV transmission in people who inject drugs.[22–25] In 2019, the US Preventive Services Task Force gave PrEP a grade A recommendation for all individuals at risk for HIV infection.[26] While sexual and drug use histories are necessary to identify a patient's risk factors for HIV, clinicians should be aware that patients requesting PrEP may minimize the disclosure of such risk factors due to stigma. This should not prevent the clinician from initiating PrEP. Provision of PrEP does not require specialist experience and can be readily integrated into general medical practice. Offering PrEP within general medical practice may reduce the burden of specialty referrals for adolescents in foster care who already have barriers to care.[13]

Disclosure of HIV Infection in Pediatrics

Disclosure of HIV infection to a child is complex and should be considered a process, not a one-time event. Some children are unaware of their HIV diagnosis due to family of origin or foster parent preference. The World Health Organization and the AAP recommend that children should be informed about their infection between the ages of 6 and 12 years.[27,28] When children are aware they are living with HIV, this can increase treatment adherence, alleviate frustration with taking medication, result in fewer emotional difficulties in adolescents, and lead to acceptance of the diagnosis, which yields positive long-term psychological effects; furthermore, it allows for better self-care, leading to durable viral suppression.[29–31] Disclosure of HIV infection has also been associated with higher self-esteem, better coping skills, and a better understanding of HIV and how to minimize its transmission.[32] Those with a durably undetectable HIV viral load (known as *undetectable = untransmittable*, or U=U) cannot transmit the virus to their partners.[33]

Pediatricians can ask adults who are privy to knowledge of a child's HIV status what the child or adolescent knows about their HIV diagnosis. If the child or adolescent is not aware of their diagnosis, discussing the benefits of disclosure and inquiring about potential barriers to disclosure can occur within the child welfare system if local laws allow. The creation of a disclosure plan for children in foster care must consider the complexities of the child being in the foster care system and who is legally allowed to be notified of their HIV status.

Key Takeaways

- Children and adolescents in foster care face a heightened vulnerability to HIV infection, largely attributable to the influence of social drivers of health and the prevalence of adverse childhood experiences.
- Pediatricians play a crucial role in caring for children and adolescents living with or at risk for HIV infection, including providing education on prevention, implementing screenings, and facilitating disclosure.
- HIV PrEP serves as a valuable resource for pediatricians to assist all young individuals who are at an elevated risk of HIV infection. It is essential for pediatricians to engage in discussions with these youth to understand the various risk factors associated with HIV, mitigate stigma, foster a supportive atmosphere, and enable them to make informed and healthy choices regarding their sexual health.

CHAPTER 33

Unaccompanied Immigrant Youth

Keith J. Martin, DO, MS
Lisa Ayoub-Rodriguez, MD, FAAP
Karla Fredricks, MD, MPH, FAAP

Background

Foreign-born children represent 3% of the US child population, approximately 2.5 million children.[1] Unfortunately, like US-born children, immigrant children may experience abuse, neglect, and other situations that lead to their entry into the foster care system. Importantly, there is also a subset of foreign-born children who interact with the foster care system after coming to the United States without a parent or legal guardian. These children have a unique set of circumstances that require understanding by medical and mental health professionals in order for them to receive the best quality of care. Immigrant children arriving in the United States without a parent or legal guardian typically fall into one of 2 categories upon initial classification (see **Table 33–1**): (1) unaccompanied refugee minors or (2) unaccompanied children.

Unaccompanied Refugee Minors

The Unaccompanied Refugee Minors (URM) program was started in 1980 and has served more than 13,000 children since its inception. Unaccompanied refugee minors have typically fled violence, abuse, or persecution and are placed in foster homes (or, occasionally, group homes) through the same state or local agencies that coordinate foster care for US-born children. For unaccompanied refugee minors, these placements are facilitated by the Lutheran Immigrant and Refugee Service and the US Conference of Catholic Bishops. Although the URM program works through state and local foster care agencies, it is financially supported by the Office of Refugee Resettlement (ORR), under the auspices of the US Department of Health and Human

Table 33–1. Definitions

Term	Description
People	
Unaccompanied refugee minor	A child (<18 years old) who fled abuse, violence, or persecution in their country of origin, entered the United States with refugee status but without a parent or legal guardian, and is placed in the URM program[2]
Unaccompanied child	A person who has no lawful immigration status in the United States, is <18 years old, and does not have a parent or legal guardian immediately present and able to care for them when they arrive in the United States[3]
Unaccompanied immigrant youth	Umbrella term used in this article to cover both unaccompanied refugee minors and unaccompanied children
Refugee	Any person outside their country of nationality who is unable or unwilling to return to their country of origin due to a well-founded fear of persecution based on race, religion, nationality, political opinion, or membership in a particular social group[4]
Sponsor	Person to whom an unaccompanied child is released after Office of Refugee Resettlement custody, usually a parent or other family member[5]
Governmental Entities	
Customs and Border Protection	Law enforcement agency within the US Department of Homeland Security, charged with border management and control[6]
Office of Refugee Resettlement	US government office within the Department of Health and Human Services; oversees resettlement services for refugees as well as the URM and UC programs
Division of Unaccompanied Children's Services	Division within Office of Refugee Resettlement that provides temporary care and custody of unaccompanied children[7]
Placements	
Residential treatment center	A live-in health care facility for unaccompanied refugee minors or unaccompanied children that provides therapeutic services for behavioral issues, mental illness, and/or substance use, in a secure and/or restrictive setting for youth who, because of the severity of their issues, are unable to adjust to other placements but do not require inpatient psychiatric hospitalization[8,9]
Group home	A therapeutic or transitional placement option for unaccompanied refugee minors. Therapeutic group homes serve unaccompanied refugee minors with significant emotional or behavioral problems who do not require placement in a residential treatment center. Transitional group homes focus on independent life skills for unaccompanied refugee minors as they prepare to exit the program.[9]

Table 33–1 *(continued)*

Term	Description
	Placements
Short-term foster care	An initial Office of Refugee Resettlement placement option for unaccompanied children <13 years old with special health care needs, who are pregnant or parenting, or who are part of a sibling group with at least one sibling <13 years old[8]
Long-term foster care	Office of Refugee Resettlement–funded, community-based foster care placements and services to which eligible unaccompanied children are transferred after a determination is made that the child will be in Office of Refugee Resettlement custody for an extended period of time[8]
Shelter	Program funded by Office of Refugee Resettlement that provides residential care for unaccompanied children (including coverage of their basic needs as well as offering medical and mental health services, education, recreation, and legal services)[8]

Abbreviations: UC, Unaccompanied Children; URM, Unaccompanied Refugee Minors.

Services. This monetary structure not only allows unaccompanied refugee minors to receive services offered to all children in foster care in their state but also provides additional resources to unaccompanied refugee minors focused on integration into US communities, preservation of heritage, English language learning, educational achievement, immigration assistance, and eventual transition to independent living.[10]

When established in 1980, the URM program was limited to unaccompanied immigrant youth entering the United States with a legal status of refugee. Over time, the program has expanded to offer eligibility to certain other categories of unaccompanied immigrant children, including asylees (those granted asylum), Cuban and Haitian migrants, those with Special Immigrant Juvenile Status (those who have been abused, neglected, or abandoned by one or both parents and have applied for and obtained this status), victims of trafficking, those with U nonimmigrant status (commonly known as U visa; victims of crime in the United States who cooperated with law enforcement and later obtained this status), and, as of 2023, paroled Afghan and Ukrainian migrants. Children who enter the URM program with a legal status of refugee are placed through the US Department of State, while other children must apply to ORR for entry (**Figure 33–1**).[10]

There are 25 URM programs in 14 states (AZ, CA, CO, FL, MA, MI, MS, ND, NY, PA, TX, UT, VA, and WA) plus Washington, DC.[2] Although 40% of unaccompanied refugee minors speak Spanish, approximately 50 different nationalities are represented from regions around the world. Males and those aged 17 years at entry comprise the majority of unaccompanied refugee minors (68% and 62%, respectively). The program typically ends when an unaccompanied refugee minor reaches 21 years of age, but they may continue to be eligible for certain services.[10]

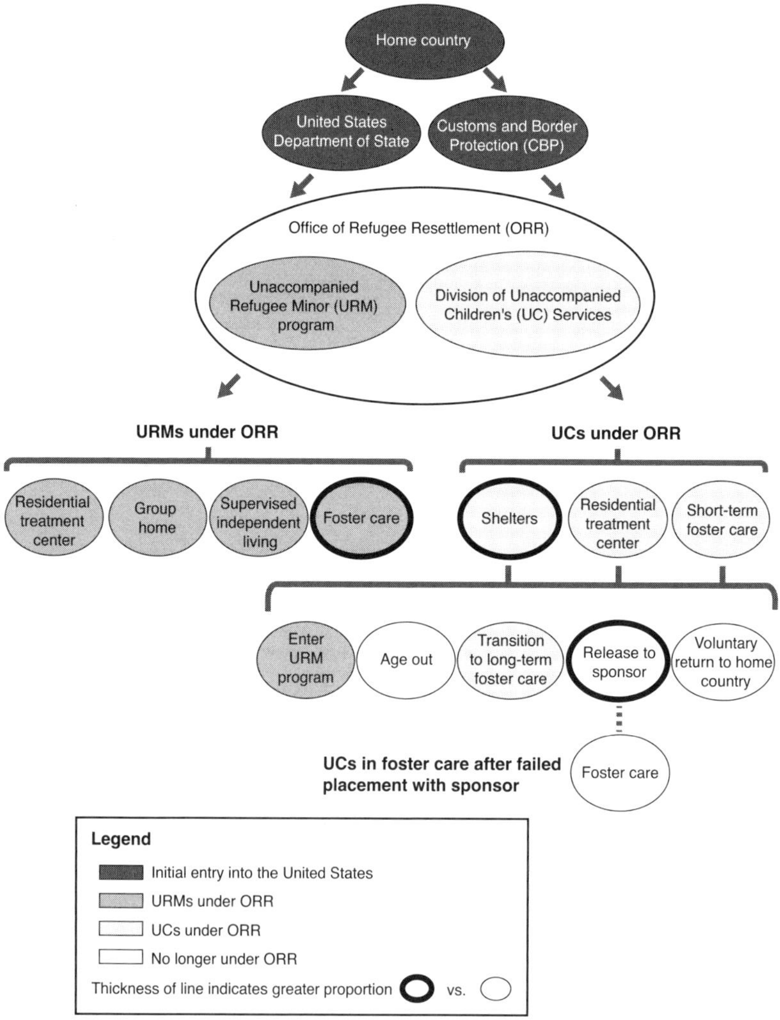

Figure 33–1. Flow of unaccompanied immigrant youth in the United States.

Unaccompanied Children

Like unaccompanied refugee minors, unaccompanied children are often fleeing harm in their country of origin and enter the United States without a parent or legal guardian. However, in contrast to unaccompanied refugee minors, unaccompanied children arrive at the US border with no lawful status. They typically undergo initial processing by Customs and Border Protection before being transferred to ORR custody (which should occur within 72 hours). Within ORR, the Division of Unaccompanied Children's Services—separate from the URM program—is responsible for unaccompanied children until such time that a suitable sponsor (typically, a family member already in the United States) can be vetted or the unaccompanied child turns 18 years old.[7] ORR assumed the care of unaccompanied children in 2002 and has since received over 800,000 children.[11] Typically, nearly three-quarters of unaccompanied children are 15 to 17 years old (although all ages are represented in the unaccompanied child population), and two-thirds of these children are male. Unaccompanied children are mostly from Guatemala, Honduras, and El Salvador, with a small proportion from other countries. The average length of stay in ORR custody is approximately 1 month.[12]

Upon transfer from Customs and Border Protection, most unaccompanied children are initially placed in shelter-type settings. Some unaccompanied children are determined to need placement in residential treatment centers for mental health concerns, and others are placed in short-term foster care.[11] Foster care is more often used for children age 12 years or younger, those who are pregnant or parenting, children with special health care needs, and sibling groups with a child aged 12 years or younger.

There are 5 possible outcomes for unaccompanied children after initial placement with ORR: (1) release to sponsor, (2) "aging out," (3) voluntary return to country of origin, (4) long-term foster care, or (5) transfer to the URM program (**Figure 33–1**). Most commonly, unaccompanied children are released to a sponsor (usually a parent or other close family member, as noted above) within a few weeks to months. Those who are close to their 18th birthday will be unified with sponsors before then, if possible, or they may "age out"—either released from ORR custody "on their own recognizance" or transferred to adult immigrant detention on their 18th birthday. Unaccompanied children may also choose to return to their country of origin, but only a small number elect to do so. Children 17 years or younger who have no viable sponsor in the United States may enter long-term foster care through ORR or, if they have one of the qualifying immigrant statuses, apply and transfer to the URM program.

A small but significant subset of unaccompanied children released to sponsors will enter the US foster care system. If a child living with a sponsor in the United States is removed from the home due to abuse and neglect, they may be placed in the US foster care system instead of returning to the care of ORR.

Caring for Unaccompanied Immigrant Youth in the Foster Care System

Consent

Foster parents of unaccompanied refugee minors and unaccompanied children who are age 17 years or younger have the authority to provide consent for medical and mental health care. In addition, these youth have the same rights as other minors to consent for care that would be confidential, based on the laws of the state in which they reside. It is also possible (especially for unaccompanied children) that there is a living parent (or close family member) with whom it would be appropriate to discuss any health conditions and treatment plans. Physicians should ask the foster care or shelter program about the appropriateness of speaking to family members and obtain assent from the youth for communication with the family as well as for the treatment plan itself (as developmentally appropriate). Although not required, consent for procedures should also be obtained (when possible) from a living parent, even if they reside in another country. If it is not possible to obtain consent from a biological parent or foster parent, ORR may provide consent.

Physical Health

Nearly all unaccompanied immigrant youth arrive from countries with limited health care infrastructure. Because of this, few unaccompanied immigrant youth have received routinely recommended preventive care, including typical newborn screening, dental care, or regular health supervision visits. This lack of preventive care can lead to a delay in or lack of diagnosis of asymptomatic conditions.[4] In addition, some unaccompanied immigrant youth may have known medical conditions that could not to be treated in their country of origin. However, despite limited past health care, most unaccompanied immigrant youth are generally physically healthy.

Medical Services for Unaccompanied Children

Upon transfer to ORR, unaccompanied children receive an initial medical examination within 2 business days.[13] This examination consists of a medical history, physical examination, psychological assessment, vaccinations, and laboratory testing.[13] While unaccompanied children in shelters, residential treatment centers, and short-term foster homes usually receive the initial medical examination and sick care through an ORR-contracted clinician who sees them in the shelter space, a subset will have primary care in the community. Further, those with additional medical needs may interact with pediatric subspecialists, emergency care providers, and hospitalists, as needed. Unaccompanied children in long-term foster care, as well as those who transfer to the URM program, typically receive all health services outside of ORR facilities, making it more likely that community primary care and mental health clinicians will interact with them.[4] ORR requires testing of all unaccompanied children for tuberculosis. All females age 10 years or older receive urinary pregnancy testing, children younger than 6 years are tested for lead, and those age 13 years or older are tested for HIV.[4] Other testing is performed according to symptoms and exposure-based risk factors, with no presumptive treatment given. Unaccompanied children have likely received several routine childhood vaccines in their country of origin, but it may not be possible to acquire a copy of those records. ORR provides the first and, possibly, subsequent rounds of vaccinations (depending on how long the child is in custody), and records can be obtained from ORR if the foster family does not bring proof of immunization.[11]

Medical Services for Unaccompanied Refugee Minors

Unaccompanied refugee minors are eligible for federally funded refugee resettlement health screening, which may be performed through the local health department, federally qualified health centers, or academic medical centers. This encounter typically consists of a history and examination, laboratory testing with or without presumptive treatment (according to the Centers for Disease Control and Prevention [CDC] Guidelines for Domestic Evaluation of Refugees), and vaccinations. Unaccompanied refugee minors should also have received testing for tuberculosis and hepatitis B, as well as presumptive treatment for certain parasitic and mosquito-borne illnesses (depending on country of departure), prior to travel to the United States. Unaccompanied refugee minors are expected to access all other primary and specialty care with community providers. If the laboratory test results and/or evidence of presumptive treatment from the resettlement health screening cannot be obtained, testing and treatment should be repeated. CareRef, a useful tool for community physicians, incorporates the CDC guidelines into individualized recommendations for this purpose.[14] In addition to immunizations given at any resettlement visits, unaccompanied refugee minors typically have received some vaccinations prior to travel to the United States. These can be found summarized in a document from the US Department of State that these children should possess as part of their records from the International Organization for Migration (if they entered the United States through the formal refugee resettlement program). That record should be accepted as valid, with only necessary routine or catch-up vaccinations given going forward.

Mental Health

In contrast to the relatively low prevalence of physical health concerns in unaccompanied immigrant youth, mental health conditions are common. Multiple studies have found that, compared with the general population of youth in the United States, unaccompanied refugee minors and unaccompanied children have increased rates of mental health concerns, particularly post-traumatic stress disorder (PTSD), major depressive disorder (MDD), and suicidal ideation.[15,16] This is likely due in large part to trauma exposure, similar to that experienced by most children in foster care.[17]

Unaccompanied refugee minors receive mental health assessments soon after placement and are subsequently referred for therapy and medications as needed.[18] Unaccompanied children, similarly, have a psychological evaluation within 2 days of placement in ORR custody. All unaccompanied children receive routine individual and group counseling while in ORR custody, and those who need higher levels of mental health care (including medication management) are referred to a psychiatrist. When caring for current or former unaccompanied youth in the community, screening for mental health concerns—particularly, anxiety, depression, and PTSD—should be done at the first visit and annually, with more frequent screening as needed. A tool such as the Refugee Health Screener-15 (RHS-15)[19] is one option (validated in several languages) to screen for PTSD, MDD, and anxiety in individuals age 14 years or older. Screening for trauma-related symptoms should also be done, recognizing the likelihood of traumatic events having occurred prior to, during, or after migration. Referrals to trauma-informed and culturally sensitive mental health specialists should be made as warranted.

Social Drivers of Health

Insurance

While low-income children with refugee or a similar status are universally eligible to receive Medicaid and the Children's Health Insurance Program (CHIP), the state of residence after ORR release determines eligibility for unaccompanied children. As of 2025, only 13 states (CA, CO, CT, IL, MA, ME, NJ, NY, OR, RI, UT, VT, WA) plus Washington, DC, offer eligibility to low-income children regardless of immigration status. Although unaccompanied children have coverage for health services through a third-party underwriter while in ORR custody, those who transfer to the URM program or who are released to sponsors may not have insurance.[20] In those cases, offering financial assistance for health care costs or referrals to programs that can provide a sliding-scale fee structure is crucial to ensure affordable access to care.

Legal

Children in the URM program typically have a pathway to citizenship established, so referral to legal services for immigration purposes is not usually warranted. Unaccompanied children, on the other hand, often do not yet have permanent legal status in the United States (although they may have applied for asylum, Special Immigrant Juvenile Status [for children who have been abused, neglected, or abandoned by one or both parents], or other types of humanitarian relief). Assessing their needs and referring to pro bono or low-cost legal resources may be beneficial.

Employment

Unaccompanied immigrant youth, especially those who are older teenagers, frequently desire to work. This is often motivated by the desire to send money to family in their country of origin and/or a need to pay debts incurred by their journey to the United States.[21] While most unaccompanied refugee minors have work authorization, unaccompanied children (including those who transfer to the URM program) may not. This can be a significant source of stress for unaccompanied children and is important to address. It is possible that accompanied children who were living with sponsors before entering foster care were working in inappropriate and/or unsafe conditions. Although it is highly unlikely that those situations would continue while in foster care, screening for past traumatic work experiences (in both unaccompanied children and unaccompanied refugee minors) is necessary.

Education

Unaccompanied immigrant youth may have experienced disruptions in their education before coming to the United States. Asking about any educational gaps or learning challenges in countries other than the United States and any current concerns with adaptation and integration into the US school system can help determine if additional support should be provided by the local school system.

Food Insecurity

Although food insecurity should not be an issue in foster homes, screening for it should not be neglected. Furthermore, assessing past food insecurity is important to determine if micronutrient deficiencies may be present and warrant laboratory testing.

Environmental Exposures

Similar to food insecurity, environmental exposures should be part of routine screening for all patients, even if the child is placed in a certified foster home. Questions should focus on both current exposures and those prior to relocation to the United States, and any areas of concern should be addressed.

Key Takeaways

» Most immigrant children who enter the United States without a parent or legal guardian are considered unaccompanied children or unaccompanied refugee minors, with much larger numbers of the former. Through 2 separate programs, ORR is responsible for the care of both populations.

- Ask all new patients, "In what country was the child/were you born?" as part of birth, past medical, or social history. If they are foreign born, ask who accompanied them the United States. If they came without a parent, ask if they were ever in a shelter or foster care. This will help identify unaccompanied immigrant youth.

» Unaccompanied children in ORR custody have coverage for health services that terminates upon their release. After release, their eligibility for Medicaid and CHIP depends on state-specific guidelines, but most will become uninsured. Unaccompanied refugee minors, no matter in what state they reside, are eligible for Medicaid or CHIP until age 21 years (with some exceptions).

- Check the medical record for insurance status. If the youth is uninsured, consider consultation with a social worker or benefits specialist to determine their eligibility for public health insurance. If eligible, help them apply. If they are not eligible, refer to local resources that offer sliding-scale discounts for health services.

» While unaccompanied immigrant youth are generally in good physical health upon arrival in the United States, some have chronic conditions and others present with acute concerns; all have experienced trauma to a certain degree. Both populations receive some type of medical and mental health evaluation soon after placement with ORR. Unaccompanied refugee minors who are formal refugees also receive a health assessment and physical examination prior to departure for the United States. However, none of these evaluations include all the components of a comprehensive health supervision visit.

- Inquire about any medical visits or health assessments conducted before or after arrival in the United States and obtain the records. If not yet completed, a health supervision visit should be performed (including history, physical examination, age-appropriate developmental and mental health screening, laboratory testing, vaccinations, and treatment and referrals as needed). Involvement of parents or past guardians (including those not in the United States) may be necessary to obtain a complete history and ensure that loved ones who know the child and can advocate in their best interest are involved in decisions regarding the child's care.

» The physical and mental health of unaccompanied immigrant youth is affected by their culture as well as circumstances in the United States, in their country of origin, and during migration.

- Complete trainings focused on trauma-informed care, cultural sensitivity, and implicit bias, and use the techniques learned with encounters involving unaccompanied immigrant youth. Remember that immigration status is also a social driver of health, and inquire about premigration, migration, and postmigration factors when conducting social drivers of health screening.

Part 5. Additional Health Care Delivery Considerations

CHAPTER

34

Medical Consents

Mary V. Greiner, MD, MS, FAAP
Kristine Fortin, MD, MPH, FAAP
Moira Szilagyi, MD, PhD, FAAP

This chapter is not designed to be an exhaustive discussion of medical consents for children and adolescents in foster care, but rather an introduction and a guideline. This is an important area for discussion because youth in foster care can sometimes be restricted from accessing needed medical services, particularly sensitive services; but it is also a complex topic, as it is governed by defined legislation and regulations that vary from state to state and sometimes county to county. In addition, foster care agencies have developed individual policies interpreting these laws and regulations. Local policies and procedures related to consent may consider factors, including the nature of the proposed care (routine, nonroutine, emergency), age of the patient, and status of parental rights. Clinicians are advised to become familiar with the policies of their particular state and county and contact an administrative or legal official of their state or county when questions or concerns about consents arise. If agencies have a health care management team, the administrator of that team should be able to offer clinicians guidance on consent issues.

Consent issues can delay delivery of important health care services. The following may help overcome access barriers related to consent:

- Clinician awareness of state and local policies and procedures related to consent
- Clinician awareness of key child welfare contacts
- Clear communication with the appropriate party about the child's medical needs and proposed treatment
- Documentation of pertinent consent information and related contacts in the medical record

General Principles Governing Medical Consents

Children and adolescents in foster care are in the care and custody of local or state child welfare agencies. The family of origin maintain legal guardianship unless parental rights have been terminated. Adolescents in foster care have a right to the same confidentiality protections and ability to consent to sensitive health care services as their peers in the general population. It is critical that the health care team understands the key information related to each child's legal status and is aware of relevant county and state policies.

Routine Care

Generally speaking, the child welfare agency has the ability to consent for routine medical care (eg, American Academy of Pediatrics Bright Futures[1] preventive care, evidence-based care for minor illnesses) for children and adolescents in foster care. In situations where child welfare agencies have the authority to consent for medical care, the person designated to sign the consent can vary by jurisdiction. Generally, caseworkers would have to seek at least supervisory authority for any medical procedure requiring written consent. Often child welfare agencies authorize foster and kinship caregivers to provide verbal consent for routine medical care, such as registering to be seen for a medical appointment. Foster caregivers do not have the authority to provide written consent for medical procedures.

Nonroutine Care

Definitions of nonroutine care can vary by child welfare agency but may include procedures, surgeries, admissions, mental health services, and prescriptions for certain medications, such as psychiatric medications. Child welfare agencies are committed to the principle that, whenever practical or possible, the family of origin of the child or adolescent should make all important medical decisions on behalf of their child. At individual agencies, policies usually are in place requiring the agencies to ask the family of origin to give consent for nonroutine medical care to involve them in the health care needs of their children. Depending on local and state rules, the child welfare agency or the birth family may sign the consent form. If the family of origin chooses not to or are unavailable to give consent for a medical treatment that is believed to be medically necessary, some states allow child welfare agencies to proceed with providing consent, while others require a court order from a judge to proceed. Best practice is to verify that the child welfare agency and family of origin are aware of and have specifically consented to medical procedures requiring informed consent.

Emergency Care
In emergencies, consent is generally not required.

Frequently Asked Questions
The information provided in this section varies across states and counties; clinicians are urged to contact their state and county child welfare agencies to determine the guidelines applicable to them.

Who May Give Medical Consent for Children and Adolescents When Parental Rights Have Been Terminated?
When the court has terminated parental rights of the family of origin, the local or state child welfare agency becomes their legal guardian. Only child welfare agency personnel can consent for medical procedures on behalf of children or adolescents who have experienced termination of parental rights. In many cases, they will seek the input of the child's primary physician, the foster care physician, and/or a child welfare medical team (when available) before providing consent.

Who May Give Consent for Sensitive Health Care Services for Adolescents in Foster Care?
The age at which adolescents can consent for medical care services varies across states. Within each state, the age of consent can also vary by type of medical service (such as dental care, mental health care, substance use treatment, testing for HIV and other sexually transmitted infections, treatment and preventive care, and contraceptive care).[2] The adolescent should also have capacity to consent. In general, if a young person can legally consent directly and confidentially for a specific type of care in a specific situation in the local jurisdiction, a young person in foster care can do so as well. See Chapter 9, Sexual and Reproductive Health Care; Chapter 21, Substance Use; and Chapter 22, Pregnant and Parenting Teens, for further discussion of this topic.

Who May Give Consent for a Child Voluntarily Placed in Child Welfare Custody?
In some states, the family of origin can voluntarily enter an agreement with child welfare agencies to place a child outside of the home. However, the ability to voluntarily place a child varies widely by state, and clinicians need to understand state and local policies. In such situations, child welfare agencies may have obtained a general medical consent at the time of placement and may be able to consent on behalf of children, if necessary. However, child welfare agencies should attempt to seek consent from the family of origin whenever possible.

Are There Situations in Which Consent of the Family of Origin or the Child Welfare Agency Is Not Required?

The consent of the family of origin or the child welfare agency is not required if the time necessary for seeking consent would present a danger to the life, health, or immediate welfare of a child or adolescent or if a clinician believes this to be the case (emergency medical treatment). Consent of the family of origin or the child welfare agency may also not be required when confidential care is being provided in an area where minor adolescents are permitted to directly provide consent (see Chapter 9, Sexual and Reproductive Health Care, and Chapter 21, Substance Use).

What Qualifies as Nonroutine Care That May Require Written Consent?

Specifications of nonroutine care may vary by county and state. Many child welfare agencies consider the following to be nonroutine care that will require written consent:

- Nonurgent or elective medical care, described as elective medical and dental services that are not customarily given as part of preventive health care. This includes any service or intervention requiring informed consent (such as surgery, chemotherapy, contrast agents, genetic testing, and anesthesia).
- The prescription of psychotropic medications requires written consent.
- Mental health agencies may require written consent for performing evaluations and providing services.
- Some child welfare agencies require written consent for certain immunizations.

What If a Child or Adolescent in Foster Care Needs Medical Intervention Requiring Consent After Hours or While on a Holiday?

There should always be someone available at child welfare agencies 24 hours a day, 7 days a week. Clinicians are advised to contact the child welfare agency at the after-hours emergency number.

Who Is the Consenting Party for the Medical Care of the Offspring of Adolescents in Foster Care?

If an adolescent is in foster care and has custody of their child who is not in foster care, the adolescent is the consenting party.

Who Has Legal Guardianship When Children or Adolescents Are Placed With a Relative?

In this case, children may be in the legal custody of their family of origin, their relatives, or the child welfare agency. It is important that the clinician understand the child's legal and custody status before obtaining consent for treatment.

Are There Any Particular Safeguards That Clinicians Should Undertake Concerning Consent for Medical Care for Children and Adolescents in Foster Care?

Pediatricians and other clinicians should be aware of the current legal and custody status of the child at the time of seeking informed consent to ensure proper consents are obtained. It is prudent to document any specific discussions about medical consent for a procedure or intervention in the patient's medical record. Pediatricians should contact their state and county child welfare agencies to determine the guidelines applicable to them.

CHAPTER
35

Supports for Foster and Kinship Caregivers and Families of Origin

Colleen E. Bennett, MD, MSHP, FAAP
Robin van der Merwe

Background

Foster and kinship caregivers play a critical role in ensuring a child's health and safety. In fact, they are the major therapeutic intervention of the child welfare system. As discussed in Chapter 17, Childhood Trauma and Resilience, safe, stable, and nurturing relationships with caregivers are healing after traumatic experiences. Therefore, it is essential that pediatricians understand the unique challenges encountered by foster and kinship caregivers and identify resources to support them in their caregiving roles. Reunification is often the goal, and it is also crucial to support families of origin. This chapter describes the unique challenges encountered by, and discusses supports and resources for, foster and kinship caregivers as well as families of origin.

Factors Promoting Retention, Stability, and Permanency

Several types of out-of-home placement exist and are discussed in detail in Chapter 18, Out-of-Home Placements. Two major categories of placement type are kinship care and nonrelative foster care. Kinship care can be further categorized into the following: 1) private kinship care, where an arrangement has been made without child welfare agency involvement, 2) informal kinship care, where a child has been removed from their family of origin and placed in kinship care without the child welfare agency taking custody, and 3) formal kinship care, where the child welfare agency has taken formal custody of the child and placed them in kinship care. Type of placement can have implications on resources available to children and caregivers. Both foster and kinship caregivers take on a significant role in a child's life, not only providing a safe home and basic needs but also supporting that child's health and social and emotional development in the context of what is often a traumatic experience of being removed from their family of origin. While foster caregivers make the autonomous decision to pursue becoming a foster parent, kinship caregivers may step into this role in the setting of a family crisis or emergency. It is not surprising that characteristics between foster and kinship caregivers may differ. Although a few studies support that foster caregivers in general are commonly middle-aged and female,[1,2] one study found that kinship caregivers were more likely to be 60 years of age or older, have a lower household income, and have a shorter length of fostering than nonrelative caregivers.[1]

Recruitment and retention of caregivers can be challenging for a multitude of reasons. For instance, caregivers may encounter financial challenges or difficulties accessing care and managing appointments for children with complex medical needs and/or significant behavioral or mental health concerns. Some factors have been identified that influence retention, including relationship with the child welfare system; material resources such as finances, child care, and respite care; personal attributes; initial and ongoing training; being involved in decision-making; and access to social and emotional support.[3,4] These factors represent opportunities for improvement to support caregivers in their roles. Specific resources are discussed in the next section, and several are summarized in **Table 35–1**. Recruitment may be influenced by the relationship with the family of origin in that extended family or friends may be uncomfortable accepting placement of a child due to potential contact or conflict with family of origin.

Caregivers, whether kinship or foster, can have a profound impact on a child's trajectory, including long-term placement and permanency, while in the child welfare system. Chapter 19, Factors Associated With Placement Stability and Permanency Outcomes, discusses these topics in full. Vanderwill et al[5] identified 16 caregiver-related factors associated with permanency and/or placement stability. The most common factors were access to support systems, access to sufficient economic resources, attentiveness to the caregiver–child relationship (caregiver can create a secure, nurturing environment; provide empathy; and meet the child's needs), caregiver recognition of value in the child's connection with their birth family/family of origin, and healthy family functioning. Other factors included understanding the effects of trauma, positive parenting/effective discipline, and participation in lifelong learning, training, and education.[5] These factors highlight areas where pediatricians can support foster and kinship caregivers to promote placement stability and permanency.

Table 35–1. Key Support Programs for Kinship and Foster Caregivers to Address Financial, Nutritional, and Medical Needs

Program	Website
Title IV-E Foster Care Maintenance Payments	https://www.acf.hhs.gov/cb/grant-funding/title-iv-e-foster-care
Temporary Assistance for Needy Families (TANF)	https://www.acf.hhs.gov/ofa/map/about/help-families
Supplemental Nutrition Assistance Program (SNAP)	https://www.fns.usda.gov/snap/supplemental-nutrition-assistance-program
Special Supplemental Nutrition Program for Women, Infants, and Children (WIC)	https://www.fns.usda.gov/wic
Medicaid and Children's Health Insurance Program (CHIP)	https://www.medicaid.gov/state-overviews/state-profiles/index.html

Caregiver Licensing and Training

It can be a daunting process to become a foster caregiver. Although requirements vary by state, they usually include criminal and child abuse registry background checks, home safety inspection, home assessment, and assessment of financial stability.[6] Most states require that foster caregivers are licensed by the state; however, there are varying regulations by state for kinship caregivers. There are no universal training programs for foster or kinship caregivers. Foster care agencies adhere to individual agency requirements in accordance with local county and state guidelines. Agencies may require a minimum number of training hours for initial licensure followed by maintenance hours over a period of time. Some training requirements may be related to reasonable and prudent parenting, child development, medical needs of children in foster care, and trauma-informed care. Federal law requires that state agencies consider giving preference to adult relatives over nonrelated caregivers when determining a child's placement.[7] For kinship caregivers, most states have policies that allow children to be placed with family members or close family friends before the caregiver meets full licensure requirements. States also have policies that allow for modification of licensing standards for kinship caregivers.[8]

Support for Foster and Kinship Caregivers

Financial Support

Several programs exist to provide monetary support to caregivers and children. The Temporary Assistance for Needy Families (TANF) program is a federal program that provides funding to states (including the District of Columbia, US territories, and federally recognized American Indian tribes and Alaskan Native organizations) to support low-income families with children. States use TANF funds to provide monthly cash-assistance payments to such families as well as to support a variety of other programs that promote the mission of TANF. Foster and kinship caregivers may be eligible for these programs.[9]

Additionally, foster family homes may be eligible to receive Title IV-E foster care maintenance payments to cover the cost of food, clothing, shelter, daily supervision, school supplies, and travel for visitation. Legislation was passed in 2023 that allows states to have different sets of standards for licensing and approval of kinship foster family homes compared to nonrelative foster homes, allowing for greater payment eligibility for kinship caregivers.[10]

Nutritional Support

Caregivers may be eligible for the Supplemental Nutrition Assistance Program (SNAP). This federal program provides nutrition benefits to low-income families so that they may purchase healthy and nutritious foods at local grocery stores.[11] Households must meet certain eligibility requirements; each state has its own application process for SNAP benefits.[11] The Special Supplemental Nutrition Program for Women, Infants, and Children (WIC) is an additional nutritional support for infants and children up to age 5 years who are at nutritional risk and for low-income pregnant, postpartum, and breastfeeding women. WIC is a federal program that provides grants to states. WIC provides food benefits including iron-fortified infant formula, baby food, fruits, vegetables, and milk. Eligible participants in WIC also can receive nutrition education, breastfeeding support, and other health care referrals.[12]

Health Care Coverage and Access

Most children and youth who are in foster care are eligible for Medicaid, with multiple pathways through which they may meet eligibility requirements.[13] Additionally, youth formerly in foster care, age 18 to 26 years, may be eligible for Medicaid based on certain criteria. If children do not meet criteria for Medicaid, they may meet state requirements for Children's Health Insurance Program (more commonly known as CHIP). Pediatricians can support caregivers in applying for health care coverage for children and adolescents who do not have insurance.[13] At times, children may have health insurance coverage but caregivers may not have access to the correct information, such as insurance card or insurance identification number. Clinicians can also support caregivers in identifying the child's insurance information as coverage transitions at the time of placement. When insurance coverage changes, the child's current pediatrician might not participate in the new insurance, creating a barrier to care because the pediatrician who knows and has cared for the child will no longer be able to do so while the child is in foster care. This offers a meaningful opportunity for pediatricians to support caregivers. Pediatricians can help identify a new pediatrician and provide care coordination support, communicate with the child's new pediatrician for continuity of care, and ensure that caregivers and child welfare agencies are aware of the child's medical needs.

Foster and kinship caregivers also encounter challenges when accessing health care for children in out-of-home placement. They report needing to advocate persistently for health care for the child, relying on others such as caseworkers and friends/family for support and information, difficulty accessing specialty services for children with chronic health conditions, and challenges attending appointments and understanding clinicians' instructions.[14,15] Pediatricians should be aware of these barriers and identify opportunities to help caregivers overcome them. Consent is detailed in Chapter 34, Medical Consents. Foster parents often accompany children to medical visits but are not authorized to consent for specific types of care, which can lead to delays in accessing important services, such as behavioral health treatment. Inability to support caregivers with behavioral health issues could affect placement stability. See Chapter 12, Mental Health, for a detailed discussion on mental health.

Kinship Navigator Programs

From 2020 to 2022, over 2.5 million children were in kinship care; most of these children were not placed through the child welfare system.[16] As noted earlier, kinship caregivers often begin to care for a child in the setting of a crisis or emergency and may have different motivations and needs compared to nonrelative foster caregivers. Additionally, kinship caregivers who are not involved with a child welfare agency may have limited supports and resources. One solution to address their unique needs is kinship navigator programs, which connect caregivers with resources and support at the local level. Most states have kinship navigator programs.[17] These programs can support kinship caregivers in applying for TANF and SNAP benefits. They can also help provide education to caregivers and help connect caregivers with resources and programs to support the needs of their children. Kinship navigator programs can receive federal funding through the Family First Prevention Services Act if they meet certain criteria.[17] Pediatricians can become familiar with kinship navigator programs in their area to guide kinship caregivers to appropriate resources.

Additional Training Programs

A variety of training programs are available to foster and kinship caregivers. Positive parenting programs offer one avenue through which caregivers can receive support. Child Adult Relationship Enhancement (known as CARE) demonstrated efficacy in improving parenting behaviors and reducing anxiety in children.[18] Another intervention, Keeping Foster and Kinship Parents Trained and Supported (commonly known as KEEP), demonstrated fewer reported child behavior problems and increased placement stability.[19] Additionally, the National Child Traumatic Stress Network has a Resource Parent Curriculum with a series of online learning modules, available at https://www.nctsn.org/resources/resource-parent-curriculum-rpc-training-modules. A meta-analysis of training programs showed that foster parents who completed these programs reported improved knowledge and skills and reduced child behavioral problems.[20] Since training program availability and eligibility will vary locally, pediatricians can collaborate with their local child welfare agencies and build relationships with community partners to identify training program opportunities. Pediatricians can then develop and share educational materials with caregivers. They can also support caregivers in accessing these programs through care coordination and direct referral processes. See **Box 35-1** for practical steps pediatricians can take to support foster and kinship caregivers.

Navigating Transitions

Children in out-of-home placement may encounter frequent transitions. Transitions can include beginning or cessation of visitation with the family of origin, transition to a new foster or kinship placement, reunification, and adoption. Pediatricians can encourage foster and kinship caregivers, the family of origin, and case workers to prepare children for these transitions. They can also encourage consistency in routines and expectations across the various care environments.[21] These transitions may ignite feelings of grief or sadness for foster and kinship caregivers. Pediatricians can provide referrals for caregivers to mental health and grief support services. One study found that foster caregivers experience difficulty letting go of children they fostered, express that their feelings were not taken into consideration in the transition, and wonder and worry about the children they fostered.[22] This study also emphasized that preparation, support systems, continued relationships with

Box 35-1

Practical Steps for Pediatricians to Support Foster and Kinship Caregivers in Accessing Resources

1. **Collaborate with local child welfare agencies.** It is critical that pediatricians understand the local child welfare system and what resources the local child welfare agency provides. Pediatricians should have up-to-date contact information for these agencies.
2. **Build connections with community partners.** Pediatricians should establish strong relationships with local schools, behavioral health clinicians, child advocacy centers, other health care providers, food banks, financial assistance programs, and other community partners. Pediatricians can work with these partners to provide resources to caregivers. Pediatricians can also develop care coordination support or scheduling assistance and direct referral processes for community programs.
3. **Develop a community resource directory.** Pediatricians can create a list of local community resources that can be shared with caregivers to assist with financial, educational, medical, or behavioral health needs. This should be reviewed frequently to ensure it is current. Alternatively, pediatricians may have knowledge of resource websites or materials that could be shared with caregivers as well.
4. **Offer educational sessions.** Pediatricians may consider offering training sessions to caregivers on how to navigate medical appointments and what to expect for children in foster or kinship care.
5. **Continue to support and follow up.** Pediatricians should establish an open line of communication with caregivers to build trust and ensure caregivers feel supported. Pediatricians can schedule routine follow-up visits whether virtually or in person to provide caregivers the opportunity to ask questions and share any concerns. This may help ensure that caregivers understand medical recommendations and further support caregivers in navigating resources.

the child they fostered, and knowledge that "it comes with the territory" facilitated "healthy loss." Caregivers also reported that they would benefit from grief counseling.[22] Pediatricians can support foster and kinship caregivers by validating their feelings of grief, offering words of support, and identifying resources for support (such as counseling and peer support groups).[22,23] One study demonstrated that children had a higher likelihood of reunification when caregivers regularly spoke with their caseworker about the child. This study also found that children had a higher probability of reunification if caregivers received respite care.[24] **Table 35–2** describes key aspects of the foster caregiver experience that pediatricians should understand.

Table 35–2. Things Every Pediatrician Should Know About Foster and Kinship Caregivers From the Perspective of a Current Foster Caregiver

Concerns	Caregiver Perceptions	Actions Pediatrician Can Take
Emotional concerns	Feeling they (the caregiver) are not okay Stress and anxiety Coping with visitation with the family of origin is hard, heartbreaking, and emotionally exhausting at times	Ask how they are doing
Lack of social support	Limited family or friends who can relate to their experience Respite care is not always available nor in the best interest of the child Babysitters are unavailable due to child welfare requirements	Identify additional supports
Feelings of judgment	Opinions of nonfoster caregivers Viewed as poor parents or incompetent Multiple points of judgment (assumed or otherwise) from caseworkers, attorneys, CASAs, school, birth parents, friends, family, etc	Offer words of encouragement
Lack of knowledge/education	Caregivers do not automatically know how to care for substance-exposed infants or children with behavioral problems such as trauma symptoms, ADHD, and ODD, and behavioral health is difficult to access	Ask questions about prior experience Ask what a good or rough day looks like Provide trauma-informed parenting education Provide resources
Need for further advocacy	Caregivers advocate on many levels—school, medical, legal Attending therapy and medical appointments Report to foster care agency, child protective services, CASA, birth family, etc	Listen intently Advocate for improved services (see Chapter 42, Advocacy and Public Policy)

Abbreviations: ADHD, attention-deficit/hyperactivity disorder; CASA, Court Appointed Special Advocate; ODD, oppositional defiant disorder.

Supports for Family of Origin

Involvement in Medical Care

For most children in out-of-home placement, reunification with their biological parent or family of origin is the goal.[25] Therefore, it is important to engage and support the family of origin. From a health care perspective, biological parents usually retain medical decision-making power for their child when the child is placed in foster or kinship care unless parental rights were terminated by the court or voluntarily. It is important to assess who the appropriate consenting party is for patients when they present for health care visits. Child welfare professionals assigned to a patient's case may aid in providing pediatricians with information on who can consent for the child's medical care including any court orders that exist, whether for routine or nonroutine care. See Chapter 34, Medical Consents, for a detailed discussion of consent issues. Because most biological parents will retain medical decision-making power, pediatricians should try to engage them in the child's care in a manner that is safe and healthy for the child. In general, the child welfare agency has the ability to consent for routine medical care and to authorize foster and kinship caregivers to provide verbal consent for components of routine care such as checking into medical visits. However, more significant decisions, such as for surgical or other procedures, psychotropic medications, or mental health therapy may require biological parent consent or court order. This can be challenging to navigate, especially for children with medical complexity.[26] Pediatricians can support biological parents in making informed medical decisions by providing effective and clear communication.

Ideally, foster/kinship caregivers and family of origin should be included in the child's medical visits when it is safe to do so because both can provide key information and will be important for ensuring adherence to medical recommendations.[21] Therefore, pediatricians may encounter challenging situations where both foster/kinship caregivers and the family of origin are present either in person or virtually during a medical visit. Pediatricians can prepare for potential conflict ahead of time by ensuring that they are aware of who will attend the appointment and setting expectations for all caregivers. Pediatricians should also be sensitive to the family of origin's cultural beliefs and practices. In these interactions, pediatricians can facilitate a calm, professional, and respectful dialogue with a focus on the child's medical needs. It can be helpful for the pediatrician to guide the appointment and ensure that all parties have the opportunity to share information and ask questions about the child's medical care. Additionally, pediatricians can ensure that both foster/kinship caregivers and the family of origin have appropriate access to medical information and, if they do not, identify barriers and solutions.

Emotional Support

It is important to recognize that the family of origin may experience trauma and intense feelings of grief or loss when a child is removed from their care. Studies have shown that family of origin may also experience a sense of threatened identity as parents.[27] Pediatricians should consider identifying support groups or counseling services for birth parents and families of origin when they identify these concerns. Additionally, parents may struggle to navigate child welfare, school, and health care systems; pediatricians can inquire about challenges and provide support.

Connection With Siblings

The Fostering Connections to Success and Increasing Adoptions Act of 2008 requires that state agencies make efforts to place siblings together and, when this is not possible, to ensure visits or ongoing contact between the child and their sibling(s) unless their safety or well-being is at risk.[7]

Sibling relationships have been shown to affect resilience and internalizing behaviors.[28,29] Placement with siblings has been associated with improved school performance and a higher likelihood of reunification.[30,31] Thus, when pediatricians encounter children in foster or kinship care, it is important to determine if siblings are also in placement and if there are opportunities to support siblings. Siblings in large sibling groups are more likely to be separated. Occasionally, siblings are placed separately because of major challenges in their relationship. Pediatricians can refer siblings for mental health support or sibling programs when locally available.[32]

Conclusion

Foster and kinship caregivers encounter unique challenges in their role caring for children. Some of these challenges are shared by birth parents and/or the family of origin. It is critical that pediatricians not only recognize these difficulties but also have knowledge of the resources available in their communities.

Key Takeaways

- Caregivers need knowledge of and access to available support programs and resources.
- Forming connections with caregivers through conversation can often identify areas of need.
- Supporting caregivers aids in their ability to help the children in their care.
- Building strong relationships with community partners can help identify local resources for caregivers.

CHAPTER

36

Privatization of Child Welfare

Valerie Borum Smith, MD, MPH, FAAP
Rachael J. Keefe, MD, MPH, FAAP

Introduction

As state child welfare systems work to meet the complex needs of children and families, they often partner with private organizations to provide services for system-involved families. *Privatization* is the process through which state or local child welfare agencies contract with nongovernmental agencies to provide specific services related to the care of children involved in the child welfare system.[1] States may choose to privatize aspects of their child welfare system for various reasons, but typically efforts are intended to improve outcomes, create innovation and efficiency within systems, and introduce risk- or performance-based payment within a system.[2] While privatization is not new to the US child welfare system, recent efforts encompass a wide spectrum of programs and services including support services, health care, placements, and case management.

Privatization is increasing within many child welfare systems across the United States, and pediatricians must be mindful of how these system changes affect the children they care for. As with any system change, there are pros and cons. Those in favor of moving toward privatization of child welfare systems highlight the benefits, including innovation and the availability of care close to home, while those opposed note some serious concerns including lack of accountability and increased rates of child abuse and neglect within a system whose mission is to keep children safe.[3]

History of Privatization of Child Welfare in the United States

Chapter 16, History of Child Welfare in the United States and Issues of Disproportionality, Inequity, and Injustice, provides a general history of the development of the child welfare system; a brief history of the transition from a private to public system and current trends toward privatization of the system is provided here. Private nonprofit child welfare organizations originated in 1874 and spread across the country; within 50 years, there were 300 such organizations in the United States, though the network often excluded rural areas and many children either were left unprotected or were aided by family and friends.[4]

Because of the patchwork nature of the private child welfare system and the gaps in its ability to care for all children in need of protection, there were calls to move child welfare from the private sector to government agencies in the early 20th century. By the 1970s, the transition to a fully governmental system was essentially complete.

During the next 20 years, the public child welfare system faced increases in reports of child abuse and in the volume of families involved in the child welfare system, which led to overwhelmed state and local systems. In response, public systems began to look for ways to partner with private agencies to contract some of their services, creating the current form of privatization within the child welfare system.

Current State of Privatization

The extent to which states lean on private agencies to provide services has always varied across the country.[5] In the 1990s, states began to increase their dependence on private agencies, with a particular leaning toward utilization of the nonprofit sector. This trend toward privatization was reported to be due to 3 key factors: efforts to downsize government, improve service quality, and decrease costs.[6]

A 2018 report by the National Conference of State Legislatures notes that as of 2011, only 2 states, Kansas and Florida, had statewide privatization of all case management services, while 7% of states had large-scale and 18% had small-scale privatization of case management services. At that time, 71% were not currently privatizing case management.[7]

Currently, all states maintain control over child investigations, while there is great state-to-state variation in what services within their child welfare systems have been transferred to the private sector.

Types of Privatization in the Current Child Welfare System

While all states contract out at least some child welfare services to private agencies, the type and scope of privatization varies widely across jurisdictions.[2] Types of privatization include support services, health care, placement, and case management.

Support Services

Support services are historically the most commonly privatized services within the child welfare system.[8] These can include foster parent recruitment, parenting classes, substance use disorder treatment, and other supports frequently needed by families involved in the child welfare system.

Health Care

Medicaid Managed Care

Perhaps the aspect of privatization that affects pediatricians caring for children in foster care the most is Medicaid Managed Care (MMC), where states contract with private, sometimes for-profit, insurance companies to provide health coverage for people enrolled in Medicaid. Title IV-E of the Social Security Act requires state Medicaid programs to provide health care for virtually all children in foster care, and many states choose to utilize MMC for at least some of those children.

A 2021 analysis of state MMC contracts and provider manuals revealed that 42 states and the District of Colombia provide Medicaid for at least some of the state's children in foster care through MMC.[9] MMC for children in foster care can include standard MMC available to all children in the state or specialized MMC that focuses on providing coverage to specific populations. These specialized MMC programs often include enhanced benefits and population-specific quality measures. One-third of states use specialized MMC for all or some children in foster care. Specialized MMC can be either specific to foster care or specific to chronic or complex diseases experienced by children in foster care. Ten states have developed foster care–specific specialized MMC plans.[9] In states that use a mix of traditional fee for service or MMC to provide care for children in foster care, the child welfare caseworker is often charged with choosing which plan a child is enrolled in. In those states, pediatricians caring for children in foster care need to be knowledgeable about both forms of care and may be able to advocate for which services best meet the needs of a particular child with their caseworker.

Behavioral Health

Because children involved with the child welfare system have higher rates of behavioral health needs, these children interact with the behavioral health system more frequently than their counterparts. Traditionally, many states have carved behavioral health services out from Medicaid services, leading them to privatize at least some aspect of behavioral health services, but the current trend in MMC is to integrate behavioral health and traditional medical services, especially for children in foster care. High-intensity services, such as inpatient and residential services, are the most frequently carved out of MMC and provided on a fee-for-service basis.[9]

Enhanced Services

Enhanced services for children in foster care can include physical or behavioral health care coordination and case management, targeted engagement with child welfare and behavioral health partners, specific assessments and screenings, psychotropic medication monitoring, transition services, and nonmedical services. Three-fourths of states provide at least 1 enhanced service for children in foster care, typically through MMC. For example, while all states are required to have general drug utilization reviews as part of their Medicaid system, at least 12 states have psychotropic medication monitoring programs specifically for children in foster care. This topic is discussed in more detail in Chapter 38, Psychotropic Medication Oversight. In recent years, some states have added nonmedical enhanced services, including personal hygiene supplies, Boys and Girls Club memberships, and rewards or incentives for participating in programs or completing trainings.[9]

Placements

States may implement placements managed by private agencies for some or all children in foster care. States have taken a variety of approaches to placement privatization. While some models focus on specific populations, such as children with complex needs, children in need of adoptive placements, or children with multisystem involvement, Kansas and Florida have chosen to privatize placements for all children in foster care. Private foster care placement agencies provide a wide range of services often including recruitment, training, and retention of foster parents. Many private agencies place children only with foster families while others provide a full spectrum of placement services including congregate care facilities such as emergency shelters, residential treatment facilities, group homes, and supervised independent living placements.

Case Management Services

The most extensive form of privatization occurs when a state relies on a private organization to assume child welfare case management services. In these cases, the private agency takes over day-to-day decisions regarding a child's case, including which services the child receives and where the child is placed. Privatization of case management services is also referred to as *community-based care* or *single-source continuum of care*. With case management privatization, the private agency often assumes some financial risk with contracts, including outcome incentives or per-child capitation, regardless of the intensity of services needed by an individual child. As mentioned previously, as of 2018, 12 states have privatized at least some case management services.[7] See **Box 36-1** and **Box 36-2** for examples of states that have privatized case management services and the outcomes they have observed.

Box 36-1

Florida

The state of Florida provides an example of systemwide privatization. As an early adopter, Florida began privatizing foster care in 1993 and had completely privatized child welfare services by 2005. The state contracts with lead agencies responsible for a full spectrum of child welfare services within a defined geographic region. These agencies then often contract with other private organizations to provide specific services. Privatization resulted in a significant reduction of the number of children in foster care in the state, falling from 29,000 in 2006 to fewer than 19,000 in 2010, although it is important to note that the decline in children in care should not be attributed solely to privatization. A 2013 evaluation by the state's Office of Program Policy Analysis and Government Accountability found lower rates of repeat maltreatment, increased adoptions, more efficient spending, and less reliance on congregate care.[10]

Box 36-2

Nebraska

Nebraska initially implemented privatization in 2009 but had multiple early struggles. The first 2 years of privatization cost the state significantly more than budgeted, and most of the private agencies contracted with the state withdrew from their contracts. The state legislature voted in 2012 to return case management services for most of the state to the Department of Health and Human Services, with Nebraska Families Collaborative retaining control of case management in the Omaha area. A 2014 audit compared outcomes for children served by Nebraska Families Collaborative with children served in the rest of the state by the Department of Health and Human Services and found no significant differences in outcomes. Nebraska continues to face financial challenges related to privatization efforts.

Concerns Surrounding Privatization

States' reliance on the private sector to assist with child welfare systems is mostly thought to be driven by 2 main factors: cost containment and innovation. Proponents of privatization of child welfare argue that it keeps children in care close to home. For example, at the outset of the move toward privatization of child welfare services in Texas, it was noted that 30% of the state's children were placed outside of their home county. An earlier privatization trial in a large metropolitan region in Texas was reported to lower the percentage of children placed out of region to 10%.[7] Privatization of child welfare systems is also associated with increased innovation, bringing in private companies to "shake up" the status quo of state agencies and moving models of care in a local, but also modernized, direction.

Those with concerns about privatization note that the private agencies that bid on the contracts are often out of state, which negates the claim of moving toward a private community-based model of service. There is also concern about the lack of accountability when private agencies take over public sector systems, especially an agency tasked to keep children safe and in which the stakes (including potential family disruptions) are so high. Some argue that privatization has even led to decreased tracking of child abuse and neglect of children within the foster care system.[11] The authors of one study note that their analysis revealed a correlation between heightened levels of privatization in a state's child welfare system and an increased risk of abuse and neglect of children within the privatized system.[3]

Role of the Pediatrician in Private Networks

Although intimately knowing the status of the state's child welfare system's level of privatization is ideal, pediatricians who care for children in foster care are urged to have at least a high-level understanding of the current degree of privatization in their home state. Many states divide their child welfare systems geographically into regional, county, or city jurisdictions, and it is helpful for pediatricians caring for children in foster care to identify their local child welfare leaders through state websites or databases and develop a relationship with them. Additionally, pediatricians who provide care for children in foster care may benefit from serving on local or regional advisory councils that often include private organizations involved in the child welfare system. This knowledge is especially important regarding health insurance. A pediatrician familiar with which Medicaid plans serve children in their state can advocate to improve patient outcomes. For those who wish to advocate for children in foster care, it is also important to have a high-level understanding of legislation surrounding privatization of child welfare within the state, as well as the stage and timeline of implementation. Pediatricians in states with some degree of privatization may consider partnering with the private sector agencies serving children in care to help advocate for improved health outcomes. An example of a partnership could be the standardization of communication systems, such as the creation of a standardized form to be completed by the health care system and sent to a child placement agency. In addition, many private organizations have community advisory boards on which pediatricians can serve to advocate for the health needs of children in their communities. Similarly, MMC organizations have medical advisory committees in which pediatricians can advocate for systemic improvements and provide oversight for plans providing care for children in foster care.

Key Takeaways

- States are increasingly depending on private organizations to provide at least some of the services necessary for children and families involved with the child welfare system.
- While privatization aims to bring innovation and contain costs, concerns regarding privatization of the child welfare system include child safety and accountability of private organizations.
- Pediatricians caring for children in foster care need to understand the role of private organizations in their state's child welfare system and may interact with local or regional staff from private organizations.

CHAPTER 37

Health Care Financing

Joseph S. Zickafoose, MD, MS, FAAP

Introduction

The breadth and depth of health care services needed by children and adolescents in foster care require financing that aligns with principles of the American Academy of Pediatrics (AAP),[1] including

- Coverage with quality, affordable health insurance should be universal.
- Comprehensive pediatric services should be covered.
- Cost sharing should be affordable and should not negatively affect care.
- Payment should be adequate to strengthen family- and patient-centered medical homes.
- Child health financing policy should promote equity and address long-standing health and health care disparities.
- Child health financing policy must be designed to reflect the unique characteristics and needs of children.

Fortunately, policy advances in recent years have brought those principles closer to a reality for children in foster care, but there remain many opportunities for improvement. This chapter is organized around the AAP principles of health care financing to address current relevant federal policy and how it intersects with state policy choices. States have substantial flexibility in how they interpret and implement federal health care financing policy, resulting in a wide range of state practices. It is important for clinicians to be aware of the potential influences of these policies on the care they and others can provide children in foster care and to consider advocacy to change policy. The chapter concludes with additional opportunities for federal and state financing policy to bring them closer to addressing the full needs of children in foster care.

Ensuring Universal Coverage

Nearly all children in foster care are eligible for health insurance coverage through Medicaid.[2] Most foster care placements are supported through federal Title IV-E funding. Children and youth up to age 21 years are automatically eligible for Medicaid in their state of residence if Title IV-E foster care or guardianship payments are made on their behalf or if they are under a Title IV-E adoption assistance agreement. If an adolescent in Title IV-E–funded foster placement is or becomes a parent, their child is also automatically eligible for Medicaid. Most children and adolescents who do not qualify for Medicaid based on Title IV-E will qualify for Medicaid through other eligibility pathways, including income-based eligibility (under rules that allow assessment of income for the child alone, not income for their household prior to or during foster placement).

For the small number of child welfare–involved children who do not qualify for any of these eligibility pathways for Medicaid, additional options for health insurance coverage include their state's Children's Health Insurance Program, subsidized coverage through a state or federal Health Insurance Marketplace, or a caregiver's employer-based health insurance. Immigrant children without legal documentation who are removed from their families in the United States typically do not qualify for Medicaid or other public insurance in most states, and their care must be paid for directly by the child welfare agency. Unaccompanied children detained by Department of Homeland Security immigration officials are placed in the custody of the Office of Refugee Resettlement (ORR), and ORR is responsible for facilitating and funding their health care (for more details related to unaccompanied minors, see Chapter 33, Unaccompanied Immigrant Youth).[3]

Despite the automatic eligibility for Medicaid of most children in foster care, states can vary in how quickly they get the child enrolled after foster placement. A delay in insurance coverage for a child after foster placement can lead to a cascade of delays in obtaining a comprehensive health assessment, identifying needs, placing referrals, and ultimately receiving any services that are needed for the child.[4]

Since 2014, state Medicaid programs have been required to allow young adults who "age out" of foster care at age 18 years to remain eligible for Medicaid in their state until their 26th birthday. As of January 2023, this mandatory eligibility for former foster youth applied to any state, regardless of which state foster placement occurred in.

Coverage of Comprehensive Pediatric Services

The health care needs of children in foster care require a comprehensive health insurance benefits package that includes the full range of pediatric services recommended by the AAP, including

> prenatal and newborn care; postnatal home visits; preventive and wellness services; urgent and emergency care; acute, inpatient, and chronic care services; medically necessary and developmentally appropriate habilitative and rehabilitative therapies and devices; dental and oral health services; vision services; behavioral and mental health services; transition to adult care services; reproductive health and pregnancy-related services; gender-affirming care; treatment of tobacco use and substance use disorders; home-based care, including private duty nursing and personal care services; palliative and hospice care services; durable medical equipment to include mobility, seating, and positioning equipment such as adaptive car seats; interpreter services; specialty formulas; and recommended medications from the US Pharmacopeia in formulations appropriate for children.[5]

Medicaid's benefit package for children, known as Early and Periodic Screening, Diagnostic and Treatment (EPSDT), is considered the standard for comprehensive pediatric health services because of its coverage mandate for all medically necessary services.[6,7]

The EPSDT Benefit in Medicaid and Foster Care

The EPSDT benefit in Medicaid is held up as a standard because state Medicaid programs are required to provide comprehensive services and "furnish all...Medicaid coverable, appropriate, and medically necessary services needed to correct and ameliorate health conditions."[6] This broad medical necessity standard is unique in its comprehensiveness compared to other health insurance standards for pediatric care. This means that Medicaid has to cover any medically necessary treatment (physical, emotional, developmental, or behavioral) identified by a clinician during a visit. This is true even if the services are not routinely covered by an individual state's Medicaid benefit package. For example, the enhanced standards for children and adolescents in foster care published by the AAP and the Child Welfare League of America should be covered under EPSDT as services deemed medically necessary.

However, states vary widely in their implementation and enforcement of EPSDT benefits, including medical necessity criteria. Most states continue to fall short of goals for EPSDT benefits for children in general[8] and for children in foster care specifically.[9] In recognition of these challenges, the Centers for Medicare and Medicaid Services released guidance in September 2024 that includes updated best practices for states to adhere to EPSDT requirements.[7] Even within this new guidance, home- and community-based services, such as intensive services for children with serious emotional disturbances, are not always considered part of EPSDT and might be covered under separate state benefit programs that can have waiting lists. When coverage is denied for services for a child in foster care enrolled in Medicaid, foster parents, birth parents, clinicians, caseworkers, attorneys, health care managers, or other interested parties might need to advocate through Medicaid appeals processes and other legal channels to ensure access to the services for the child based on medical necessity under the EPSDT standard.

Medicaid Managed Care for Children in Foster Care

Most children in foster care are enrolled in Medicaid, and most state Medicaid programs administer benefits for children, including children in foster care, through some form of managed care.[10] Broadly defined, managed care is a system for delivering health care that is organized to manage cost, use, and quality. Within Medicaid, this commonly involves contracts between the state Medicaid agency and managed care organizations (MCOs) for a set (capitated) payment per month per beneficiary to deliver necessary services with provisions incentivizing improvements in access and quality of care.[11] The MCOs in turn must contract with the wide range of clinicians needed to deliver covered services. This contrasts with the historical approach of fee for service (FFS), in which states paid clinicians directly, with no specific requirements for managing access, quality, or costs.

As of 2021, 42 states and the District of Columbia used some form of managed care for some or all children in foster care.[9] Most states enroll children in foster care in their standard MCOs for other Medicaid beneficiaries, but 14 states and the District of Columbia use specialized MCOs specific to children in foster care or include them in MCOs for broader groups of beneficiaries with complex needs.

When the system is working well, Medicaid managed care has potential benefits in making MCOs accountable for reaching access and quality goals through incentives and penalties within contracts. MCOs have more flexibility in setting payment rates for clinicians that are different from a state's FFS rates, giving them the opportunity to set higher rates to meet their goals, and they typically have care management staff assigned to identify and address beneficiaries with complex needs. However, managed care's role in managing costs can lead to barriers to care, such as requiring prior authorization, denying claims, and creating narrow clinician networks, which can be especially problematic for children in foster care with complex needs. To help address this, some states (for example, Washington) require MCOs to remove limits on services, such as health supervision visits, for children in foster care without regard to the standard periodicity schedule.[12]

About three-quarters of states provide some types of enhanced services for children in foster care, primarily through managed care.[9] These services can include care coordination and case management, targeted engagement with child welfare and behavioral health partners, foster care–specific assessments and screenings, psychotropic medication monitoring, dedicated services for transitions between foster placements and to care once youth leave foster care, and nonmedical supports, such as personal supplies and Boys and Girls Club memberships.

Behavioral Health Services

States take different approaches to financing behavioral health services for children in foster care within Medicaid. Most states include behavioral health care in their managed care programs. This is especially true within specialized MCOs that cover children in foster care, which frequently include enhanced community-based behavioral health services, such as intensive wraparound services with care coordination, crisis stabilization, and therapeutic foster care.[9] Some states continue to provide some or all behavioral health services through FFS, especially inpatient and residential services.

Strengthening Medical Homes and Promoting Equity

Medicaid provides nearly universal coverage for children in foster care, but the value of that coverage can be blunted by Medicaid's historical challenges with access to services, driven in large part by the low payment rates in the program. Medicaid FFS base payment rates are generally substantially less than Medicare or private insurance rates for the same service. According to the most recent national comparisons, using data from 2019, Medicaid FFS rates for 27 common primary care, obstetric, and other physician services were 72% of the rate Medicare paid for the same services on average; this ratio was largely unchanged from 2008.[13] Although MCOs have more flexibility in payment rates, MCOs have historically based clinician payment on the FFS rate.

Given the complexity and urgency of needs for many children in foster care, some states (for example, Maine,[14] South Carolina,[15] and Washington[11]) have implemented enhanced payment rates for services to children in foster care, such as for initial health screens and routine health supervision visits. These enhanced rates are intended to incentivize clinicians to provide access to children in foster care, especially for the initial and comprehensive assessments soon after placement, and to compensate clinicians for the time needed to address complex needs. However, little is known about how effective these enhanced rates are at increasing the number of clinicians willing to provide care for children in foster care overall and especially for timely assessments soon after placement.

Other Sources of Financing

Given the typically low Medicaid reimbursement rates, clinics serving children in foster care often need to identify other sources of financial support. These can include direct contracts with child welfare agencies, other sources of state or local government funding, hospital or health system funding, grants, and philanthropy.[16,17]

Key Takeaways

Health care financing for children and adolescents in foster care should be designed to improve these children's overall physical, emotional, developmental, and behavioral health. In doing so, it should support the child welfare goals of health, safety, and permanency for children and adolescents. Substantial progress has been made in recent years in financing services for the often complex needs of children in foster care, but many opportunities for improvement remain, including:

- Health insurance coverage for children entering foster care that is immediate, universal, portable, and ongoing during the stay in foster care to avoid delays in care
- Financing models in Medicaid FFS and managed care that include enhanced services tailored to meet the needs of children in foster care
- Enhanced reimbursement rates for services for children in foster care that are sufficient to incentivize timely and ongoing access to the full complement of pediatric services

CHAPTER 38

Psychotropic Medication Oversight

Wynne Morgan, MD
Christelle Tan, MD, FAAP
Raul J. Martinez-McFaline, MD, PhD

Overview

Youth in the child welfare system are at risk for inappropriate use of psychotropic medication stemming from several factors, including care fragmentation, incomplete medical and developmental histories, challenges with communication, and system silos, as well as a lack of trauma-informed diagnosis and treatment planning. Data show the rates of psychotropic medications are significantly higher in youth in foster care. Child welfare placements also influence the rates of psychotropic medications. Youth in congregate care settings are more likely to be on psychotropic medications than youth placed in the community. Children in foster care receive psychotropic medications at a range of 13% to 37%[1–6] in community settings and up to 67% in therapeutic foster care and 77% in group homes,[7] compared to about 4% in the general population.[8] Overall, when compared with other Medicaid-eligible youth, children in foster care can have 2 to 8 times the rates of psychotropic use.[9]

The cause of the high rates of psychotropic medication use among youth in foster care is likely multifactorial. In some cases, these children may be appropriately prescribed more psychotropics due to their higher rates of mental health disorders, gaining access to Medicaid insurance, and being systematically screened for mental health disorders.[9] Children in foster care access outpatient mental health resources, including psychological services, at higher rates than do other Medicaid-insured children.[10,11] Furthermore, having insurance and any general medication or outpatient mental health specialist use is positively correlated with psychotropic prescribing.[3,12] However, rates of medication use among children in foster care have wide geographic variations, with rates of any psychotropic medication use ranging from 0% to 40% and rates of polypharmacy (concomitant regimens of 3 or more classes of psychotropic medications) ranging from 0.5% to 13.6%, suggesting both underprescribing and overprescribing across regions.[2,12] This variability in prescribing rates supports findings that factors other than clinical need influence prescribing practices.[3,13] Racial and gender disparities raise further concern, with white males being prescribed psychotropics at higher rates.[1–3,6,14] African American children in foster care have lower rates of psychotropic medication use, which could reflect underprescribing when also considering their lower utilization of mental health services.[1,3,9]

Among children in foster care who are prescribed psychotropic medications, 38% to 86% are prescribed medications from more than one psychotropic medication class concomitantly. The overall rate of children in foster care prescribed multiple psychotropic medications concomitantly is about 5-fold greater than the rate seen in their peers not in foster care who receive Medicaid benefits.[15] Children are also prescribed multiple psychotropics starting as young as age 4 years.[12] Antipsychotics with attention-deficit/hyperactivity disorder (ADHD) medications are the most common psychotropic class combination in this population.[6]

Prescribing rates of antipsychotics are particularly concerning because of the limited safety and efficacy data for individuals younger than 18 years, particularly for indications not approved by the Food and Drug Administration.[16] The side-effect profiles of these medications are also concerning, particularly metabolic side effects, such as a 3-fold risk of developing type 2 diabetes[17] and significant weight gain among youth treated with second-generation antipsychotics.[18] The increase in antipsychotic prescribing rates for children and adolescents, including those in foster care, peaked in the mid to late 2000s before national attention and concerted quality improvement efforts supported a gradual reduction in prescribing rates.[11,19,20] Children in foster care are prescribed antipsychotics at higher rates and numbers than other Medicaid-insured children, even after controlling for psychiatric diagnoses, health care utilization, and demographic factors.[21,22] Children in foster care are prescribed antipsychotics primarily for conduct disorders.[13] Among children in foster care who are prescribed 4 to 5 concomitant medications, antipsychotics are the most prescribed medication.[6,14] Although children in foster care who are prescribed antipsychotics are more likely to obtain appropriate metabolic monitoring compared to other Medicaid-insured children, rates of monitoring are low overall, at 28% for children in foster care compared to 18% for children not in foster care.[11]

With decades of data highlighting the high rates of psychotropic use, including antipsychotic medications, in this population, there are policies and best practice standards that pediatricians working with youth in the child welfare system should know. This chapter outlines efforts to ensure appropriate prescribing through systems-level oversight programs, an overview of the importance of medication consent, clinical practice efforts to ensure appropriate psychotropic medications through deprescribing, and the utilization of child psychiatric consultation.

Psychotropic Oversight Programs

Pediatric psychotropic oversight programs have emerged nationally since 2014, with a wide variability in how the programs are implemented. Psychotropic oversight grew out of public concern for the high rates of psychotropic medications in children in foster care, which led to policy changes nationally.[9] The Child and Family Services Improvement and Innovations Act of 2011 requires states to develop protocols for appropriate use and monitoring of psychotropic medication for youth in state custody.[23] Following this legislation, stakeholders including the Children's Bureau,[24] the Annie E. Casey Foundation,[25] and the American Academy of Child and Adolescent Psychiatrists[26–28] published resources to help guide state implementation of oversight programs. The documents outline best practices for creating successful psychotropic oversight programs in pediatric patients (see **Box 38–1**).

Considering these guidelines, states have developed several different oversight program types using both prospective and retrospective review strategies. Prospective review of psychotropic medication occurs before the child starts a medication. One type of process for prospective review involves collegial secondary review, where the request for the medication is reviewed by a second clinician prior to consenting.[29] The state of Illinois currently utilizes this model through an academic–state partnership between the University of Illinois at Chicago and the Illinois Child Welfare Agency. In this model, the prescriber must complete a medication request form and submit that form for medical review. The medication review must approve the medication prior to consent and subsequent authorization of the medication. The medication cannot be dispensed at a pharmacy until this approval is received.[30] Another form of prospective review is judicial review, where a judge authorizes consent to use of a psychotropic medication for a child in state custody. California has a judicial review requirement for all psychotropic medications prescribed to a child in state custody. The prescriber must seek authorization from the court prior to initiating treatment with any psychotropic medication.[31] Prior authorizations are another form of prospective review that occur after consent is issued through an administrative tool by a health plan that requires the prescriber to obtain approval from the health plan prior to the medication

Box 38-1

Best Practices for Child Welfare Oversight Programs

1. Comprehensive Mental Health Screening, Assessment, and Treatment Planning
   - Structured, trauma-informed process to identify mental health needs
   - Developmentally informed approach to prescribing that includes psychosocial interventions
   - Communication pathways between medical, mental health, and child welfare systems
2. Consent and Assent
   - Process for shared decision-making among youth, caregivers, prescribers, and child welfare workers
   - Review process for psychotropic medications to help identify high-risk prescribing
3. Psychiatric Expertise and Consultation
   - Access to a child and adolescent psychiatrist to provide consultation around appropriate prescribing practices that are trauma informed
4. Access to Data for Monitoring and Continuous Quality Improvement
   - Monitoring process at both a systems level and child/family level
   - Establish consensus statewide on type of data collected and reviewed
5. Guidance, Education, and Information Sharing
   - Provide resources for children, families, and child welfare workers that address mental health and trauma
   - Disseminate information to caregivers and child welfare staff to empower their understanding of psychotropic medication benefits and side effects

being covered. Massachusetts is an example of an oversight program that requires prior-authorization approval for what the state Medicaid program defines as high-risk psychotropic prescribing in pediatric populations. This program covers all youth in the state Medicaid program, including youth in the child welfare system.[32]

Retrospective reviews occur when the child has already received the medication and presumably started taking it. One retrospective strategy involves database review to identify high-risk prescribing. Other forms may happen during social work case review, where the case worker may raise concern about the prescribing of high-risk medications. There also can be retrospective judicial review, where the psychotropic medications the youth is taking are reviewed by the court. Texas's state oversight program includes pharmacy claims data review and also requests from child welfare teams and courts to flag cases that require further review. Texas has defined parameters for high-risk prescribing that requires further review.[33]

Prospective reviews have the most potential to prevent children from starting a psychotropic medication and to ensure safety; however, these strategies often cause added administrative burden on the prescriber as well as risk for additional barriers to accessing medication and subsequent treatment that may be needed. Retrospective oversight strategies have less of an administrative burden and are easier to implement in a child welfare population but are associated with greater safety risks because the child has already started the medication at the time of review. It is important that any oversight processes balance timely access to medication with ensuring safety.[29]

Medication Consent

An important piece of psychotropic oversight for youth in the child welfare system is medication consent because this process points to how a medication is agreed upon and started. There are unique issues for pediatricians to consider when prescribing psychotropic medications for youth in the foster care system. These include involving the youth and all relevant stakeholders responsible for them.[34] See Chapter 34, Medical Consents, for more details.

Deprescribing

Following concerns about inappropriate prescribing for youth in foster care, there have been efforts in the field of child and adolescent psychiatry to incorporate deprescribing practices into clinical work. *Deprescribing* is a structured approach to drug discontinuation, with the goal of parsimonious use, or use that provides the minimum effective dose and number of medications.[35] Deprescribing is part of good prescribing and essential in pediatric mental health because it provides a framework for reassessing medication over time. When working with children, the clinical need for medications changes over time because of age, development, disease course, cognitive abilities, coping skills, and patient and family preferences. Deprescribing is one tool to help prevent inappropriate prescribing.[36]

Current guidance on time frames to stop medications for mental health disorders is limited. Discontinuation of medications for anxiety disorder may be considered after 12 months of remission and should occur in periods of low stress. For depressive disorders, medication discontinuation may occur after 6 to 12 months in remission during low-stress time periods.[37,38]

Child psychiatrists have made efforts to outline best practice guidelines for deprescribing. A comprehensive assessment of the child with their caregiver is the first step. The second step is medication reconciliation, and the third step includes identifying and stopping medications that have the highest risk and lowest benefit. This also may include medications without a clear indication, that are ineffective, or that have no evidence to support ongoing use. Medications that are prescribed outside of clinical guidelines or have the greatest risk of adverse effects may also be candidates for dosage decreases or discontinuation. Prescribing cascades, where one medication is being used to counteract the side effect of another medication, should also be identified for potential discontinuation. The fourth step is for trauma-informed psychosocial supports to be incorporated into the treatment plan, as well as additional behavioral or academic supports that may be needed in the school setting. Continued communication with the school, caregiver, social worker, and child about the medication changes is also a key component to stopping medications because it is important to know any changes in functioning across multiple settings. Once tapering has started or a medication is stopped, the fifth and final step of implementation—monitoring and management—may require more frequent follow-up appointments to assess for withdrawal symptoms and relapse. Stopping psychotropic medications can cause withdrawal symptoms; therefore, it is generally best for the patient to slowly taper off medications.[35,36,39–42] This process is summarized in **Box 38-2**.

Collaboration With Child and Adolescent Psychiatry

Pediatricians are faced with the challenges of polypharmacy and are sometimes tasked with the decision to streamline psychotropic medication use, especially in patients involved in the foster care system. This may necessitate collaboration with psychiatrists and other clinicians in the psychotherapeutic management of these individuals.[42]

Given the high rates of mental health concerns in this population, it is of the utmost importance that children involved in the foster care system have a medical home, and that is usually located with the pediatrician. A pediatrician should be well qualified to begin a mental health encounter and perform a psychosocial assessment of the child when a mental health concern and psychotherapeutic intervention may be warranted. During the encounter, brief pediatric interventions can be implemented, such as additional screening, brief interventions, or referrals to mental health clinicians. If there does seem to be a need for psychotropic medications, then a full diagnostic assessment should be completed by the pediatrician or medical home clinician.

Box 38-2

Practical Steps to Deprescribing

1. Comprehensive Assessment
   - ▲ Key parties: caregiver, child, child welfare workers
   - ▲ Collateral information from other caregivers or clinicians
   - ▲ Administration of standardized tools/scales
   - ▲ Incorporation of trauma and adversity into clinical assessment
   - ▲ Impact of culture and race on clinical presentation
2. Medication Reconciliation and Assessment of Effectiveness
   - ▲ Obtain comprehensive list of *all* current medications
   - ▲ Diagnosis should align with medication treatment
   - ▲ Assess effectiveness of medication
   - ▲ Review past medication trials
   - ▲ Identify symptoms that may be related to medication side effects (eg, sedation or insomnia)
3. Medication Discontinuation
   - ▲ Prescribed without clear indication
   - ▲ Least evidence case
   - ▲ Ineffective medication
   - ▲ Prescribed outside of current guidelines
   - ▲ Insufficient benefit to justify harms
   - ▲ Greatest risk of adverse effects
   - ▲ Part of a prescribing cascade
4. Incorporate Medication Changes Into a Comprehensive Treatment Plan
   - ▲ Ensure caregiver and child understand risks and benefits of medication cessation
   - ▲ Include psychosocial interventions in treatment plan
   - ▲ Advocate for appropriate school supports
   - ▲ Continue to support health and well-being
5. Implementation, Monitoring, and Management
   - ▲ Follow-up appointments may be more frequent
   - ▲ Provide anticipatory guidance about withdrawal symptoms and how to manage
   - ▲ Gather feedback from youth, caregiver, and other collaterals
   - ▲ Monitor for clinical worsening and relapse
   - ▲ Have plan to address concerns for clinical worsening and relapse

Understanding the impact of developmental trauma and the importance of relational health is another key aspect of the mental health assessment for children in foster care. During this time, the clinician should triage for psychiatric emergencies, and emergency referrals should be made.[43–45]

When a clinician decides that a full diagnostic assessment is warranted, either for medication or further diagnostic workup, they can proceed to perform the assessment themselves or make a referral to a mental health clinician. Of note, the American Academy of Pediatrics has outlined considerations for prescribing in pediatrics, including the prescriber having regularly encountered the disorder for which the medication will be prescribed. These disorders include ADHD, depression, anxiety disorders, and substance use. Prescribing psychotropic medications for trauma-related disorders should always incorporate psychosocial interventions prior to initiation of medications. Considerations should be made according to the clinician's comfort level with further assessments and treatments. When a clinician determines the assessment and management are outside the scope of their practice, they can refer to associated mental health clinician or seek collaboration with other physicians.[42,43] One type of referral that could be made is via a telephone consultation program. Modeled after the Massachusetts Child Psychiatry Access Program, hotlines have been developed nationwide to help primary care clinicians with psychiatric consultations, psychotropic medication oversight, and referral to other mental health services if necessary.[46]

Conclusion

Pediatricians, whose relationships with patients often span the course of childhood, are poised to help ensure appropriate use of psychotropic medications in youth in the child welfare system. It is important to understand the multitude of factors that may affect high-risk medication use in the foster care population, including care fragmentation, unknown medical histories, and lack of trauma-informed diagnoses.[9] Psychotropic oversight programs are one type of intervention that can create an added safety net for these children, but they should not be implemented in isolation of other factors, such as access to therapeutic supports, placement stability, bridging system silos, and trauma-informed care, that can help prevent high-risk prescribing and increase access to appropriate care.[47] Integration of the therapeutic supports provided by the child-serving systems of care is essential to consider because medication is only one component of a mental health treatment plan, and it is critical that systems of care (medical, judicial, mental health, juvenile justice, and school systems) communicate to support youth in the child welfare system. For a pediatrician working with this population and their families, it is important to understand the child- and family-serving systems of care that help support the mental health care needs of vulnerable families. Informed consent and assent processes are important to ensure there has been a risk–benefit discussion that includes the patient, caregiver, family of origin (when appropriate), and child welfare agency in the decision to start a medication. Deprescribing is a clinical practice tool to help ensure that when psychotropic medications are needed, they are appropriate and used at the lowest effective dose for the shortest length of time. To aid in determining best practices, pediatricians should have access to psychiatric consultation to ensure that concerns or questions around the appropriateness of prescribing are reviewed with a child and adolescent psychiatrist.

These current strategies are a start, but more information is needed regarding research into and guidelines about ways to prevent inappropriate prescribing and, once children are on medication, how best to discontinue these medications. The work of ensuring appropriate use of psychotropic medications takes time, and clinicians are often faced with limited resources and reimbursement rates that do not allow the flexibility to do the work that is needed for this vulnerable pediatric population. System supports are needed to ensure best practices in prescribing, including shared decision-making tools for assent and consent, elective psychiatric consultation, and continuous quality improvement and learning collaboratives.[25] Systems delivery is another area of need because access to appropriate therapeutic supports that are trauma informed is essential to reducing the use of psychotropic medication. Public reporting on rates of psychotropic medications and accountability is another step that can be taken to ensure youth in the child welfare system are receiving appropriate medications.

Key Takeaways

- Repeated studies have shown that youth in the child welfare system are at risk for the inappropriate use of psychotropic medications.
- Psychotropic oversight programs have been implemented in states across the country to help ensure appropriate prescribing for youth in foster care.
- The use of informed consent in child welfare, implementation of deprescribing in clinical practice, and access to child and adolescent psychiatric consultation are other tools to help ensure appropriate psychotropic use in this population.

CHAPTER 39

Improving Care, Expanding the Field

James G. Kaferly III, MD, FAAP
Sara J. Hills, PhD, IMH-E

Research plays an essential role in discovering better and more innovative ways to promote health and improve outcomes among all children, including young people in kinship, foster, and congregate care (hereafter referred to as *foster care*). Given that foster care placement is common and associated with worse health and social outcomes across an individual's life course,[1,2] quality improvement, quantitative (numbers-based), qualitative (information that cannot be represented by numbers), and mixed-methods (both quantitative and qualitative) research efforts are well suited to advancing high-quality, evidence-based care, reducing health inequities, and amplifying health priorities among youth in foster care. However, research inclusive of and specific to young people in foster care lags that of peers not involved in the foster care system. Barriers in accessing accurate and reliable data, establishing shared short- and long-term outcome measures, engaging young people and communities with lived experience, and obtaining informed consent have impeded the development of a robust evidence base to diagnose, intervene in, and improve health disparities prevalent among young people in foster care.[3]

Achieving the best possible outcomes for young people who experience foster care requires more efficient, unified, and effective research. This chapter briefly summarizes extant literature and highlights potential areas and important considerations for pursuing research relevant to young people placed in foster care. This chapter is not an exhaustive list of essential research questions or of the methodological approaches available to pursue research with young people in foster care. Similarly, it provides an incomplete summary of regulatory requirements. As with all research, adherence to ethics, laws, and regulations is paramount. Therefore, pediatric clinicians and researchers must be familiar with federal, state, agency, and institutional regulations and ethical guidelines, as currently implemented, and monitor for potential modifications in the future. Despite these limitations, the text may serve as a helpful guide toward understanding both the need for and considerations necessary to expanding research to improve care for young people in foster care.

Improving Care Through Research

The American Academy of Pediatrics identifies young people in foster care as a population with special health care needs due to higher prevalence of health conditions and greater unmet health needs compared to peers not in foster care.[4] Extant literature highlights the increased frequencies of physical, developmental, behavioral, and chronic health conditions as well as all-cause mortality risk among young people placed in foster care compared to peers not in foster care.[5–8] Counteracting these health inequities requires a more expansive description of health conditions among youth in foster care. Epidemiology, comorbidity, and long-term outcomes need to be assessed by race, ethnicity, age, and health complexity. This research can inform the identification and treatment of health problems and facilitate collaboration between individuals and communities with lived experience and stakeholders in health care, child welfare, health policy, and other systems.[7–9]

Seeking to address these questions, researchers require accurate and reliable data. Yet, investigators must frequently rely on data sources with important methodological limitations—select health conditions, reported versus confirmed diagnoses, and divergent study populations—that may limit investigation (**Table 39–1**). Prior research examining Adoption and Foster Care Analysis and Reporting System (AFCARS) data to determine the prevalence of special health care needs among young people in foster care found wide state-by-state variation, suggesting discordance in both how and when child health assessment occurs.[5] Furthermore, the National Survey of Child Health and National Survey of Child and Adolescent Well-Being include young people in foster care but determine child health status through caregiver reports and examine limited health conditions.[7] This approach is problematic for 2 reasons. First, young people in foster care often reside with nonrelative caregivers who may not know their health history or may not identify health concerns.[10] Second, reporting only select health conditions restricts investigation of broader health problems, age of onset, and condition severity—information that is required for long-term, population-based research designed to understand health needs and inform responsive, evidence-based strategies.[7,11]

Federal legislation and health care reform in the 2000s and 2010s established requirements for increased accountability among health care and child welfare systems for the health outcomes of children in foster care.[12–17] The success of such efforts requires effective collaboration between child welfare and health care systems to assess individual and population health metrics. Given near-universal Medicaid coverage for young people in foster care, Medicaid administrative claims data are well suited to address critical research gaps among this population but require better linkage and integration with child welfare data.[18] Recently, a promising new linkage of Medicaid and child welfare data sets is available for researchers to examine child-centered outcomes,[19] and growing literature highlights health and child welfare system partnerships to improve health among children in foster care, though significant barriers remain.[9,11]

While data linkage is promising, electronic health record (EHR) data are a more accessible resource for most pediatricians. EHRs contain a variety of information collected in health care delivery—clinical conditions, laboratory results, diagnoses, and treatments—which provide a "real-world view" valuable to health research, intervention assessment, and quality improvement efforts.[20] However, pediatricians should be aware of both the benefits and

Table 39–1. Benefits and Limitations of Select Data Sources

Data Source	Benefits	Limitations
Survey data	Data collection options: in person, telephone, mail, and electronic	Administration can be costly and time consuming
	Reach large sample	Nonresponse rate can impede sufficient power
	Established methodology	Subject to recall bias
Administrative data	Access to large population	Accuracy identifying young people in foster care
	Assess longitudinal trends	Only describes individuals who use service
	Analyze less frequent conditions or outcomes through aggregated data	Available data variables may not match research goals
	Assist with local, state, and national evaluation	Incomplete and/or irregular data
Electronic health records	Includes clinical, laboratory, treatment, and billing data	Potential for poor data quality
	Assess feasibility	Bias with data capture or toward population subsets with barriers to accessing care
	Assist with recruitment	Incomplete and/or irregular data
	Streamline data collection	Ethical concerns for confidentiality and privacy

limitations of EHR data and guidelines[21] for reporting EHR-based investigation when considering EHRs as a data source.

Cross-system partnerships and data linkages are beneficial to research relevant to young people in foster care.[11] Yet, success of these initiatives would be further strengthened through the development of a core set of mutually agreed upon short- and long-term outcomes and measures pertinent not only to health care, child welfare, and other stakeholder systems but also to young people placed in foster care and their families, caregivers, and communities. Such efforts require dedication to the meaningful inclusion of individuals and communities with lived experience related to foster care as well as flexibility when considering what measures should be prioritized for mutual learning and impact (further described in the section Approaching Research With Communities and Across Systems, later in this chapter). As shown in **Box 39–1**, previous work provides a guide for these efforts, with well-being outcome domains relevant across the lifespan.[22]

Designing and Delivering Health Care

At the practice level, pediatricians and other clinicians must be prepared to attend to the complex health and social needs found among young people in foster care. Literature outlines the ideal characteristics of care for these young people, including expert guidelines on how high-quality care should be delivered.[4] The current literature is less robust regarding how to implement and disseminate high-quality care principles across different settings and systems—health, child welfare, education and public health—to more broadly support well-being and promote health.[23] Results from previous research indicate that the pediatric medical home model facilitates positive outcomes among youth in foster care.[24] More recent primary care initiatives, such as population health–based and value-based payment efforts, offer additional opportunities to improve access to and use of primary care services, reduce the use of antipsychotic medications, and incentivize individualized wrap-around services.[25] Further research is necessary to evaluate health care design, delivery, and payment models relevant to young people in foster care and account for short- and long-term outcomes.

Examining Policies Seeking to Preserve Families and Prevent Removal

Structural racism, as well as social and structural drivers of health, produce significant racial, ethnic, socioeconomic, and disability disproportionalities

Box 39–1

Well-Being Life Domains

Educational and economic: Gain access to quality early learning, schools, job training, and learning that promote the skills and ability to attain employment, self-sufficiency, and personal fulfillment.

Social and emotional: Maximize individual growth and development and promote well-being by cultivating resilience and supportive, nurturing relationships.

Mental health and wellness: Support and manage mental health and wellness through appropriate, timely, accessible, and quality services, supports, and activities.

Physical health: Maximize physical health, strengths, and functioning through access to green spaces, active environments, nutritious food, safe water, adequate housing, and effective preventive and curative health care.

Safety: Be physically, mentally, and emotionally safe and free from violence, fear of harm, abuse, and neglect.

Spiritual: Establish a state of harmony with oneself and others while appreciating the diversity of beliefs and cultures that enrich the community in which they live.

Justice: Gain access to a sensitive, fair, financially accessible justice system to ensure that individuals can thrive in communities and engage with organizations that understand the implications of inequities and injustice and intentionally support practice and policy efforts designed to eliminate both.

Equity: Live in an environment free of discrimination that provides equal access to services, opportunities, and resources; promotes self-determination; and allows individuals to realize their full potential.

Reproduced from Casey Family Programs. The Path to Transformation: A Framework to Promote Family and Child Well-Being. 2021.

within the child welfare system.[8,26,27] Empowering families to provide safe, stable, and nurturing environments through supportive social, health care, and child welfare policies is not only an attractive method to prevent placement in foster care but also an essential component for equity, justice, and respect. Public benefit programs, which provide defined economic and resource supports, are social policy levers to support families while reducing child welfare involvement and maltreatment.[28] Increasingly, states have implemented public benefit programs; however, adoption of such programming varies by state. Expanding evidence relevant to socioeconomic policy, health care, and child welfare systems is a critical area for further study.

Many states, tribes, and territories have opted for Title IV-E waivers for flexibility in testing innovative approaches to child welfare service delivery and financing. An assessment of Title IV-E waivers demonstrated fewer out-of-home placements and, for those children who were removed, increased placement stability, kinship placement, and permanency with less time in foster care.[29] More recently, the Family First Prevention Service Act (FFPSA) enables use of Title IV funds to support families with preventive services prior to a child's removal in addition to reducing the use of congregate care.[30] Many states have enacted legislation and implemented practices and programs to align with FFPSA requirements. The Title IV-E Prevention Services Clearinghouse, created by the Administration for Children and Families and the US Department of Health and Human Services to conduct rigorous and transparent evaluation of programs and services, provides useful evidence-based recommendations as states enhance support for children and families and prevent foster placement.[31] Research that examines child and family health outcomes in the context of policies, practices, and programs that seek to prevent maltreatment and preserve families is crucial to assess the impact of FFPSA, as is prioritization of family-setting placements and permanency for young people who enter foster care.

Approaching Research With Communities and Across Systems

Research that seeks to benefit the health and well-being of young people placed in foster care is strengthened by including individuals, families, and communities who have lived experience, defined as direct effects from placement in foster care.[32] Often, marginalized individuals and communities have been excluded from and express mistrust of research.[33] Much of the current literature centered on young people in foster care reflects the interests of the multiple child-serving agencies and systems involved, including health care, child welfare, court, and educational systems. However, the obligations and priorities of these parties may not reflect the priorities and goals of the young people they serve.[7,34]

Increasingly, greater value and importance have been placed on engaging those with lived experience as experts who can inform the creation and evaluation of interventions, services, and policies (**Figure 39–1**).[35,36] Expert individuals and communities provide diverse perspectives and voices according to culture, race, ethnicity, socioeconomic class, geographic setting, sexual orientation, and gender identity. Engaging lived-experience experts in research is advantageous not only for investigators but also for the young experts themselves.[22,32,34,35] First, engagement increases equity, advances knowledge, and engenders trust. Next, early and ongoing conversations with experts allows investigators to ensure research efforts are both relevant to and disseminated among communities with lived experience. Finally, engagement can impart knowledge and build skills among individual and community participants.[37]

Additional work is needed to understand how agencies and systems incorporate research involving lived-experience experts into practice, programming, and policy.[22,32] Community-based participatory research and youth-led participatory action research are two action research frameworks that include communities and young people as genuine partners through meaningful participation across the research continuum.[34,35,37] **Figure 39–2** offers a process example of engaging and partnering with individuals and communities who have lived experience relevant to foster care research endeavors.[38] **Table 39-2** provides potential research topics and approaches relevant to research involving young people in foster care.

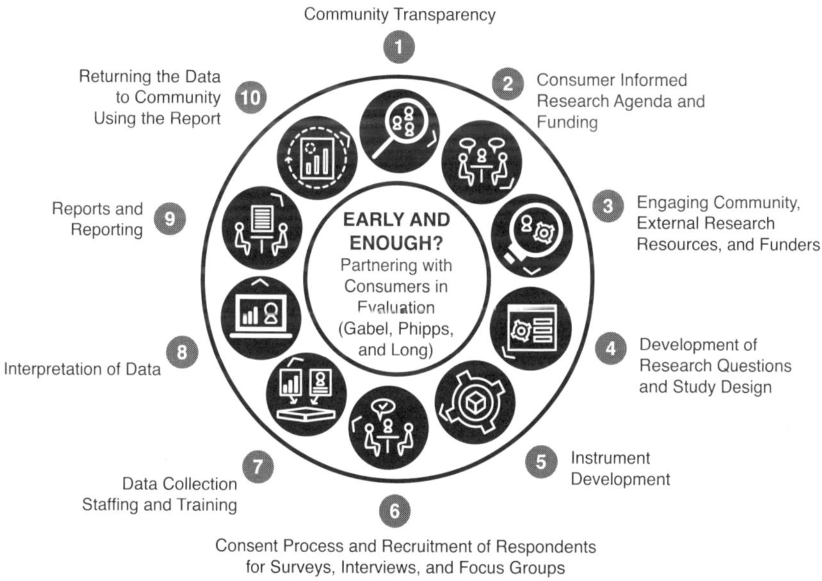

Issues Throughout:

- Respect (scheduling, compensation, acknowledgement)
- Trauma practice
- Race, gender, diversity must be considered
- Full representation, not tokenism (inc. training of consumers)
- Pragmatic schedule and budget
- Researcher capability and readiness

Figure 39–1. Opportunities to partner with lived-experience experts during research.

Reproduced with permission from George G, Long T, Phipps T. Early and enough? Partnering with consumers in evaluation processes. KEMPE Center National Conference. October 6, 2020.

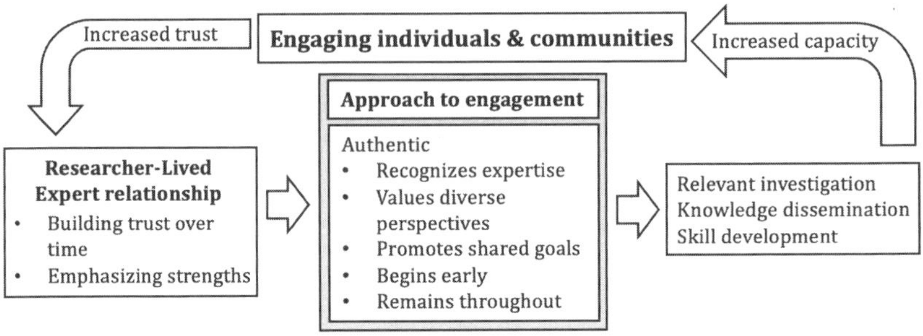
Increased trust
Engaging individuals & communities
Increased capacity
Approach to engagement
Researcher-Lived Expert relationship
• Building trust over time
• Emphasizing strengths
Authentic
• Recognizes expertise
• Values diverse perspectives
• Promotes shared goals
• Begins early
• Remains throughout
Relevant investigation
Knowledge dissemination
Skill development

Figure 39–2. Approach to engaging lived experience experts with research.

Adapted from Seekamp S, Ey LA, Tsiros MD. Partnering with families known to child protection in an interprofessional context. *Child Abuse Negl.* 2023;145:106426.

Understanding Regulations and Protections

Federal requirements provide guidance for research involving children. Subpart D of the Health and Human Service regulations at 45 CFR part 46 also contains additional conditions for research involving children who are wards of the state (ie, placed in foster care).[39] Federal requirements differentiate research according to risk and benefit. Minimal risk is defined as "the probability and magnitude of harm or discomfort anticipated in the research are not greater in and of themselves than those ordinarily encountered in daily life or during the performance of routine physical or psychological examinations or tests."[40] For children, including young people in foster care, research participation may or may not represent greater than minimal risk. Youth in foster care may participate in research with minimal risk contingent on securing informed consent (further described in the section Considering Consent and Assent, later in this chapter). With research involving greater than minimal risk, results must (1) have direct benefit to the child or contribute to the child's well-being or (2) produce generalizable knowledge relevant to a child's health or social condition. Any research including children in foster care that exceeds minimal risk without direct benefit carries 2 additional requirements. First, most enrolled children must be external to foster care and the research must relate to their placement in foster care. Second, a child-specific advocate must be appointed. Independent from both the study team and the child welfare agency, the appointed advocate must have sufficient expertise and agree to act in the child's best interest for the duration of the child's participation in the research.

Table 39–2. Sample Health Research Topics for Children Who Experience Foster Care

Topic	Example Research Question	Potential Research Approaches
Principles of care	How are high-quality care principles implemented and disseminated across clinical settings?	Effectiveness–implementation hybrid design
Population health	How might physical and behavioral health status change among youth following entry into foster care?	Observational cohort study with time-series analysis
Placement type and stability	How might long-term health outcomes differ by placement type? How do service factors (eg, time to service, continuity of services) affect placement stability?	Longitudinal observational design with latent class analysis Observational design with time-to-event analysis
Emancipation	What are health and well-being priorities among young people preparing for, and following, emancipation from foster care? What is the most effective strategy or combination of strategies to facilitate adolescent-to-adult health care transition for young adults emancipating from foster care?	Community-based participatory research survey or questionnaire Mixed-method qualitative-quantitative framework
Systems	What data sources, tools, and resources are needed to strengthen collaboration between health care, child welfare, and public health systems to improve health outcomes?	Mixed-method qualitative-quantitative framework
Policy	How might programs such as Chafee and extended foster care influence health outcomes among young people emancipated from foster care? Among evidence-based programs and services available to states, territories and tribes through Family First Prevention Service Act, what programs and services produce the best health and social outcomes for children and families?	Observational case-control study; mixed methods Prospective observational study with quasi-experimental analysis
Financing	What Medicaid payment models result in the highest quality care and best health outcomes among children placed in foster care?	Comparative effectiveness analysis

Institutional review boards (IRBs) review and monitor biomedical research involving human subjects to ensure that the rights and welfare of participants are adequately protected both before and during the research. To achieve this aim, an IRB reviews research protocols and related material to approve, require modifications in, or deny a research proposal. While familiarity with federal requirements for additional protections specific to youth in foster care is helpful, investigators should have early and ongoing discussion of proposed studies with their local IRB. Following initial approval, an IRB will monitor to ensure that sufficient protections remain for human subject participants through periodic reviews of the study.

Considering Consent and Assent

If young people are involved with research activities, informed consent is required. Informed consent and youth assent are key materials reviewed by an IRB, because federal regulations require parental consent and child assent for research involving children. These concepts are defined as follows:

- *Informed consent* is the process through which an individual can voluntarily indicate their willingness to participate in a research study after receiving and understanding research-related information.
- *Assent* is "a child's affirmative agreement to participate in research."[40] Assent is required when a child is not yet legally able to give consent. Most often applicable to young people age 7 to 18 years, the child's age and developmental and psychological status are considered when determining if a child is capable of providing assent.

Informed consent must be completed prior to recruiting and including young people in foster care for participation in research. Frequently, young people in care do not have traditional caregivers who can provide consent. Greiner and colleagues[3] found 14 different combinations of individuals—biological parents, judges, caseworkers, and caregivers with youth assent—identified to obtain informed consent for minimal-risk research among minors in foster care. Inconsistent approaches to seeking informed consent result in the unnecessary exclusion of young people in care from research overall, as well as from research on foster-specific topics such as placement stability and health outcomes. The adoption of a standard, universal consent approach would clarify which individual(s) have authority to provide consent and serve as a resource in shared decision-making and communication. Pediatricians can advocate for such an approach through education and collaboration with agencies, courts, and other organizations serving young people in foster care.[3,6]

Role of the Pediatrician

Pediatricians are uniquely positioned to support and lead research relevant to youth placed in foster care. Opportunities exist across the research continuum, such as

- Reviewing literature
- Organizing a journal club at their clinic
- Encouraging young people to participate in research
- Reviewing health data to inform clinical interventions and quality improvement efforts
- Collaborating with researchers to support projects as a coinvestigator
- Leading research efforts as a primary investigator

Conclusion

Establishing and expanding a robust evidence base that improves care for and outcomes among young people in foster care is essential. Pediatricians and child health advocates can accelerate this critical work by advocating for, supporting, and leading research that addresses the needs of this population.

Key Takeaways

- Research is a valuable tool for understanding the lived experience of young people in foster care and their caregivers while aiming to improve care.
- Interprofessional and community partnerships offer opportunities for authentic, meaningful research processes and outcomes informed by young people in foster care and their caregivers.
- Researchers must be familiar with local and federal regulations and protections specific to including young people in foster care.
- Pediatricians are uniquely positioned to advance research relevant to young people in foster care.

Part 6. Cross-Systems Collaboration

CHAPTER

40

Systems Involved in the Life of a Child in Foster Care: An Overview

Adrienne W. Carmack, MD, FAAP
Molly Curtin Berkoff, MD, MPH, FAAP

It is helpful for the pediatrician who is working with youth and families involved in the foster care system to understand both child welfare, including the source of child welfare funding and associated policy or legislative requirements, and the systems influencing the delivery of care to this population. Becoming familiar with the funding requirements for families involved in child welfare as well as the many different systems will help avoid delays in accessing care, including medication and other treatments. Gaining a general understanding of the court, juvenile justice, and school systems, as well as placement types, will ensure clarity of roles and expectations. This chapter provides an overview of child welfare funding and legislation as well as several of the systems most frequently encountered by clinicians caring for this population. State legislation varies and may be more specific than federal legislation. The Child Welfare Information Gateway (www.childwelfare.gov) is a good resource for further information.

Overview of the Child Welfare System

The goal of child welfare is to promote the safety, permanency, and well-being of children and families. Child welfare systems typically take the following actions:

- **Investigate reports:** Receive and investigate reports of possible child abuse and neglect.
- **Support families:** Provide prevention services to families that need assistance protecting and caring for their children to prevent entry into foster care.

- **Provide temporary safe shelter:** Arrange for children to live with kin (including fictive kin) or foster families or another placement type when they are not safe at home.
- **Seek to return children to their families when safety has improved or find other permanent arrangements:** Arrange for reunification, adoption, or other permanent family connections for children leaving foster care.
- **Prepare youth for independent living when other permanency options have not been identified.**

Service delivery for child welfare systems in the United States varies by state, but each state must comply with federal legislation. The federal government determines the funding and the regulatory guidelines, and the states determine how the programs will be implemented. The majority of states have a state-administered child welfare agency.[1] Nine states use county-administered service delivery: California, Colorado, Minnesota, New York, North Carolina, North Dakota, Ohio, Pennsylvania, and Virginia. Nevada and Wisconsin are hybrid, including service administration at both the state and county levels.

The following is a brief overview of federal legislation that has significantly influenced current child welfare work:

- In 1974, the **Child Abuse Prevention and Treatment Act** (CAPTA)[2,3] was passed to allow federal funds to support the development of a variety of functions for child welfare treatment. CAPTA legislation has been reauthorized multiple times with amendments and further requirements for funding.
- The **Adoption and Safe Families Act (ASFA)** of 1997 (PL-105-89)[4] refocused the foster care system on the rights of children to health, safety, and permanency. It mandated that a permanency plan must be made no later than 12 months after the child's entry into care and that states begin termination of parental rights once a child had been in foster care for 15 of the previous 22 months as long as there was no compelling reason not to do so. It also provided increased adoption subsidies.
- With the passage of the **Fostering Connections to Success and Increasing Adoptions Act (FCSIAA)** of 2008 (PL 110-351),[5] states were required, among other provisions, to address educational stability and ensure all school-age children in foster care were enrolled in school. Additionally, it required all states to develop a state health care plan to coordinate health care of the youth in care, and to work with pediatricians to develop these plans.
- In 2011, the **Child and Family Services Improvement and Innovation Act**[6] required states to not only develop a child's health plan but also submit a

plan for oversight of the use of psychotropic prescription medications. States also are expected to address the developmental needs of young children in foster care and the emotional needs of all youth from the effects of the trauma they have experienced.

- In 2018, the **Family First Prevention Services Act (FFPSA)** was passed. This act has a primary focus of keeping children and youth out of foster care and maintaining them safely in their homes.[7] Mental health and substance use treatment as well as in-home parenting skills programs can be covered by Title IV-E funding.[8] The legislation also included a goal to decrease the use of congregate care or group homes for children in custody and, when this type of care is used, to decrease the duration of time a youth requires placement in the facility.[9]

The compliance of states is monitored by federal plan approvals, audits, and reviews. Most of the federal child welfare programs are administered by the Children's Bureau, which is within US Department of Health and Human Services.[10] When a federal law is passed, it is the the role of the Children's Bureau to determine what actions are needed by states and tribes to meet the new requirements of a federal statute and to determine the funding requirements for distribution to the states and tribes. The overall focus of the Children's Bureau is to do the following:

- **Strengthen families** and prevent child abuse and neglect
- **Protect children** when abuse or neglect has occurred
- Ensure that every child and youth has a **permanent family** or family connection

The funding grants from the Children's Bureau that support and permit child welfare operations at the local level include the following[11]:

- IV-E Foster Care
- IV-E Adoption and Guardianship Assistance
- IV-E Prevention Services
- Chafee Services for Youth Formerly in Foster Care
- IV-B and CAPTA funding

Each of the federal grants comes with requirements. For instance, to maintain eligibility for Title IV-B services, states, tribes, and territories must develop a comprehensive 5-year child and family services plan (CFSP).[12] The CFSP outlines initiatives and activities the state, tribe, or territory will carry out in administering programs and services to promote the safety, permanency, and well-being of children and families. In years between CFSP submissions, states and tribes must submit an annual progress and services report.[12] Knowledge of these plans can help to identify the focus of a local child welfare agency in addition to other community and state partners. For example, North Carolina's plan includes a priority of alignment with the state's *Early Childhood Action Plan*[13] and *Opioid Action Plan*[14] in addition to descriptions of community agencies that help guide child welfare well-being and foster care permanency priorities.[15] While child welfare can identify the risk factors and gaps in services that led to children and youth coming into contact with the system, the services and treatment programs to help prevent further involvement with child welfare are done in partnership with community agencies. These service and treatment programs include health (physical and behavioral), education, law enforcement, early intervention, and home visiting.

Much attention has been placed on reshaping the child welfare system so that there is a larger commitment to access to equitable services and a focus on maintaining children safely in their homes.[16] It is helpful to think of child welfare agencies as part of a larger system of care in their state or county. A national focus includes developing, organizing, and restructuring systems to focus on the prevention of child abuse in addition to the prevention of removal of children and youth from their homes of origin. Funding from both the FFPSA and Title IV-B support evidence-based programs that intervene with services to families at risk for separation, in the hope of preventing a child from entering foster care, when possible. Knowledge of the child welfare system as part of a larger "well-being" system has grown. This has permitted the promotion of concepts such as strengthening of families to support the safety and well-being of children to include the prevention of abuse and neglect. Some states have created well-being plans or agencies to help with ensuring a new focus on prevention and a goal of avoiding foster care placement. Examples are as follows:

- **Division of Child and Family Well-Being with the North Carolina Department of Health and Human Services.**[17] A primary function is to ensure oversight of the state's systems that help to serve families. The division monitors the challenges faced by families that lead to an interaction with the child welfare system and helps to invest in solutions to avoid out-of-home placement. Services included in this division include a state psychiatric access line to help improve support for the primary care physician caring for children and youth with behavioral needs, as well as investing in parental substance use treatment and recovery teams.[18]
- **Maine Child Safety and Family Well-Being Plan.**[19,20] This plan outlines key strategies for legislative bills and outlines specific budget priorities with a goal of reducing the need for out-of-home care and involvement

with child welfare. The original plan focused on efforts to promote keeping children safe in their homes of origin, the subsequent version provides opportunities for all members of the community to consider how to support the well-being of children and families.

Foster Care and Placement

A role of the medical home is to ensure child welfare has a clear understanding of the well-being needs of the child, to ensure the ability of the potential placement to meet those needs. Additionally, the medical home can assist with a caregiver's knowledge of the child's well-being needs upon initial placement. This can help ensure clear expectations, identify needed supports, and build strong relational health, which can set the foundation to promote a child's resilience.[21] Placement stability is critical for children in foster care and strongly associated with improved outcomes.[22]

The decision of where a child can be placed upon entering foster care rests with the child welfare agency. The following is a brief overview of placement types (see also Chapter 18, Out-of-Home Placements):

1. The priority is for children to be placed with relatives when possible (ie, kinship care; may also be a close family member, or "fictive kin"). Kinship placement can include children in the formal custody of child welfare. However, not all children placed in kinship care are in child welfare custody.
2. Family foster care is provided by caregivers who have received formal training on the caregiving needs for children in child welfare custody. The amount may vary, as some elect to receive extra training in order to provide care for children with more specialized health care needs (therapeutic or treatment foster care).[23] They receive formal monitoring from child welfare agencies.
3. Residential or group homes generally provide care to larger groups of children who live in a congregate setting and do not have individual caregivers but are staffed by trained professionals. Some provide specific behavioral or psychiatric treatment for the children or youth at the facility.

Foster Care and the Court

Children in foster care are affected by several different types of court hearings.[24] Understanding the stage of the case will assist in identifying who has the ability to consent to medication and treatment as well as understanding if there is an ability to provide education to the court to ensure appropriate identification and treatment of well-being needs.

- **Adjudication.** Occurs after the child is removed and placed in foster care. The hearing is to determine if the child has been abused or neglected. If the judge does not find evidence to support a ruling of abuse or neglect, the child may be returned to their home of origin. If they are returned to their home of origin, it generally means the child is no longer in foster care.
- **Disposition.** Determination of ongoing placement if the child has been adjudicated abused or neglected. Additionally, the service plan will be set at this hearing. It is helpful for the court to understand any unique well-being needs at this time so the appropriate consent and understanding of priority of needs is set.
- **Review.** Addresses progress of the case and can address well-being issues for the child. This is another opportunity for the court to be aware of any unmet needs or changes to the youth's well-being needs.
- **Permanency.** Addresses ongoing needs of the child and family and if reasonable efforts have been made by the agency and caregivers of origin. A court hearing or administrative review will occur at least once every 6 months for children in foster care.[25]

For court proceedings, youth are represented by both an attorney and a guardian ad litem (GAL) or Court Appointed Special Advocate (CASA). The purpose of the GAL and/or CASA is to advocate for the children's best interests in a court hearing.

Foster Care and Juvenile Justice

It is well known that interaction with the child welfare system for a youth increases the chance for involvement in the juvenile justice system.[26] Unfortunately, most states do not have administrative integration of youth involved in both systems. This means a youth who is dually involved may have separate social workers for both systems and information about their well-being needs may not be shared in a consistent fashion. Advocating for the needs of youth who are dually involved is therefore an opportunity for their medical home provider, who can frame those needs in the context of both youth development and traumatic stress. Pediatricians can work to improve collaboration between health care professionals (physical, developmental, and behavioral health) caring for both groups of youth to ensure comprehensive care is provided and duplication is avoided. Sharing of health care information between systems should be prioritized, so access to care is continuously provided, well-being needs are met, and information is updated accurately. Assistance with prioritization of health care needs should be provided to avoid missed evaluation and treatment of urgent conditions.

Foster Care and the School System

In 2015, the Every Student Succeeds Act (ESSA), a new federal education law, was signed.[27] A particular focus of ESSA was to ensure educational stability for youth in foster care to achieve improved educational outcomes.[27] Specifics include prioritizing that a child is maintained in their school of origin and, when that is not possible, to avoid delays in enrollment at a new school, including the requirement for the school of origin to enroll a youth in foster care at a new school without the typically required documents. Additionally, the school of origin must prioritize and immediately transfer records for that child to their new school.

Key Takeaways

- » To help build successful relationships, know the well-being priorities for the child welfare agency. Understanding and meeting the needs for child welfare will help promote strong relationships and better understanding of the needs of the children, youth, and families.
- » Be familiar with the systems interfacing with children, youth, and families to achieve better outcomes for this population. While many systems operate independently of each other, the medical home can be the bridge for communication.
- » Identify the physician-led care teams from the different systems that are involved in a youth's care so as to ensure quick and reliable communication.

CHAPTER

41

Privacy and Information Sharing

Mary V. Greiner, MD, MS, FAAP
Nathan M. Lutz, PhD
Eric S. Hall, PhD, MBA, FAMIA

Introduction

Caring for children in foster care presents unique challenges, particularly when it comes to sharing and managing health information. Clinicians, child welfare professionals, families of origin, foster and kinship caregivers, and youth themselves must navigate complex privacy laws and regulations to ensure the best care. This chapter discusses the intricacies of health care privacy laws, including the Health Insurance Portability and Accountability Act (HIPAA)[1] and the 21st Century Cures Act,[2] as well as their implications for children and adolescents in foster care. It also reviews the role of electronic health records (EHRs), health information exchanges (HIEs), data-sharing platforms, and patient portals in managing and sharing health information. It is critical to access and disclose information to provide timely and comprehensive health care while also protecting privacy and confidentiality for youth in foster care and their caregivers. By skillfully navigating privacy and confidentiality laws and policies using available technologies, clinicians can offer optimal care for children in foster care, who often face substantial inequities that can lead to poor health outcomes.

Understanding EHRs, HIEs, Data-Sharing Platforms, and Patient Portals

EHRs

EHRs[3] are digital versions of patients' medical records that store information such as medical history, diagnoses, medications, treatment plans, and test results. EHRs aim to streamline and improve the quality of patient care by allowing clinicians to store, access, and share patients' medical information more efficiently and securely.

HIEs

HIEs[4] facilitate electronic sharing of health information among health care organizations. Using nationally recognized standards, these exchanges enable improved care coordination and communication while maintaining patient privacy and information security. HIEs enable clinicians to access and exchange patients' medical information, such as medical history, laboratory results, and medication lists.

Data-Sharing Platforms

A variety of data-sharing platforms have been designed to improve interoperability of data and create a more comprehensive and multisystem view of a child's well-being.[5] Such platforms have demonstrated time savings and improved care delivery for health care systems[6] and child welfare systems.[7] These data exchanges incorporate information from multiple sources that may include health care systems, child welfare organizations, education, and more.

Patient Portals

Patient portals[8] are secure online platforms that allow patients to access their personal health information, such as medical records, test results, and medications. For patients under the age of 18, proxy access (ie, allowing an individual to view the medical records of another person), is often granted to a parent or legal guardian. These portals provide greater control over health information and facilitate communication between patients/caregivers and their clinicians, including direct messaging. Adolescents can often access their own patient portals and may be able to designate proxy access. Institutional policies vary on who is eligible for proxy access (eg, foster/kinship caregivers, child welfare professionals, families of origin) and the level of information that is shared with proxies, taking local adolescent confidentiality laws into consideration.

Overview of Health Care Privacy Laws

HIPAA

HIPAA[1] was established to set standards for protecting sensitive patient information, particularly that which is stored electronically.[9] Title II of HIPAA includes 5 rules to enforce administrative simplification, 2 of which have direct implications on clinical practice: the privacy rule and the security rule.

HIPAA's privacy rule governs the use and disclosure of protected health information (PHI) and applies to clinicians, health plans, and health care clearinghouses. It requires clinicians to disclose PHI under specific circumstances (for example, suspected child abuse or when ordered by a court). However, for any other disclosure, written authorization must be obtained, and clinicians are advised to share only the minimum necessary information. The privacy rule also includes patients' *right to access*, which grants individuals the right to their own health information and requires clinicians to release information to the patient or an authorized third party upon request. The security rule introduces 3 additional types of security safeguards for PHI that is stored electronically: administrative (eg, training, development of procedures), physical (eg, controlling access to equipment, placement of computer monitors), and technical (eg, network access and configuration).

21st Century Cures Act

The 21st Century Cures Act[2] (commonly known as the Cures Act) is a federal law enacted in 2016 that aims to accelerate medical product development and bring innovations to patients more quickly and efficiently. The Cures Act encourages the seamless and secure exchange of electronic health information among clinicians, patients, and other stakeholders, while maintaining the privacy and security of individuals' health information. A key aspect of the Cures Act is preventing information blocking, which occurs when a health care entity prevents or materially discourages access, exchange, or use of electronic health information. By preventing information blocking, the Cures Act aims to improve transparency and the flow of health information to patients and other authorized individuals. However, restrictions on information blocking may result in releasing information to patients that has not yet been reviewed by their clinician and creates new challenges in protecting adolescent confidentiality.[10]

Implications for Children and Adolescents in Foster Care

Confidentiality

When a child is removed from their family of origin and placed in protective custody (foster care), several issues related to the delivery of health care services may arise.[11] Among these are issues related to consent for services and confidentiality of medical information. After a child is removed from the home, legal custody is granted to the county or state, and these children live with adults who do not have custody of them. These caregivers, who often bring the children to their medical appointments, do not have the ability to provide medical consent, and they sometimes are not authorized to receive confidential medical information. To ensure that the rights of children in foster care are protected, it is important that clinicians keep records of medical decision-making and health information-sharing abilities as well as limitations for each individual involved in the child's care (eg, child welfare professionals, caregivers, guardians ad litem [GALs]) by adhering to appropriate documentation (eg, court orders).

Access to Medical Information

Pediatricians should allow reasonable access to custodians (child welfare professionals) and court-appointed attorneys (ie, GALs) to the medical information within the confines of applicable federal and state law and privacy regulations. Although the caregivers of children in protective custody (eg, foster or kinship care providers) are not their legal guardians, they are responsible for day-to-day caregiving responsibilities, many of which can only occur if they have access to relevant health information. While caregivers may not be granted access to the complete medical record, they must be able to communicate about appointments, manage medications, and access the minimal amount of information necessary to manage the health of children in their care. It is also important to consider that when a child is in the temporary custody of child welfare, the family of origin typically maintains rights to receive medical information, may need to provide consent for certain medical decisions (such as surgeries), and is often encouraged to attend medical appointments when safe and appropriate.

Special Considerations for Adolescents

Adolescents in foster care may have special confidentiality and consent considerations related to sexual and reproductive health (eg, contraception, pregnancy, sexually transmitted infections), mental health, and substance use.[12] In these cases, minors with the capacity to consent have the right to limited confidentiality. There may be other circumstances, such as gender diversity, that require special consideration of privacy and confidentiality within the confines of state regulations. Adolescents should be able to access their confidential information in a safe and secure manner through the patient portal. Depending on state regulations, consent of the minor may be required for sharing confidential information with child welfare professionals, foster and kinship caregivers, or family of origin. Limits to adolescent confidentiality include concerns for abuse or neglect or risk of harm to self or others. Clinicians should review the rights of minors with capacity to consent in their states. Due to the social complexity for youth in foster care, typically with multiple adults serving in different roles (such as custodian or caregiver), respecting the adolescent in foster care's right to consent to sensitive services and be afforded confidentiality may be difficult but is critically important. Notably, one study found that more than half of adolescent accounts with outbound patient portal messages have been accessed by guardians[13]; however, it is unclear if youth in foster care also have caregivers accessing their portals, making confidential care more challenging. Adolescents in foster care may also be parents themselves and may have rights to medical information for their child (see Chapter 22, Pregnant and Parenting Teens).

Best Practices for Information Sharing

As children remain in foster care longer, they tend to experience multiple placement changes. To optimally serve children in foster care, clinicians must have access to ongoing documentation of complex and dynamic family and living structures. They also must know who can make decisions for the child and who can receive information about that child, and they must have a historical record as living circumstances change. It is important for clinicians to communicate about medical decision-making and health information sharing with each individual involved in the child's care (eg, child welfare professionals, caregivers, GALs) with appropriate documentation (court orders, for example). These tasks can be very challenging in complex social circumstances, and ensuring clarity, accuracy, and consistency in practice requires collaboration and communication between the multiple systems serving these children (for example, between the health care system and the child welfare system).

Sharing Information With Child Welfare

As the child's custodian, child welfare professionals have the legal right to access the child's medical information. Finding ways to share information in efficient and clear mechanisms that can verify the child's legal status, such as through data-sharing platforms,[5] is an important part of health care delivery for children in foster care.

Sharing Information With Foster Caregivers

Clinicians should share relevant medical information with foster and kinship caregivers to ensure proper care and support for children in foster care. This may include information about medical conditions, treatments, medications, and any necessary follow-up care. It is essential to maintain open communication with caregivers while respecting the privacy and confidentiality of the child and family of origin.

There are challenges when it comes to granting foster caregivers access to medical information. In some health care systems, patient portal proxy access is not permitted for foster caregivers for several reasons, including

- An inability to monitor a patient's entrance into and exit from foster care, making it difficult to manage information access effectively
- Frequent placement changes, which are difficult to manage and keep track of in terms of information access
- The presence of sensitive information related to the family of origin in clinic notes, which should be kept confidential from foster caregivers

Overcoming such challenges requires careful implementation of patient portals specifically designed for use by caregivers, with appropriate limitations on the duration of access (ensuring access is terminated when the child leaves the placement) and sufficient authentication methods to prevent inappropriate access. Data-sharing platforms with child welfare organizations can support these limitations by providing up-to-date information on custody and legal status.

This underscores the importance of clear communication between clinicians and foster and kinship caregivers, as well as adherence to legal and compliance guidelines when sharing medical information. Clinicians should work closely with their legal and compliance teams to ensure that they are sharing necessary information with foster and kinship caregivers while maintaining privacy and confidentiality standards.

Access to Medical Information by Family of Origin

Families of origin must be considered in information sharing in patient portals, as families typically maintain rights to medical information and participate in medical decision-making. Access to health information can be an important mechanism to support the parent–child relationship and efforts toward reunification. Access must therefore be provided in a safe manner and implemented in such a way that allows flexibility for change. For example, if a safety concern arises or the child's legal status changes (such as reunification with the family of origin or termination of parental rights), changes in access will be necessary. It is of the utmost importance that clinicians protect potentially confidential information, such as the name and contact information of the foster family or placement location.

Access to Medical Information by GALS and Court Appointed Special Advocates

GALs and Court Appointed Special Advocates have a court appointment that supports access to health information, including access to medical records, in order to represent a child's best interest to the court. They may only access confidential medical information for children in foster care through a subpoena or written consent from authorized persons. Clinicians should seek guidance from their health information management and legal and compliance teams when faced with requests for medical information from these parties.

Sharing Information With Clinicians

When referring a child in foster care to another clinician, it is crucial to share pertinent medical history and other relevant information to facilitate proper diagnosis and treatment. This may include records of previous medical evaluations, treatments, medications, and any known allergies or medical conditions. Because children in foster care often have disruptions in clinicians, this information exchange is particularly important to prevent omissions or duplications in care (such as trialing a medication that has previously not worked well for a child).

Sharing Information With Other Entities

In some cases, clinicians may need to share medical information with other entities involved in the child's care, such as foster care placement agencies, schools, or other support services. This should be done in compliance with applicable privacy laws.

Improving data interoperability to allow cross-sector automated data-sharing between systems including health care and mental health systems, child welfare systems, educational systems, juvenile justice, and others offers an opportunity to break down silos and support coordinated assessments, planning, and execution of care, thereby improving foster care outcomes.[14]

Conclusion

Caring for children and adolescents in foster care presents unique challenges for clinicians, particularly when it comes to managing privacy and confidentiality concerns. Clinicians can be at risk of disclosing confidential information that causes harm or failing to share information that prevents effective health care delivery. Familiarizing oneself with relevant health care privacy laws, including HIPAA, the 21st Century Cures Act, and state and local policies, can provide a solid foundation for understanding the implications of these laws on the care of children in foster care. By employing best practices for information sharing, clinicians can support these children by coordinating care and improving the health outcomes of this vulnerable population. By maintaining communication and collaboration with all parties involved in the child's care, clinicians can help create a supportive environment that fosters the child's well-being and success.

Key Takeaways

- Following local and state laws, pediatricians and other clinicians must access and disclose information to provide timely and comprehensive health care, while also protecting privacy and confidentiality for youth in foster care and their caregivers.
- Information sharing regarding youth in foster care requires collaboration and communication between the multiple systems involved in the care of the child, such as the health care system, the child welfare system, and others.
- Adolescents in foster care require special privacy and confidentiality considerations.
- Technology, through EHR portals, HIEs, and data-sharing portals, can support information exchange for youth in foster care.

Part 7. Legislation, Policy, and Advocacy

CHAPTER 42

Advocacy and Public Policy

Zach Laris, MPH
Keri Hope Richmond
Jeff Hudson, MA

Advocacy plays a crucial role in shaping child welfare policy. This chapter highlights the pediatrician's role in advocating for the health and well-being of children in foster care at the local, state, and federal levels. After a look back at child welfare policies over the years, the discussion proceeds to the current policy landscape, ideals for systems reform, and the pediatrician's role in advocating for changes that support children and their families and caregivers equitably.

Overview of the Pediatrician's Role in Child Welfare Policy and Advocacy

Advocacy is simple: it is speaking up on behalf of children and caregivers on issues that affect their health and well-being. Advocacy is also speaking up on behalf of fellow pediatricians when issues arise that affect the practice of pediatrics. From advocating in the halls of Congress to change child welfare policy to meeting with local school boards to discuss access to physical education, advocacy can improve the lives of children and their caregivers. As part of the natural course of the practice of medicine, pediatricians advocate for their patients. For example, pediatricians advocate by educating parents about vaccine safety and efficacy, discussing sensitive health topics with adolescent patients, and ensuring that insurance will cover the care patients need. Pediatricians occupy a unique role in the lives of children and their caregivers. Not only do caregivers rely on them to provide optimal medical care to their children, but they also know that the clinic is a safe place to discuss issues and seek guidance. Pediatricians' lived experience positions them as experts to local, state, and federal policymakers on children's health and well-being issues. This position allows pediatricians to influence policymaking decisions and raise awareness of issues in the clinic or community to policymakers. (See **Box 42–1**)

The same reasons that pediatricians are effective in those forms of advocacy also make them compelling messengers on child welfare policy issues at the local, state, and federal levels. Pediatricians with direct experience caring for children in or at risk of entering the child welfare system intuitively recognize that so many factors that affect their health and well-being go beyond the practice of clinical medicine. As mandated reporters, even those who do not yet care directly for children in foster care carry daily the responsibility of evaluating and reporting concerns about maltreatment. These experiences make pediatricians critical contributors to child welfare policy deliberations as experts and advocates. Understanding deeply these strengths and the unique point of view they bring will enable pediatricians to maximize the effectiveness of their child welfare policy advocacy.

Pediatricians' Child Welfare Policy Value Proposition

Effective advocacy rests on a foundation of self-understanding. Each stakeholder in any policy discussion has areas where they are either the lead voice of expertise and authentic representation, a contributing voice of validation for a perspective the lead voice is raising, or an observer of debate on a topic in which they do not have a direct stake but which may indirectly affect issues in which they do.

Pediatrician advocates can maximize their success by understanding the unique perspective pediatricians, American Academy of Pediatricians (AAP) state chapters, and the national AAP bring to child welfare policy issues. Rather than limit the pediatrician voice to purely clinical issues, this focuses pediatrician advocacy to effectively speak to the impact of policies on the health and well-being of children.

Other stakeholders may be best situated to make persuasive economic or moral arguments or to speak authoritatively on behalf of a workforce, like social workers. Pediatrician advocacy will be most effective when it is rooted in medical and public health expertise and authority. Grounding pediatrician advocacy in that perspective ensures a unique and powerful value proposition.

Box 42–1

Advocacy at Every Level of Government

Local Advocacy

Local advocacy is born out of the belief that children's health and well-being is influenced by social, economic, environmental, and political factors within a community.

Key policymakers:

- Mayor
- City council/local governing body
- School board
- Child welfare nonprofit organizations

State Advocacy

State advocacy seeks public policy change at the state level. Many issues and trends develop at the state level before making it to the national stage.

Key policymakers:

- Governor
- State legislatures
- State house/state senate committees overseeing child welfare
- State child welfare agency
- State health department

Federal Advocacy

Federal advocacy pursues public policy changes to improve children's health nationwide. Federal advocacy tends to develop more slowly but has the broadest reach and most funding.

Key policymakers:

- President
- Congress, with key committees including:
  - Senate Finance Committee
  - Senate HELP Committee
  - House Ways and Means Committee
  - House Energy and Commerce Committee
  - House/Senate Appropriations Committees
- Administration for Children and Families
- Children's Bureau

What Makes Pediatricians Effective Advocates

Pediatricians are trusted messengers. Parents, the public, and policymakers trust pediatricians. In polling, pediatricians consistently rank as highly trusted messengers. This means that policymakers take seriously what pediatricians have to say about child welfare policy.

Pediatricians ground their advocacy in science. When policymakers hear from pediatricians, they know they are discussing what the latest science says works best for children. AAP policy rests on the best available evidence, and that centers discussions on data and best practice rather than politics.

Pediatricians advocate for their patients. In advocacy, data are necessary but not sufficient. Policymakers need to see the human dimension of an issue to care. Pediatricians provide that critical perspective when they speak about the experiences of their patients in or at risk of entering the child welfare system, making abstract policy issues concrete.

The Role of Stakeholder Advocacy in Child Welfare Policy

Child advocacy movements played a crucial role in shaping all the child welfare policies discussed in this chapter. Advocacy groups, such as the Child Welfare League of America, Children's Defense Fund, and National Association of Social Workers, amplified the voices of children and advocated for their rights and well-being. These movements brought attention to issues affecting vulnerable children and influenced policy agendas, leading to legislative changes and reforms.

In all these foundational child welfare policies, the focus was primarily on protecting the children rather than protecting the entire family unit. Over time, child welfare policy expanded to encompass a broader range of services and support. There was a growing recognition that supporting families was essential to prevent the need for out-of-home placements. Programs addressing poverty, substance use, mental health, and other underlying factors were established to prevent separation, empower families, and promote their well-being.

Overview of Local, State, and Federal Advocacy

Within federal, state, and local advocacy, there are several distinct elements: the executive branch, the judicial branch, and the legislative branch of federal, state, and local governments. Advocacy targets these components at all 3 levels of government. Executive advocacy, sometimes referred to as administrative advocacy, seeks to change policies and programs run by the president, a governor, or a mayor and the agencies reporting to them. For example, the AAP routinely comments on proposed regulations at the federal level to ensure that changes in policy and programs or new policies and programs reflect AAP policy, are grounded in science, and meet the needs of children and their caregivers. Judicial advocacy involves educating judges, attorneys, and other members of the judicial system on the needs of children and their caregivers. For an example of judicial advocacy from the AAP, see **Box 42-2**. Legislative advocacy, the most common type of advocacy, involves advocating with congressional representatives, state representatives, and local elected representatives to affect a change in laws. In general, legislative advocacy focuses on the creation or reform of laws, executive advocacy focuses on the implementation and administration of existing laws, and judicial advocacy focuses on the interpretation and permissibility of laws under state and federal constitutions.

Box 42-2

AAP Joins US Supreme Court Case on the Indian Child Welfare Act

On June 15, 2023, the US Supreme Court upheld the Indian Child Welfare Act (ICWA), the 43-year-old federal law that reaffirms the rights of Tribal nations to be involved in child welfare matters and keeps American Indian and Alaska Native children connected to their community and culture. The AAP led an amicus brief from the medical community in this case defending ICWA, contributing to a comprehensive advocacy strategy organized by Tribal nations.

Local Advocacy

Advocacy at the local level seeks change in the community. It is important to remember that a community is not just a geographic location; it can also represent different ethnic, racial, and religious groups. Regardless of composition, location, and size, all communities can improve the health and well-being of children and caregivers.

Local advocacy is grounded in the economic, environmental, political, and social dynamics of the community. Access to health care, access to healthy foods, child maltreatment, exposure to violence, housing, poverty, and many more issues can be affected by these dynamics. For example, a pediatrician in a rural community sees the daily struggle of children and caregivers to secure healthy foods. The pediatrician then partners with a local community organization to purchase food and open a food pantry in their clinic, addressing some of the underlying causes of the challenges they see each day in their clinic.

State Advocacy

A state AAP chapter organizes pediatricians' state advocacy efforts, and joining a chapter provides a unified advocacy voice. State advocacy includes writing, calling, or meeting with state legislators on specific legislation; writing an op-ed for the local newspaper; partnering with other medical or social service organizations; and commenting on proposed state regulations, to name just a few activities. For example, AAP chapters continually advocate to increase access to and payment for care, such as with Medicaid expansion, and to increase immunization rates for children. **Box 42-3** describes what the New Mexico Pediatric Society advocated for in 2020.

Box 42-3

State Advocacy

In 2020, New Mexico enacted SB 168, which established its Fostering Connections program. This law extends the eligibility for foster care services to young adults up to 21 years of age. The New Mexico Pediatric Society advocated for the bill's passage.

Federal Advocacy

Federal advocacy includes writing, calling, or meeting with members of Congress on specific legislation; grassroots and social media calls to action; reviewing specific legislation and providing expert feedback and recommendations; and attending the AAP Advocacy Conference, among many other activities. For example, the AAP Federal Advocacy team routinely issues calls for action on matters being discussed in Congress, asking pediatricians to contact their members of Congress to advocate for the best interests of children and families.

Federal, state, and local advocacy are not siloed. All of these advocacy efforts are often interconnected and influence each other, and pediatrician advocacy at all 3 levels is often part of a coordinated and comprehensive strategy. For example, a local advocacy effort to improve safe areas to play may garner attention from a state legislator, who in turn introduces legislation to enact these local improvements in every community in the state. Once that state law is enacted, a member of Congress from that state may see these improvements as something that needs to be required on a national scale and introduce legislation to do just that.

A Look Back at Child Welfare Policy

The foundation of modern child welfare policy can be traced back to the Federal Aid for Dependent Children (FADC) law. Enacted in 1935 as part of the Social Security Act, FADC provided financial assistance to states to support children who were deprived of parental care. This landmark legislation marked a significant shift in societal recognition of the responsibility to protect and care for vulnerable children.

Building upon the FADC, the emergence of foster care and adoption services played a pivotal role in child welfare policy in the 1970s. Recognizing the importance of providing stable and nurturing environments for children, foster care provided temporary placements for children who could not remain with their birth families. Adoption services were also developed to provide permanent homes for children in need.

It was in the 1970s that child welfare policy really began to take shape, with the passage of the Child Abuse Prevention and Treatment Act (CAPTA). Enacted in 1974, this law aimed to address the issue of child abuse and neglect by providing federal funding, establishing reporting requirements, and promoting prevention and intervention strategies.

With FADC and CAPTA as guiding forces, early developments in child welfare policy aimed to address the needs of children who were at risk of experiencing maltreatment or deprived of a stable family environment. The focus was on ensuring that children were protected from neglect, abuse, and exploitation. State agencies were established to administer services and interventions to safeguard the well-being of children.

The Adoption and Safe Families Act (ASFA) of 1997 sought to expedite permanency for children in foster care by placing greater emphasis on timely decision-making and permanency planning. ASFA encouraged states to prioritize adoption as a permanent solution for children unable to reunify with their birth families. Child welfare policy has evolved over time to reflect growing scientific understanding of children's health and well-being. Throughout that evolution, pediatricians have been central to informing those deliberations, and pediatrician expertise will continue to be critical in this work. An understanding of the positive impacts of safe, stable, nurturing environments informed the most recent major federal policy, the Family First Prevention Services Act, discussed below.

Table 42–1 provides a timeline of key federal child welfare laws over the years.

Table 42–1. Child Welfare Policy Over the Years

Decade	Notable Child Welfare Policy
1970s	Child Abuse Prevention and Treatment Act Education for All Handicapped Children Act/Individuals With Disabilities Education Act Child Abuse Prevention and Treatment and Adoption Reform Act Indian Child Welfare Act
1980s	Adoption Assistance and Child Welfare Act Amendments of the Child Abuse Prevention and Treatment Act Omnibus Reconciliation Act of 1986 Child Abuse Prevention, Adoption, and Family Services Act
1990s	Child Abuse, Domestic Violence, Adoption, and Family Services Act Family Preservation and Support Services Act Amendments of the Child Abuse Prevention and Treatment Act Adoption and Safe Families Act Foster Care Independence Act
2000s	Promoting Safe and Stable Families Act Keeping Children and Families Safe Act Child and Family Services Improvement Act Fostering Connections to Success and Increasing Adoptions Act (Fostering Connections) Patient Protection and Affordable Care Act
2010s	Child Abuse Prevention and Treatment Act of 2010 Child and Family Services Improvement and Innovation Act RAISE Family Caregivers Act Family First Prevention Services Act Family First Transition Act Supporting Grandparents Raising Grandchildren Act
2020s	Abolishing Trafficking Act Trafficking Victims Prevention and Protection Reauthorization Act Supporting Foster Youth and Families Through the Pandemic Act Jackie Walorski Maternal and Child Home Visiting Reauthorization Act Supporting America's Children and Families Act

The Current Moment in Child Welfare

From its early beginnings to the present day, child welfare policy has evolved to encompass a more comprehensive and family-centered approach.

In recent years, a significant shift in culture has occurred, placing a renewed emphasis on keeping families together and ensuring policies that promote and incentivize child and family well-being. For years, science has confirmed that children fare best within families, which has led to an emphasis on family-based foster care placement when children are removed from their families. Now, an understanding of how closely the well-being of children is intertwined with the stability and support provided by their families of origin whenever safely possible has led to a reevaluation of traditional notions of child welfare, which often involved removing children from their homes and placing them in foster care. Instead, there is now a rising focus on providing families with the resources and support they need to overcome challenges and maintain a healthy and safe environment for their children.

An instrumental milestone in this movement was the enactment in 2018 of the AAP-championed Family First Prevention Services Act (commonly referred to as Family First). Family First marked a paradigm shift in child welfare policy, prioritizing prevention and support services over out-of-home placements and redirecting resources toward programs aimed at keeping families together.

The AAP played a critical role in advocating for Family First, helping stakeholders recognize the significance of preventing family separations and the importance of early intervention and support. The AAP worked closely with lawmakers, provided expert guidance and input on policy deliberations, and used its platform to raise awareness about the benefits of family preservation.

In this new movement, there is a growing recognition that system reforms and effective solutions must incorporate the lived experiences of individuals and address race equity. The principle of "nothing about us without us" has gained traction, emphasizing the inclusion of individuals and families with lived experiences in decision-making processes. Their insights and perspectives are crucial for designing policies and interventions designed to adequately serve and resonate with families' diverse needs.

Moreover, a more integrated approach to systems reform has emerged, acknowledging that the challenges faced by families are often interconnected and influenced by systemic inequities. Recognizing and addressing racial disparities is a critical aspect of this approach. Communities of color have historically faced disproportionate challenges in accessing resources and support, leading to a greater risk of family separations and adverse outcomes for children, particularly for Black and Indigenous children.

By centering race equity and adopting a comprehensive approach to systems reform, policymakers and practitioners can work toward dismantling systemic barriers that hinder family well-being. This involves implementing culturally responsive programs, ensuring equitable access to resources, and addressing the root causes of disparities. By doing so, we can create communities that support and uplift all families, regardless of their racial or ethnic background.

To promote family well-being effectively, a comprehensive set of solutions is needed. This includes strengthening support systems for families, providing accessible mental health services, addressing economic inequalities, and investing in quality education and child care. By adopting a preventive approach, these solutions can help families overcome challenges and promote resilience.

Additionally, community-based organizations and nonprofits play a vital role in supporting families and implementing effective interventions. By collaborating with these organizations, policymakers can tap into their expertise and leverage their connections within communities to ensure that solutions are tailored to meet the unique needs of diverse populations.

The shift in culture toward prioritizing family preservation and child well-being is a significant milestone in child welfare. The enactment of Family First and the advocacy efforts of organizations like the AAP have propelled this movement forward. By embracing a more comprehensive approach to systems reform, prioritizing lived experiences, and addressing race equity, we can create a future where all families have the support and resources they need to thrive. It is through collective efforts that we can build a brighter future for children and families, ensuring their well-being remains at the forefront of our society's priorities.

Core Tension Points in Child Welfare Policymaking

A truism of advocacy is that "where you sit is where you stand." In other words, the policy positions one takes are very often a function of their experiences, affiliations, and relationship to the policy itself. What can seem like an obvious solution to someone based on their proximity to the issue can be nonintuitive to someone without those experiences. When one sees advocating their preferred outcome as the only reasonable position to take, it is likely that they cannot see all of the factors motivating those with different positions on the issue.

A clear understanding of the trade-offs inherent in policymaking is essential to supporting pediatrician advocacy. To an advocate, it can feel frustrating to see slow progress on a policy reform that feels obvious. It can also be confusing to find that there is significant opposition to something that appears to be a moral issue of fairness and justice.

Learning to explore the contours of these trade-offs will equip pediatrician advocates with additional advocacy skills, enabling them to effectively analyze different stakeholders' perspectives on a topic. That in turn will better support pediatricians' ability to work effectively in coalition with diverse partners.

Child welfare policy heightens the tension in analyzing these trade-offs because the issues are foundational to the safe raising of children. Foundational to these policy deliberations are questions about what makes a good parent, what value system informs this decision, and who gets to decide. The child welfare policy issues policymakers grapple with influence the approach a child welfare system will take, decisions about where to prioritize resources, and how to determine who receives help or a punitive response.

With an impact that is so consequential, it can be difficult to see why there might be multiple perspectives on a child welfare policy issue. Often, these differences emerge from different philosophical approaches to work, alternative priorities, underlying assumptions, or unique lived experiences from proximity to an issue. When feeling stuck in the analysis of an issue, coming back to these core trade-offs can be illuminating. The following sections discuss some of the key tensions and trade-offs in child welfare policy.

Balancing Family Preservation and Child Safety

Families come to the child welfare system during times of crisis. Pediatricians know the power of relational health and how transformative it can be for a child to have safe, stable, nurturing relationships. The connection to culture, history, and a network of loving families underscores how valuable it is for children to have their families receive the support they need to be at their best. Advocates prioritizing family preservation point to the importance of family and promote policies that minimize removals and focus on keeping families safely together.

Conversely, a core component of the child welfare system is promoting child safety and preventing harm. Children can experience serious injuries and death from abuse and neglect. When the person responsible for loving and protecting a child is causing them harm, the child welfare system exists to intervene and protect the child. Advocates prioritizing child safety point to the importance of preventing and stopping harm to children.

Often, child welfare vacillates between these 2 ends of the spectrum over time, with the swinging of the pendulum occurring in reactive patterns. A jurisdiction may find that they have high numbers of children in foster care and "aging out" of the system. As they examine the reasons children are entering the system, they find that many are related to unmet parental service and support needs. They make reforms to the system to prioritize family preservation. Then, a highly publicized child death may occur because the system missed a real safety risk. New calls for reform emerge and the cycle begins again. Understanding the child welfare system's constant role in navigating and balancing these trade-offs is essential to making lasting reforms.

Finding the Appropriate Role of the Child Welfare System

Increasingly, child welfare policymakers are interested in taking a public health approach to child welfare policy. Also, there is ongoing discussion of the role of concrete and economic support in reducing unnecessary child welfare system involvement. As policymakers look at these upstream policy solutions, they are engaging with questions about the appropriate role of the child welfare system and how to balance supporting families effectively with not inadvertently bringing more families into the child welfare system unnecessarily.

There are diverse perspectives on the appropriate role of the child welfare system, ranging from being focused on child protection and supporting families in and at risk of entering the system, to promoting families' access to services that can prevent abuse or neglect from ever happening. In addition, the punitive powers of the child welfare system to remove children from their families and terminate parental rights cause many communities to have a complicated relationship to the child welfare system. Erosion of trust among families can also place limits on the roles the child welfare system can effectively assume.

The Role of Systemic Racism and Poverty

There is growing recognition that the impact of the child welfare system is not evenly distributed across the population. In nearly three-quarters of cases in which children are removed from their families, it is for reasons of neglect, which are often tied to poverty and economic deprivation. Like all areas of public policy in the United States, historical issues of injustice and systemic racism create the inequities that generate racial disproportionality in the child welfare system, with Black and American Indian/Alaska Native children removed from their families at rates far higher than those for white children.

The AAP continues to grapple with the role pediatricians can play in addressing these inequities. For example, this was a key consideration in the organization's Reimagining Child Welfare policy proposal. For pediatricians, these issues most concretely arise in their role as mandated reporters, balancing potential implicit bias and challenges that are more connected to unmet parental need with the legal duty to protect children from potential harm. This includes considering factors including implicit bias and what services and supports exist in a community to help families. These complex issues, without any easy answers, are at the heart of the practice of pediatrics. See Chapter 16, History of Child Welfare in the United States and Issues of Disproportionality, Inequity, and Injustice, for additional discussion.

Conclusion

Child welfare policy has evolved over time, with pediatricians playing a vital role in its development and advocacy. Pediatricians bring unique value to the table, extending beyond clinical care to advocate for the well-being of children and families. Their expertise and perspectives have a significant impact on shaping effective policies and ensuring positive outcomes.

Pediatricians' advocacy efforts are rooted in their position as trusted messengers. Parents, the public, and policymakers hold pediatricians in high regard, valuing their insights and expertise. This trust gives weight to their advocacy, making policymakers take their opinions seriously when it comes to child welfare policies. Pediatricians' grounding in scientific evidence further enhances their credibility, ensuring policy discussions are guided by the latest research and best practices in child health.

Advocacy at the local, state, and federal levels allows pediatricians to address child welfare issues comprehensively. At the local level, they can collaborate with community organizations, identify community needs, and work with local leaders to improve child well-being. State-level advocacy involves engaging with state chapters of the AAP, meeting with legislators, and influencing state-level policies. Federal advocacy provides an opportunity to affect national child welfare policies by engaging with policymakers, participating in advocacy days, and providing feedback on draft legislation. In all these roles, the expertise of pediatricians is invaluable.

For pediatricians who are new to the realm of advocacy, the AAP has created an advocacy guide (https://www.aap.org/en/advocacy/aap-advocacy-guide/advocacy-building-blocks) that details effective strategies and tactics used in state and federal policy. The guide was created for pediatrician advocates at all levels and is a comprehensive toolbox for AAP members who are looking to develop their skills or teach others.

By actively engaging at various levels, pediatricians can shape policies that protect and promote the health and happiness of children and families. Through collective efforts and a focus on family preservation, holistic approaches, and equitable solutions, pediatricians can create a brighter future for all children, ensuring that their well-being remains a top priority.

Key Takeaways

» Pediatricians have the knowledge and expertise to effectively advocate for the health and well-being of children involved in the child welfare system.

» Pediatricians are a trusted voice to policymakers at the local, state, and federal levels.

» Pediatrician partnership with those who have lived experience in the child welfare system has the potential to create powerful change for children and families.

Suggested Readings

- American Academy of Pediatrics. AAP Advocacy Guide: Building Blocks. AAP.org. Updated 2023. Accessed July 29, 2023. https://www.aap.org/en/advocacy/aap-advocacy-guide/advocacy-building-blocks
- American Academy of Pediatrics. AAP Advocacy Guide. AAP.org. Updated 2009. Accessed July 29, 2023. https://downloads.aap.org/AAP/PDF/aap_advocacy_guide.pdf?_ga=2.196224236.13076941.1685982138-1025446989.1661864354
- The United States Census Bureau. Quick Facts: Los Angeles. Updated May 18, 2023. Census.gov. Accessed July 23, 2023. https://www.census.gov/quickfacts/fact/faq/losangelescitycalifornia/PST045222
- State of Indiana. Stats Indiana: Floyd County. States.Indiana.edu. Accessed July 23, 2023. https://www.stats.indiana.edu/profiles/profiles.asp?scope_choice=a&county_changer=18043
- American Academy of Pediatrics. Reimagining Child Welfare: Recommendations for Public Policy Change. Updated April 16, 2021. Accessed July 17, 2023. https://www.aap.org/en/advocacy/child-welfare-report
- Family First Prevention Services Act, Pub. L. No. 115–123, 132 Stat. 232. February 9, 2018. Accessed July 17, 2023. https://familyfirstact.org/sites/default/files/PLAW-115publ123_FFPSA%20.pdf

Index

Page numbers followed by *f* indicate a figure; by *t,* a table; and by *b,* a box.

A

B

E

F

I

N

O

Q

R

S

U

V

W

Y